# Clinician's Handbook of Preventive Services

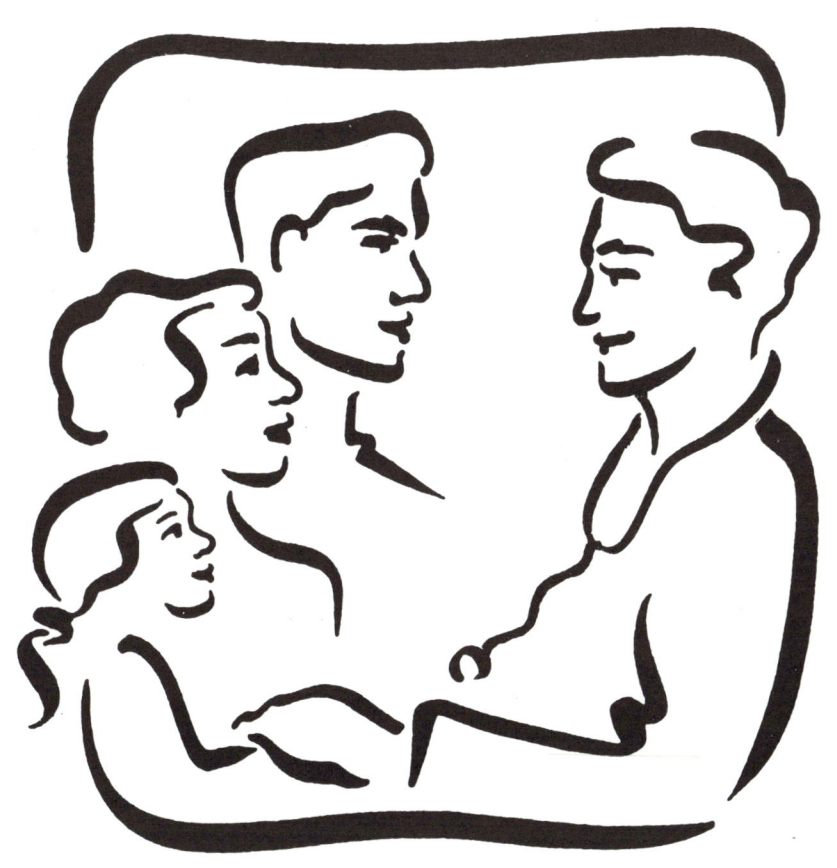

## PUT PREVENTION
## INTO PRACTICE

U.S. DEPARTMENT OF HEALTH AND HUMAN SERVICES
PUBLIC HEALTH SERVICE
OFFICE OF DISEASE PREVENTION AND HEALTH PROMOTION

For sale by the U.S. Government Printing Office
Superintendent of Documents, Mail Stop: SSOP, Washington, DC 20402-9328
ISBN 0-16-043115-8

# Clinician's Handbook of Preventive Services

## Foreword

Americans want preventive care. A recent Gallup poll found that 50 percent of adults would change their doctor if they felt they were not getting appropriate clinical preventive services—screening tests, immunizations, and especially counseling and health advice.

Providers—physicians, nurses, nurse practitioners, and physician assistants—consider these services important as well, but several barriers have deterred their optimal delivery. One important barrier has been a simple lack of authoritative information on preventive care. Because these services have not been a prominent part of training curricula for providers, there is a need for a practical, comprehensive, "how-to" guide for preventive services.

The *Clinician's Handbook of Preventive Services* was designed to fill this need. In 60 concise chapters, a wide range of preventive care is covered, with information on how to perform each particular preventive service; how to obtain patient education materials; and where to turn for further references.

The *Clinician's Handbook* is both an excellent reference for the practicing clinician and a useful text for health professions students of all disciplines. Although it can be used by itself, it is also an integral part of the U.S. Public Health Service's Put Prevention Into Practice national preventive services education campaign. The campaign is designed to improve the preventive care that all Americans receive. Educational materials for patients and office system tools for office staff members complement this book for providers; together, they comprise the *Put Prevention Into Practice Education and Action Kit*.

We hope that clinicians will find this book helpful in their daily activities. The *Clinician's Handbook of Preventive Services* and the Put Prevention Into Practice campaign are important stepping stones on our march to better health care and, ultimately, better health for all Americans.

                    Philip R. Lee, M.D.
                    Assistant Secretary for Health
                    U.S. Department of Health and Human Services

# Clinician's Handbook of Preventive Services

## Table of Contents

Page

**Foreword** .................................................. iii

**Overview**

   i. Introduction ........................................... xi
  ii. Implementing Preventive Care ............................ xvii

**Children/Adolescents**

*Screening*

1. Anemia ............................................... 1
2. Blood Pressure ........................................ 5
3. Body Measurement ..................................... 9
4. Cholesterol ........................................... 13
5. Depression and Suicide ................................. 17
6. Hearing .............................................. 21
7. Lead ................................................ 25
8. Newborn Screening .................................... 31
9. Tuberculosis (Including Prophylaxis and BCG Vaccination) ... 39
10. Urinalysis ........................................... 45
11. Vision .............................................. 49

*Immunization/Prophylaxis*
(*See also* Chapter 48: Influenza; Chapter 49: Pneumococcus, and Appendix C: Varicella Immunization)

12. Diphtheria, Tetanus, and Pertussis ...................... 55
13. *Haemophilus influenzae* Type b ........................ 61
14. Hepatitis B .......................................... 65
15. Measles, Mumps, and Rubella .......................... 73
16. Poliomyelitis ........................................ 79

*Counseling*

17. Alcohol and Other Drug Abuse ......................... 85
18. Dental and Oral Health ............................... 89
19. Nutrition ........................................... 93

# Table of Contents

**Children/Adolescents**—Continued
*Counseling*—Continued

    20. Physical Activity ................................................. 97
    21. Safety ........................................................... 103
    22. Sexually Transmitted Diseases and HIV Infection ...................... 109
    23. Tobacco ......................................................... 115
    24. Unintended Pregnancy ............................................ 119
    25. Violent Behavior and Firearms .................................... 125

**Adults/Older Adults**

*Screening*

    26. Anemia and Hemoglobinopathies ................................... 131
    27. Blood Pressure .................................................. 135
    28. Body Measurement ............................................... 141
    29. Cancer Detection by Physical Examination ......................... 147
        Breast ........................................................ 147
        Oral Cavity ................................................... 150
        Pelvic Organs ................................................. 152
        Rectum and Prostate ........................................... 153
        Skin .......................................................... 155
        Testis ........................................................ 156
        Thyroid ....................................................... 158
    30. Cholesterol ..................................................... 163
    31. Cognitive and Functional Impairment .............................. 171
    32. Depression ...................................................... 177
    33. Fecal Occult Blood .............................................. 183
    34. Hearing ......................................................... 187
    35. Mammography ..................................................... 191
    36. Papanicolaou Smear .............................................. 195
    37. Plasma Glucose .................................................. 201
    38. Prostate-Specific Antigen ....................................... 205
    39. Sexually Transmitted Diseases and HIV Infection ................... 209
    40. Sigmoidoscopy ................................................... 219
    41. Thyroid Function ................................................ 223
    42. Tuberculosis (Including Prophylaxis and BCG Vaccination) ............ 227
    43. Urinalysis ...................................................... 233
    44. Vision .......................................................... 237

*Immunization/Prophylaxis*

    45. Aspirin ......................................................... 241
    46. Estrogen and Progestin .......................................... 245
    47. Hepatitis B ..................................................... 251

## Table of Contents

**Adults/Older Adults**—Continued
*Immunization/Prophylaxis*—Continued

    48. Influenza (Including Childhood Immunization) ........................ 257
    49. Pneumococcus (Including Childhood Immunization) .................. 263
    50. Rubella ............................................................. 267
    51. Tetanus and Diphtheria ............................................ 271

*Counseling*

    52. Alcohol and Other Drug Abuse .................................... 275
    53. Dental and Oral Health ........................................... 285
    54. Injury and Violence Prevention .................................... 291
    55. Nutrition .......................................................... 299
    56. Physical Activity .................................................. 311
    57. Polypharmacy .................................................... 319
    58. Sexually Transmitted Diseases and HIV Infection .................... 323
    59. Smoking Cessation ............................................... 329
    60. Unintended Pregnancy ............................................ 337

## Appendices

    A. Major Authorities Cited ............................................ A-1
    B. Summary Risk-Factor Tables ....................................... B-1
    C. Varicella Immunization ............................................ C-1
    D. Copyright Considerations .......................................... D-1

## Index ............................................................... Index-1

## List of Figures

ii-1.   Child Preventive Care Timeline: Recommendations of Major Authorities
ii-2.   Adult Preventive Care Timeline: Recommendations of Major Authorities
ii-3.   Testing Conditions: Positive Predictive Value (PPV) and Prevalence
2-1.   Algorithm for Identifying Children and Adolescents With Hypertension
4-1.   Assessment and Follow-up of Total Cholesterol Measurements
4-2.   Assessment and Follow-up of Lipoprotein Analysis
28-1.  Body Mass Index (BMI) Nomogram
30-1.  Primary Prevention in Adults Without Evidence of CHD: Initial Classification Based on Total Cholesterol and HDL-Cholesterol
30-2.  Primary Prevention in Adults Without Evidence of CHD: Subsequent Classification Based on LDL-Cholesterol
30-3.  Secondary Prevention in Adults With Evidence of CHD: Classification Based on LDL-Cholesterol
52-1.  Alcoholism Screening Protocol
55-1.  Food Guide Pyramid: A Guide to Daily Food Choices

# Table of Contents

## List of Figures—Continued

55-2. Guide To Using the New Food Label
59-1. Benefits of Smoking Cessation

## List of Tables

ii-1. Examples of Preventive Care NOT Routinely Recommended for Asymptomatic, Normal-Risk Individuals
ii-2. USPSTF Rating System of Quality of Scientific Evidence
ii-3. National Vaccine Advisory Committee Standards for Childhood Immunization Practices
ii-4. Contraindications and Precautions for Childhood Immunizations
ii-5. National Coalition for Adult Immunization Standards for Adult Immunization Practices, 1990
ii-6. USPSTF Principles of Patient Education and Counseling
1-1. Hemoglobin and Hematocrit Cutpoints for Anemia in Children 1 Year of Age or Older
2-1. 90th and 95th Percentile Blood Pressures According to Gender and Age
5-1. Symptoms of Major Depression
7-1. Recommended Questions for Assessing Exposure Risk
7-2. CDC Recommendations for Follow-up of Blood Lead Measurements
7-3. Recommendations for Minimizing the Contamination of Capillary Blood Samples Obtained by Finger Stick
8-1. Newborn Screening by State
9-1. Medical Conditions That Increase the Risk of Tuberculosis Infection
11-1. Eye and Vision Examination Recommendations for Primary Care Physicians
12-1. Contraindications and Precautions for DTP/DTaP Vaccination
14-1. Groups at High Risk for Hepatitis B Infections
14-2. Recommended Doses for Children of Currently Licensed Recombinant Hepatitis B Vaccines
14-3. Recommended Schedule of Hepatitis B Immunoprophylaxis To Prevent Perinatal Transmission
15-1. Contraindications and Precautions for MMR Vaccination
16-1. Contraindications and Precautions for OPV/IPV Vaccination
17-1. Sample Questions Concerning Drugs for School-Aged Children
17-2. Sample Questions Concerning Drug Use for Adolescents
18-1. Daily Fluoride Dosage According to Age and Water Supply Content
20-1. Classification of Sports According to Strenuousness and Contact
20-2. Recommendations for Participation in Competitive Sports
22-1. Guidelines for Proper Condom Use
24-1. Addressing Adolescents' Common Concerns About Oral Contraceptives
26-1. Smoking Adjustments for Hb and Hct Cut Points for Anemia
26-2. Altitude Adjustments for Hb and Hct Cut Points for Anemia
27-1. Classification of Blood Pressure for Adults Aged 18 Years and Older

## List of Tables—Continued

27-2. Recommendations for Follow-Up Based on Initial Set of Blood Pressure Measurements for Adults Age 18 and Over
27-3. Situations In Which Automated Noninvasive Ambulatory Blood Pressure Monitoring Devices May Be Useful
27-4. Life-style Modifications for Hypertension Control
28-1. Height and Weight Tables for Men Aged 25 and Over
28-2. Height and Weight Tables for Women Aged 25 and Over
28-3. Desirable Body Mass Index (BMI) in Relation to Age
29-1. Leading Sites of Cancer Incidence and Death—1994 Estimates
30-1. NCEP Coronary Heart Disease Risk Factors Other Than LDL-Cholesterol
31-1. Mini-Mental State Examination
32-1. Risk Factors for Depression
32-2. Criteria for Major Depressive Disorder
32-3. Center for Epidemiologic Studies Depression Scale
33-1. Diet for Patients Using Guaiac-Based Tests
34-1. Hearing Handicap Inventory in the Elderly Screening Questionnaire
36-1. The Revised Bethesda System for Reporting Cervical and/or Vaginal Cytologic Diagnoses
37-1. Criteria for Diagnosing Diabetes in Non-Pregnant Adults
39-1. Conditions That May Cause Falsely Reactive Syphilis Tests
39-2. Pre- and Post-Test Information for HIV Testing
42-1. Criteria for Determining Need for TB Preventive Therapy by Category and Age Group
43-1. Prevalence of Asymptomatic Bacteriuria in Adults and Estimated Positive Predictive Values of Nitrite and Leukocyte Esterase Dipstick Tests
43-2. Causes of Inaccurate Nitrite Dipstick Tests
43-3. Causes of Inaccurate Leukocyte Esterase Dipstick Tests
44-1. Visual Impairment Questionnaire
46-1. Relative Risk of Selected Conditions for a 50-Year-Old White Woman Treated With Long-Term Hormone Replacement
47-1. Groups at High Risk for Hepatitis B Infections
47-2. Recommendations for Hepatitis B Prophylaxis Following Percutaneous and Mucosal Exposure
48-1. Groups at Increased Risk for Influenza-Related Complications
48-2. Groups That Can Transmit Influenza to Persons at High Risk
49-1. Groups at Increased Risk for Pneumococcal Disease
51-1. Summary Guide to Tetanus Prophylaxis in Routine Wound Management
52-1. CAGE Questionnaire
52-2. Alcohol Use Disorders Identification Test (AUDIT)
52-3. Trauma Questionnaire
53-1. Oral Effects of Selected Drugs
53-2. Cardiac Conditions for Which Endocarditis Prophylaxis Is and Is Not Recommended
53-3. Standard Antibiotic Prophylaxis Regimens for Dental or Operative Procedures in the Oral Cavity of Patients Subject to Bacterial Endocarditis

# Table of Contents

## List of Tables—Continued

54-1. Proper Safety Belt Use
54-2. Home Safety Checklist for Older Adults
55-1. Determining Your Nutritional Health: Checklist for Older Adults
55-2. Examples of Foods To Choose or Decrease for the NCEP Step I and Step II Diets
56-1. Heart Rates According to Age
56-2. Major Coronary Risk Factors
56-3. Major Symptoms and Signs Suggestive of Cardiopulmonary or Metabolic Disease
56-4. ACSM Guidelines for Medical Examination and Diagnostic Exercise Testing Prior to Beginning an Exercise Program
56-5. Overcoming Barriers to Exercise
57-1. How To Simplify the Medication Regimen
58-1. Examples of Questions for Taking Clinical Histories About Sexual Behavior and Drug Use
59-1. Smoking Assessment Form
59-2. Information About Nicotine Gum Use
59-3. Information About Nicotine Patch Use
60-1. Percent of Women Experiencing an Accidental Pregnancy in First Year of Use of Contraceptives
60-2. Complications, Side Effects, and Benefits of Major Methods of Contraception
B-1. Summary Risk Factors: Ethnic and Geographic Origin
B-2. Summary Risk Factors: Family History
B-3. Summary Risk Factors: Medical History
B-4. Summary Risk Factors: Occupational and Recreational History
B-5. Summary Risk Factors: Sexual History
B-6. Summary Risk Factors: Social or Living Situation
B-7. Summary Risk Factors: Substance Abuse History

# Clinician's Handbook of Preventive Services

# Overview

# OVERVIEW

## i. Introduction

The *Clinician's Handbook of Preventive Services* is part of a set of materials created for the U.S. Public Health Services's Put Prevention into Practice campaign. The purpose of this campaign is to enhance the delivery of preventive care in primary care practice. The *Handbook* is designed to provide primary care clinicians with a practical and comprehensive reference on clinical preventive services—screening tests for the early detection of disease, immunizations and prophylaxis to prevent disease, and counseling to modify risk factors that lead to disease.

The busy clinician may not have time to provide (or even to read about) lengthy preventive care interventions. This book provides concise discussions and strategies for brief, targeted preventive interventions in 60 short chapters. Clinicians may also have difficulty keeping up with the frequent changes in recommendations for preventive care, since knowledge and technology change rapidly. The *Handbook* brings together recommendations of major authorities on preventive care, and information has been updated through December 1993. Finally, clinicians may have difficulty learning about and acquiring useful educational resources on preventive care for themselves and their patients. Each *Handbook* chapter provides a list of resources for the patient or family, including ordering instructions where appropriate.

The *Handbook* is intended to be both a handy reference for the practicing clinician and a useful textbook for students. Health professional education, particularly of physicians, often neglects preventive care in favor of treatment care. This, in turn, results in practicing clinicians who have little interest in or knowledge of the basics of preventive medicine. Prevention of disease and promotion of health should be a major part of all health professional educational curricula.

**Organization**

The *Handbook* is divided into four sections: chapters i-ii provide basic information on understanding and implementing preventive care; chapters 1-25 cover specific preventive care topics for children and adolescents (up to 18 years of age); chapters 26-60 include material on specific types of preventive care for adults and older adults; and the appendices provide a list of major authorities cited, tables that summarize disorders according to specific risk factors, and late-breaking information on varicella immunization.

Within the age-specific sections, chapters are grouped into subsections on screening, immunization and prophylaxis, and counseling. Each chapter is divided into five parts:

- The introduction reviews the burden of suffering of the disease, risk factors for it, and the effectiveness of the preventive intervention.

# Ch. i. Introduction                                                                 Overview

- "Recommendations of Major Authorities" summarizes recommendations on which patients should receive the preventive service and at what frequency.

- "Basics of..." presents information on how to perform each type of preventive service.

- "Patient (or Family) Resources" lists useful resources for patients or families, as well as how to obtain them. Resources are usually pamphlets, but (where noted) also include videotapes, posters, and other media. In many cases, a "Provider Resources" section is also included.

- "Selected References" lists key references used in preparation of the chapter.

## Content

The criterion for inclusion of a preventive service in the *Handbook* is a recommendation for its routine use in the care of asymptomatic persons by a major U.S. authority: Federal health agency (e.g., Centers for Disease Control and Prevention, National Institutes of Health), non-Federal expert panel (e.g., U.S. Preventive Services Task Force), national professional organization (e.g., American Academy of Family Physicians, American Academy of Pediatrics), or national voluntary association (e.g., American Cancer Society, American Heart Association). Recommendations of the Canadian Task Force on the Periodic Health Examination have also been included. Because the *Handbook* focuses on preventive care for the general population without special risk factors, the following types of preventive care have not been included: tertiary prevention (treatment to prevent progression of known disease), prenatal and perinatal care; and preventive care for certain high-risk groups. Preventive services not recommended by any major authority also have been excluded. The exclusion of a medical procedure does not reflect on its effectiveness in diagnosing and treating disease.

Every effort has been made to ensure that the listings in the "Recommendations of Major Authorities" sections accurately represent the current positions of these authorities. Recommendations are listed alphabetically by organization. Similar recommendations are often grouped together to facilitate comparisons by the reader. Appearance in the *Clinician's Handbook* does not necessarily imply endorsement of a specific authority or its recommendations by either the U.S. Department of Health and Human Services or the Public Health Service; readers are encouraged to consult the references provided to evaluate the scientific basis for individual recommendations. Similarly, the citation of a group's recommendations does not imply that the group has endorsed the *Clinician's Handbook* or its contents. A complete listing of authorities cited may be found in Appendix A.

The chapter sections on the "Basics of..." how to perform each type of preventive service have been prepared using a numerical, stepwise format that generally reflects the temporal sequence of decisionmaking in patient care, not order of importance. Thus, issues regarding whether a preventive service should be performed are addressed initially, the specifics of how to perform the service follow, and a discussion of the follow-up care and potential adverse effects conclude each chapter. Steps for the work-up of abnormalities detected by screening tests are generally not included.

In some cases, the data supporting the optimal method of performing a particular preventive procedure are scant or absent. This is especially true for some physical examination and counseling procedures. Often, expert opinion has been relied on for guidance. In these situations, conditional language is generally used, such as "some authorities believe...". The reader is urged to consider information of this type provisional in nature and subject to revision as research progresses.

The items listed in the "Patient (or Family) Resources" sections of the chapters have been selected after an extensive review of materials solicited from government agencies and professional and voluntary organizations. However, there are undoubtedly other, equally useful publications that have not been included. The materials listed here are provided as a starting point for clinicians in building a library of high-quality literature and resources for patients. The availability of these materials and correctness of ordering instructions have been verified. Appropriateness in any specific case must be determined by the individual clinician.

The publications listed in the "Selected References" sections were chosen because of their use in preparing the chapters and their potential usefulness to the clinician. These lists are not intended to be a comprehensive bibliography of the literature, but to provide a core set of references for the reader.

No single set of preventive services is appropriate for all patients in all settings. The *Handbook* is designed to facilitate the design and implementation of a preventive care program for practices of all sizes and types. Chapter ii discusses the establishment of a preventive care protocol, implementation of that protocol, and general principles of screening, immunizations, and counseling. It includes charts of core preventive services (Figs ii-1 and ii-2). This information, when combined with the more specific recommendations of authorities, relevant patient risk factors given in each chapter, and the summary risk-factor tables in Appendix B, should help readers select a set of preventive services appropriate for their patients and practice.

## Sources

The data for the *Handbook* have been obtained from a variety of sources:

- Scientific literature identified by searching computerized data bases and reference lists of primary sources

- Policy statements and position papers issued by government agencies, professional groups, and voluntary associations

- Educational brochures, booklets, and other materials from government agencies, professional groups, and voluntary associations

- Consultation with experts

## Ch. i. Introduction — Overview

**The National Coordinating Committee on Clinical Preventive Services**

Oversight of the Put Prevention Into Practice campaign is provided by the National Coordinating Committee on Clinical Preventive Services (NCCCPS). The NCCCPS was formed in 1989 to accelerate the integration of clinical preventive services into primary care delivery in the United States. The institutional members of this group also provided extensive review of the Put Prevention Into Practice materials during their development. NCCCPS member organizations include:

Ambulatory Pediatrics Association
American Academy of Family Physicians
American Academy of Pediatrics
American Academy of Physician Assistants
American Association of Colleges of Nursing
American College of Obstetricians and Gynecologists
American College of Physicians
American College of Preventive Medicine
American Hospital Association
American Medical Association
American Nurses' Association
American Osteopathic Association
American Osteopathic College of Preventive Medicine
American Public Health Association
Association of Academic Health Centers
Association of American Medical Colleges
Association of Health Services Research
Association of Schools of Public Health
Association of State and Territorial Health Officials
Association of Teachers of Preventive Medicine
Blue Cross and Blue Shield Association
Group Health Association of America
Health Insurance Association of America
Institute of Medicine
National Alliance of Nurse Practitioners
National Association of County Health Officials
National Association of Community Health Centers
North American Primary Care Research Group
Society of General Internal Medicine
Society for Public Health Education
Society of Teachers of Family Medicine
U.S. Conference of Local Health Officers

## Review

The chapters of this book have been reviewed for scientific accuracy by experts in the agencies of the U.S. Public Health Service:

Agency for Health Care Policy and Research
Centers for Disease Control and Prevention
Food and Drug Administration
Health Resources and Services Administration
Indian Health Service
National Institutes of Health
Substance Abuse and Mental Health Services Administration

## Acknowledgments

Preparation of the *Clinician's Handbook of Preventive Services* was coordinated by staff in the Office of Disease Prevention and Health Promotion, Public Health Service, U.S. Department of Health and Human Services, under the general supervision of J. Michael McGinnis, M.D., Deputy Assistant Secretary for Health (Disease Prevention and Health Promotion). Principal staff responsible for the preparation of this book were:

Larry L. Dickey, M.D., M.P.H., Luther Terry Senior Fellow (scientific editor and principal writer)
Hurdis M. Griffith, Ph.D., R.N., Senior Policy Advisor (review coordinator and writer)
Douglas B. Kamerow, M.D., M.P.H., Director, Clinical Preventive Services Staff (managing editor)

Other staff members of the Office of Disease Prevention and Health Promotion who contributed to preparation of this book were:

David R. Baker
Rachel Ballard-Barbash, M.D., M.P.H.
Elena Carbone, M.S., R.D.
Carolyn DiGuiseppi, M.D., M.P.H.
Walter H. Glinsman, M.D.
Linda D. Meyers, Ph.D.
Janice T. Radak
Susan Simmons, R.N., Ph.D.
Marilyn G. Stephenson, M.S., R.D.

Valuable research and writing contributions were made by the following preventive medicine residents from Johns Hopkins University and the University of Maryland during rotations at the Office of Disease Prevention and Health Promotion:

- Robert Beardall, M.D., M.P.H.
- Karen S. Collins, M.D., M.P.H.
- Paul Denning, M.D., M.P.H.
- Tina Farup, M.D.
- Clarice Green, M.D.
- Lana Jeng, M.D., M.P.H.
- S. Patrick Kachur, M.D., M.P.H.
- Cynthia Mobley, M.D., M.P.H.
- Peter W. Pendergrass, M.D., M.P.H.
- Donald Robinson, M.D., M.P.H.
- William Schluter, M.D.
- Suzanne Steinberg, M.D.

Material on preventive services for older adults was researched and prepared by fellows of the Multicampus Division of Geriatric Medicine and Gerontology at the University of California, Los Angeles (listed below). David B. Reuben, M.D., was supervising editor for this component of *Handbook* preparation.

- Nelson C. Apostol, M.D.
- Christopher J. Bula, M.D.
- Russel E. Hoxie, M.D.
- David Kelley, M.D.
- Michael E. Lim, M.D.
- Matthew K. McNabney, M.D.
- Alison A. Moore, M.D.
- Michael Temporal, M.D.
- Emil Yagudin, M.D.
- Michael P. Zeitlin, M.D.

Assistance in researching and preparing the chapters on sexually transmitted diseases was provided by C. Patrick Chaulk, M.D., M.P.H., Johns Hopkins School of Hygiene and Public Health.

Copy editor was Barbara Ravage.

## OVERVIEW

# ii. Implementing Preventive Care

Never has preventive health care been more important than today. Many of the most serious disorders encountered in clinical practice can be prevented or postponed by immunizations, chemoprophylaxis, and healthier life-styles, or detected early with screening and treated effectively. To an unprecedented extent, clinicians now have the opportunities, skills, and resources to prevent disease and promote health as well as to cure disease.

However, preventive care has also never been more complex. The yearly physical examination, a reassuringly simple but relatively ineffective ritual, has been supplanted by a shifting array of tests, immunizations, prophylactic medications, and counseling interventions—many of which have not been a part of traditional training curricula. In addition, differing sets of preventive services are recommended by government agencies, professional organizations, voluntary associations, and academic experts, which may lead to confusion on the part of clinicians.

In the face of these perceived contradictions, it is important to emphasize that there is basic agreement among authorities about recommendations for most types of preventive care. This is illustrated in Figs ii-1 and ii-2, in which the preventive care recommendations of major U.S. authorities are summarized in a timeline format. The dark bars in these timelines denote agreement among all major U.S. authorities; the light bars denote agreement among some, but not all, major U.S. authorities.

The delivery of preventive care, even for services on which all authorities agree, is far from satisfactory. For example, the vaccination rate of adults 65 and older against pneumococcal infections is only about 20%. Delivery rates are also low for other basic types of preventive care—often less than 50%. There are multiple reasons for these poor rates, including: lack of clinician time, often related to inadequate reimbursement; lack of clinician interest and knowledge; lack of patient involvement and knowledge; and lack of office or clinic systems to promote preventive care. Some of these factors are beyond the control of the practicing clinician, but many are not. There is much that clinicians can do to help ensure that their patients receive the preventive care they need.

This chapter briefly discusses two important aspects of the delivery of clinical preventive services—establishing a preventive care protocol and implementing it in practice—and then reviews basic principles of screening, immunization, and counseling. These general topics form a foundation for the more specific information discussed in the subsequent 60 chapters of the *Handbook*. The references at the end of this chapter have been selected as a basic bibliography on the implementation of preventive services in primary care settings.

Ch. ii. Implementing Preventive Care         Overview

**Figure ii-1. Child Preventive Care Timeline: Recommendations of Major Authorities**

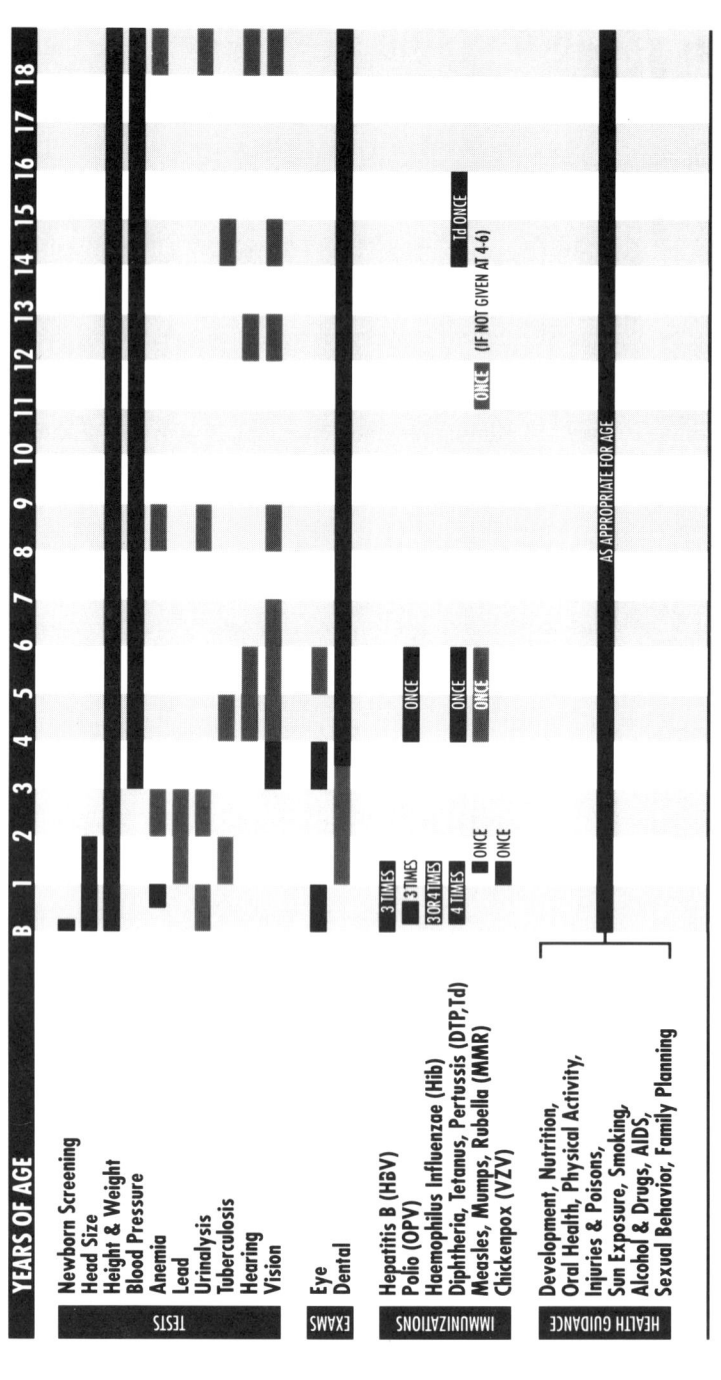

# Ch. ii. Implementing Preventive Care — Overview

**Figure ii-2. Adult Preventive Care Timeline: Recommendations of Major Authorities**

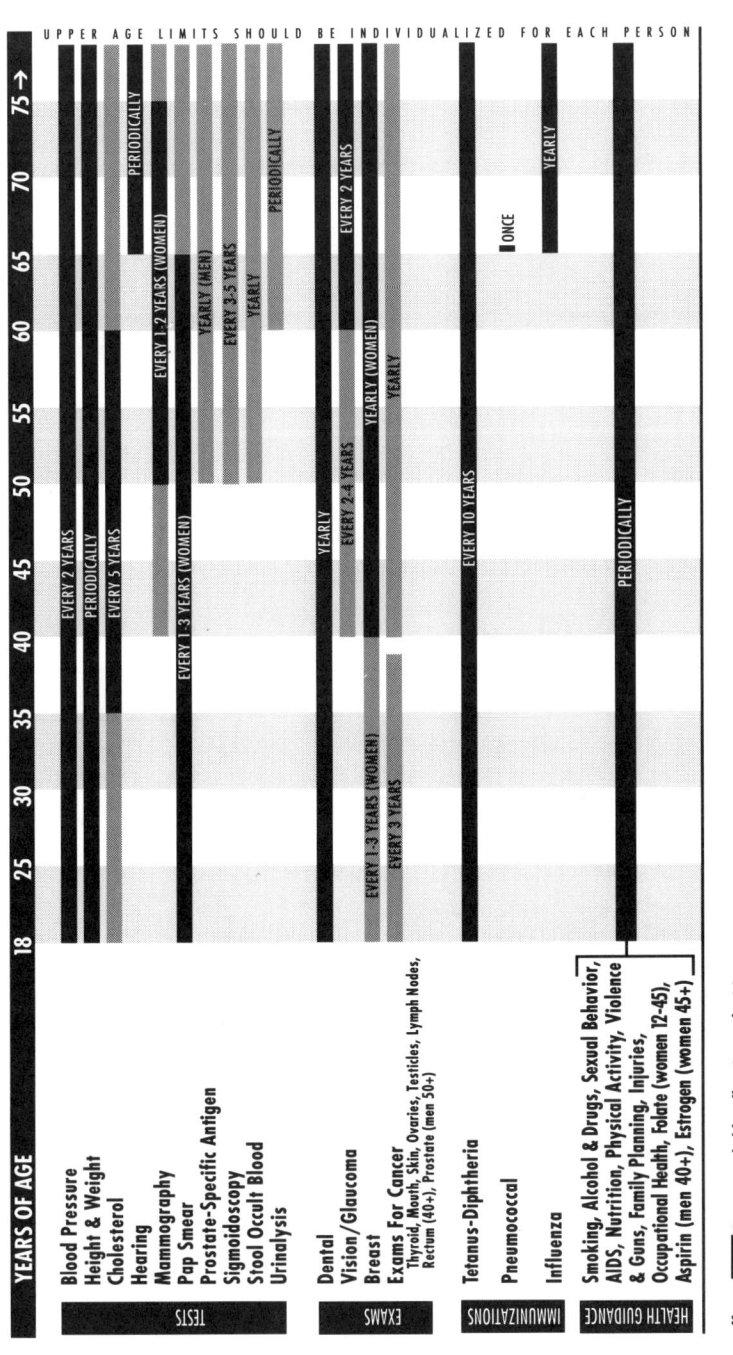

## Establishing a Preventive Care Protocol

As a first step, every clinician or practice needs to create a clear, written protocol of preventive services to be delivered to patients. This protocol must be, above all, realistic and achievable; it can be both and still be comprehensive, including screening tests, immunizations, prophylaxis, and counseling services. The set of preventive services recommended by all major U.S. authorities represented by the dark bars in Figs ii-1 and ii-2, for example, constitutes a core set of services that may be reasonably included in every clinician's protocol. Conversely, preventive services not recommended by any major U.S. authority need not, in general, be included. Table ii-1 lists examples of preventive services that are not recommended.

**Table ii-1. Examples of Preventive Care NOT Routinely Recommended for Asymptomatic, Normal-Risk Individuals**

- Chest X-ray
- Electrocardiogram
- Exercise stress testing
- Multiple blood chemistry screens
- Sputum cytology testing
- Multivitamin or megavitamin prophylaxis

Rather than simply adopt the recommendations of major authorities, clinicians are encouraged to develop a protocol of preventive care that meets the particular needs of their practice and patients. Some of the factors to consider in this selection process are discussed below.

### *Quality of Scientific Evidence*

In general, preventive interventions should not be used unless they have been demonstrated to be effective in well-designed studies. Ineffective interventions may be costly and lead to adverse effects (e.g., unnecessary work-ups with their attendant costs and risks). Although it is unrealistic to expect every clinician to assess the quality of scientific evidence for each preventive service individually, it is important that clinicians be discerning consumers of recommendations made by preventive care authorities.

Although all major authorities base their recommendations on scientific evidence, some rely to a greater degree on more rigorous forms of evidence, such as randomized controlled trials, in formulating their recommendations. The U.S. Preventive Services Task Force (USPSTF), a body of preventive care experts convened by the U.S. Public Health Service, has developed a system for rating the quality of scientific evidence used in its deliberations. The USPSTF rating system for grading scientific evidence is given in Table ii-2.

## Table ii-2. USPSTF Rating System of Quality of Scientific Evidence

| | |
|---|---|
| I: | Evidence obtained from at least one properly designed randomized controlled trial |
| II-1: | Evidence obtained from well-designed controlled trials without randomization |
| II-2: | Evidence obtained from well-designed cohort or case-control analytic studies, preferably from more than one center or research group |
| II-3: | Evidence obtained from multiple time series with or without the intervention, or dramatic results in uncontrolled experiments (such as the results of the introduction of penicillin treatment in the 1940s) |
| III: | Opinions of respected authorities, based on clinical experience, descriptive studies, or reports of expert committees |

From: U.S. Preventive Services Task Force. Task Force Ratings. *Guide to Clinical Preventive Services.* Baltimore, Md: Williams & Wilkins; 1989:388.

Although the recommendations of major authorities are cited in this book, it has not been possible to provide the scientific rationale for each group's recommendations. The reader is urged to consult the position and background papers of each authority (listed in the "Selected References" in each chapter) to understand the quality of evidence used to determine specific recommendations, or contact the authority (addresses are listed in Appendix A).

### *Risk Profile of Patient Population*

Some patient populations are at higher risk for certain preventable disorders than others. For example, medically underserved, low-income populations are at increased risk for tuberculosis (TB). Although TB screening is not recommended for the general population, it may be prudent for a clinician with a large proportion of such patients to include TB screening in the protocol of preventive care for all patients in the practice. Risk factors for the conditions discussed are given in most chapters of this book and summarized in Appendix B.

In establishing a preventive care protocol, every clinician should conduct an assessment of the risk-factor profile of his or her patient population. Local or state health departments often can provide relevant health information on specific populations, including incidence of low-birth-weight infants, immunization-preventable diseases, and sexually transmitted and other important infections.

### *Feasibility*

Although a particular type of preventive care may be desirable, the staff and other resources may not be available for its delivery. In such cases, it is reasonable to concentrate efforts on delivery of appropriate preventive care that can actually be provided. Each clinician should consider both importance and feasibility of services in establishing a protocol of preventive care, keeping the protocol simple and realistic. Since many types of preventive care currently are not delivered to most patients on a regular schedule, a concerted effort to deliver even a basic set of preventive services to all is likely to yield significant improvements in care.

*Financial Factors*

At present, some types of preventive care may not be covered by private or public health insurance, and patients may not be willing or able to pay for them. Although this problem may diminish with progress in health care reform, it is a necessary current concern. Clinicians should strive to deliver the basic set of preventive services that all major authorities have endorsed (dark bars, Figs ii-1 and ii-2); however, due to financial factors some types of preventive care may have to be excluded or delivered less frequently than usually recommended. If necessary, clinicians should make every effort to use and refer to low-cost, high-quality (and, if available, subsidized) service delivery settings to minimize the impact of financial factors on preventive care.

**Implementing the Preventive Care Protocol in Practice**

After the protocol of preventive care to be delivered is decided, the next step is to put into place interventions in the office or clinic to ensure that the protocol is carried out efficiently and consistently. Implementation of preventive care in practice requires special efforts and the use of specific tools, although these activities do not necessarily need to be complicated or high-tech. It is important to create an atmosphere in the office or clinic that encourages and reminds everyone—including clinicians, staff, and patients—to work together, each playing an active role in preventive care. The best intentions and efforts of providers alone are not sufficient without patient involvement, nursing and office staff participation, and the use of office tools.

*Patients*

Preventive care cannot be delivered effectively without active patient involvement. At the most basic level, patients must consent to receive preventive care. Most studies have found high levels of patient interest in preventive services, usually higher than clinicians expect. Studies of large public education campaigns, such as the National Cholesterol Education Program, have found that patient demand may positively influence clinician delivery of preventive care. Every effort should be made to foster patient knowledge and interest in preventive care with the use of various educational materials. These may be made available at conspicuous locations throughout the office or clinic, as well as actively distributed to patients with special needs. A list of patient resources for specific types of preventive care is provided at the end of most chapters in this book.

The valuable role that patients can play in tracking and prompting their own preventive care is often overlooked by clinicians. Studies have shown that patient- or parent-held records, such as those used to promote childhood immunizations, are well-received by clinicians and patients and are useful in tracking and prompting both child and adult preventive care. The *Personal Health Guide* and *Child Health Guide*, integral components of the *Put Prevention Into Practice Education and Action Kit*, were designed in response to this need.

## Staff

Nursing and office/clinic staff need to be involved to the maximum extent possible in both the delivery and monitoring of preventive services. Many nursing and office/clinic staff are better trained than primary care physicians in the delivery of certain types of preventive care. The success of the blood pressure screening program in the United States, for example, can be attributed largely to the involvement of nursing and other staff. All immunizations and many types of screening can be successfully provided by nursing staff. Patient counseling on many topics can be delivered effectively by well-trained staff. Several studies have demonstrated the effectiveness of staff involvement in record keeping and in prompting clinicians and patients about preventive care. Examples of staff functions in this regard include updating flow sheets or computerized data bases, issuing reminders to clinicians and patients, and following up on test results. Another important role for staff in preventive care is helping patients gain access to community resources, such as local mammography centers or smoking cessation support groups.

## Office Tools

Research has proven the ability of even simple office tools to improve preventive care. The most basic tool for tracking and prompting preventive services is a flow sheet in the patient medical record. These inexpensive paper forms provide a convenient format for display of the preventive care protocol, and they have been demonstrated in many studies to improve the delivery of preventive care. However, in order for flow sheets to be effective, data about the patient's preventive care must be consistently and promptly entered. This may prove difficult for a busy clinician. The assistance of staff in updating and maintaining chart flow sheets is very important.

Some practices use office computer systems to track preventive care. Several popular office management software packages for microcomputers now include preventive care modules, and computerized systems exclusively for tracking preventive care have been developed. These systems have several advantages over printed flow sheets; perhaps the most significant are the ability to generate reminders for both clinicians and patients at any time (not just when the patient comes in for a visit) and the ability to provide feedback quickly and accurately on the practice-wide performance of preventive care. Computerized systems, like chart flow sheets, require constant updating, although the process may be performed by office staff. Whether a manual flow sheet or computerized system is used, some type of office tool to track patient preventive care is needed.

Office tools have been shown to help perform several other important tasks as well:

- Patient risk-factor assessment may be aided by the use of patient- or clinician-completed questionnaires or history forms. Risk factors listed in most chapters of this book and in Appendix B may be helpful in preparing such questionnaires or history forms. Computerized tools are currently being developed for this purpose; most use direct patient data entry at a keyboard or onto scanable forms.

- Prompting of patients to come in for needed preventive care may be aided by the use of mailed postcards or letters. These can be created easily by the clinician or obtained preprinted from outside sources. Some computerized systems are capable of generating such mailed prompts. Telephone calls may also be used for this purpose, but in general they have been found to be less cost-effective than mailed prompts.

- Prescription pads or patient contract forms that may be completed and presented to the patient in the office or clinic may be used as patient prompts for preventive care.

- Chart stickers of various types are helpful in alerting clinicians about the special preventive care needs of individual patients.

The *Put Prevention Into Practice Education and Action Kit* is a set of paper-based office tools for preventive care that includes many of the materials mentioned above. See page xxxiii.

## *Using Every Opportunity*

Just as it is important to involve everyone (clinicians, staff, and patients) in the delivery of preventive services, it is also important to use every patient encounter as an opportunity for preventive care. Many patients, particularly young adults, visit their provider or clinic for acute care but rarely come in specifically for preventive care. Other, often older, patients with chronic medical problems (diabetes, hypertension, etc.) visit regularly but do not schedule preventive care appointments. In order to take advantage of acute and chronic care visits as opportunities to deliver preventive care, it is necessary to have a tracking and prompting system in place; this allows the clinician to determine quickly a patient's need for preventive care. If time is lacking to actually deliver the needed preventive service at the visit, the patient may at least be accurately informed of what is needed and a plan established (referral, follow-up appointment, etc.) to obtain it.

## *Getting Accurate Feedback*

Most studies indicate that clinicians substantially overestimate the amount of preventive care (particularly screening tests) they deliver to their patients. Thus, it is useful to have periodic or ongoing objective feedback on actual compliance with the preventive care protocol. One way this may be accomplished is with periodic reviews of a random sample of patient charts. Up-to-date flow sheets in patient charts greatly facilitate this process. Some health insurers currently require periodic chart audits for certain types of preventive care. Clinicians with computerized tracking systems usually have the ability to perform audits of preventive care delivery frequently and quickly.

## Principles of Screening, Immunization, and Counseling

Each chapter of this book provides information on the basics of performing specific types of preventive care. Included here are principles that underlie each of the three major types of preventive care—screening, immunization, and counseling.

## Screening

1. Certain circumstances must exist for a screening test to be useful. Frame and Carlson summarized them as follows:

   - The condition must have a significant effect on the quality and quantity of life.

   - Acceptable methods of treatment must be available.

   - The condition must have an asymptomatic period during which detection and treatment significantly reduce morbidity or mortality.

   - Treatment in the asymptomatic phase must yield a therapeutic result superior to that obtained by delaying treatment until symptoms appear.

   - Tests that are acceptable to patients must be available, at a reasonable cost, to detect the condition in the asymptomatic period.

   - The incidence of the condition must be sufficient to justify the cost of the screening.

2. The concepts of test sensitivity, specificity, and positive predictive value are important to understand when evaluating and selecting screening tests. The U.S. Preventive Services Task Force summarized the issues of sensitivity and specificity as follows:

   *Sensitivity* refers to the proportion of persons with a condition who correctly test positive when screened. A test with poor sensitivity will miss cases (persons with the condition) and will produce a large proportion of false-negative results; true cases will be told incorrectly that they are free of disease. *Specificity* refers to the proportion of persons without the condition who correctly test negative when screened. A test with poor specificity will result in healthy persons being told they have the condition (false positives).

   The use of screening tests with poor sensitivity and/or specificity is of special significance to the clinician because of the potentially serious consequences of false-negative and false-positive results. Persons who receive false-negative results may experience important delays in diagnosis and treatment. Some might develop a false sense of security, resulting in inadequate attention to risk reduction and delays in seeking medical care when warning symptoms become present. False-positive results may lead to follow-up testing that may be uncomfortable, expensive, and, in some cases, potentially harmful. If follow-up testing does not disclose the error, the patient may even receive unnecessary treatment. There may also be psychological consequences. Persons informed of an abnormal medical test that is falsely positive may experience unnecessary anxiety until the error is corrected. Labeling may affect behavior; for example, studies have shown that some persons with hypertension identified through screening may experience altered behavior and decreased work productivity.

   *Positive predictive value* is the proportion of persons with a positive test who have the condition. It is equal to the number of true positives divided by the sum of true and false positives. This is directly related to the prevalence of the disease and the specificity of the test. The relationship between positive predictive value and prevalence is illustrated in Fig ii-3. An attempt has been made to provide information on the sensitivity, specificity, and positive predictive value of the screening tests included in this book. Because most target conditions for screening are relatively uncommon and most screening tests have imperfect specificity, the positive predictive value of screening tests is often in the 10 to 30% range. Thus, many patients with positive screening tests do not actually have the disease. This necessitates careful selection of tests and counseling of patients to prevent unnecessary and potentially harmful testing and anxiety.

3. There is little value in performing screening tests without close tracking of results and needed follow-up testing. Involvement of staff in keeping track of screening and follow-up tests is crucial.

4. Laboratories used to analyze screening tests must adhere to national standards for accuracy in testing and reporting of results. Substandard sensitivity or specificity may negate the value of screening.

5. Patients should be clearly informed of the potential cost and morbidity of necessary follow-up testing and treatment, as appropriate. Some authorities now advocate that informed consent be obtained from patients before screening takes place.

## Figure ii-3. Testing Conditions: Positive Predictive Value (PPV) and Prevalence

Size of Population = 100,000
Sensitivity of Test = 90%
Specificity of Test = 90%

Cancer Prevalence = 1%

|  | Cancer Present | Cancer Absent |
|---|---|---|
| Positive Test | 900 | 9900 |
| Negative Test | 100 | 89,100 |

PPV = 8.3%

Cancer Prevalence = 0.1%

|  | Cancer Present | Cancer Absent |
|---|---|---|
| Positive Test | 90 | 9900 |
| Negative Test | 10 | 89,910 |

PPV = 0.9%

From: U.S. Preventive Services Task Force. *Guide to Clinical Preventive Services*. Baltimore, MD: Williams & Wilkins; 1989:xxxii.

## Immunization

1. Persons administering immunizations should take the necessary precautions to minimize the risk of spreading disease.

   - They should themselves be adequately immunized against hepatitis B, measles, mumps, rubella, and influenza. Immunization against tetanus and diphtheria is recommended for all persons.

   - Hands should be washed before each new patient is seen.

   - Gloves are not required when administering immunizations unless contact with potentially infectious body fluids is likely or the person giving the immunization has open sores on his or her hands.

   - Syringes and needles must be sterile and preferably disposable to minimize the risk of contamination. A separate needle and syringe should be used for each injection.

   - Needles and syringes should be discarded in labeled, puncture-proof containers to prevent accidental needlesticks or reuse.

   - Jet injectors that employ the same nozzle tip to immunize more than one person have generally been considered safe and effective for administering vaccine if used properly by trained personnel. However, certain multiple-use nozzle jet injectors may pose a potential hazard of blood-borne disease transmission. It is advisable to seek advice from sources (e.g., state or local health departments) experienced in the use of jet injectors before beginning a vaccination program in which they will be used. Jet injectors may be used in selected situations: if large numbers of persons must be rapidly immunized with the same vaccine; if the use of needles and syringes is not practical; if state and/or local health authorities judge that the public health benefit from the use of the injector outweighs the small potential risk of bloodborne disease transmission. Use of newer jet injectors that employ single-use disposable nozzle tips should not pose a potential risk if used appropriately.

2. Persons administering immunizations should comply with recommendations for proper technique and performance.

   - After inserting the needle into the injection site and before giving the injection, the syringe plunger should be pulled back. If blood appears in the needle hub, the needle should be withdrawn, reinserted into a new site, and the plunger once again pulled back. This process should be repeated until a site is found from which blood is not aspirated.

   - If more than one vaccine preparation is administered or if vaccine and immune globulin are administered simultaneously, it is preferable to give each at a different anatomic site. Ideally, it is preferable to avoid giving two intramuscular injections in the same limb. However, if more than one injection must be given in the same limb, the thigh is usually the preferred site because of greater muscle mass. The injections should be sufficiently separated (i.e. 1-2 inches) so that any local reactions are unlikely to overlap.

- Different vaccines should not be mixed in the same syringe unless specifically designed for such use. Currently, the only vaccines licensed to be mixed in the same syringe are PRP-T *Haemophilis influenzae* type b conjugate vaccine and the DTP vaccine produced by Connaught Laboratories.

- Deviations from recommendations regarding route, site, volume, number, and timing of immunizations should be avoided. Inadequate intervals between immunizations or use of inadequate volumes may lead to unsatisfactory antibody response. If such immunizations are given, generally they should be repeated using recommended technique. If medically documented concern exists that revaccination may result in an increased risk of adverse effects because of repeated prior exposure from the nonstandard vaccinations, immunity to most relevant antigens can be tested serologically to assess the need for revaccination. Immunizations that are given at greater than recommended intervals do not need to be repeated, although recommendations regarding interval and number should be followed in the future.

3. Serious or unusual adverse events occurring after immunization should be reported to the Vaccine Adverse Events Reporting System (VAERS), regardless of whether the provider thinks they are causally related to immunization. VAERS forms and instructions are available in the *FDA Drug Bulletin* (Food and Drug Administration) and the *Physicians' Drug Reference*, or by calling the 24-hour VAERS information recording at 1-800-822-7967.

*Childhood Immunizations*

The National Vaccine Advisory Committee has recently published a comprehensive list of standards for the delivery of childhood immunizations (Table ii-3). Most of these standards are directly relevant to the clinical practices of providers.

Standards 5 and 6 relate to parent and guardian education about immunizations. Beginning in April 1992, as mandated by the National Childhood Vaccine Injury Act (NCVIA) of 1986, every patient who receives a diphtheria-tetanus-pertussis, measles-mumps-rubella, or polio immunization must receive *written* information about: the nature of diseases immunized against; manifestations of adverse reactions; precautionary measures that should be taken to reduce the risk for major adverse reactions; contraindications to, and the basis for delay of, administration of the vaccine; and the availability of the National Vaccine Injury Compensation Program. The U.S. Department of Health and Human Services has developed pamphlets for this purpose. Camera-ready copies are available from each state health department; printed copies may be purchased from the American Academy of Family Physicians or the American Academy of Pediatrics. For ordering information, see the "Family Resources" sections of chapter 12, 15, or 16.

### Table ii-3. National Vaccine Advisory Committee Standards for Childhood Immunization Practices

1. Immunization services are readily available.
2. There are no barriers or unnecessary prerequisites to the receipt of vaccines.
3. Immunization services are available free or for a minimal fee.
4. Providers utilize all clinical encounters to screen and, when indicated, immunize children.
5. Providers educate parents and guardians about immunization in general terms.
6. Providers question parents or guardians about contraindications and, before immunizing a child, inform them in specific terms about the risks and benefits of the immunizations their child is to receive.
7. Providers follow only true contraindications.
8. Providers administer simultaneously all vaccine doses for which a child is eligible at the time of each visit.
9. Providers use accurate and complete recording procedures.
10. Providers co-schedule immunization appointments in conjunction with appointments for other child health services.
11. Providers report adverse events following immunization promptly, accurately and completely.
12. Providers operate a tracking system.
13. Providers adhere to appropriate procedures for vaccine management.
14. Providers conduct semi-annual audits to assess immunization coverage levels and to review immunization records in the patient population they serve.
15. Providers maintain up-to-date, easily retrievable medical protocols at all locations where vaccines are administered.
16. Providers operate with patient-oriented and community-based approaches.
17. Vaccines are administered by properly trained individuals.
18. Providers receive ongoing education and training on current immunization recommendations.

From: National Vaccine Advisory Committee. *Standards for Pediatric Immunization Practices*. Atlanta, Ga: Centers for Disease Control and Prevention; 1993.

Standard 7 is particularly important. Many opportunities to immunize children are missed because clinicians withhold immunizations from children for invalid reasons. The National Vaccine Advisory Committee has issued guidelines on the contraindications and precautions for childhood immunizations. Table ii-4 gives these guidelines for childhood immunizations in general; guidelines for specific immunizations are given in the relevant chapters of this book.

Standard 9 stresses the importance of accurate and complete record keeping. The NCVIA requires for each of the vaccines covered by the act (DTP or component antigens, MMR or component antigens, IPV, and OPV) that the vaccine recipient's permanent medical record (or

## Ch. ii. Implementing Preventive Care — Overview

**Table ii-4. Contraindications and Precautions for Childhood Immunizations***

| True Contraindications and Precautions | NOT Contraindications (vaccines may be given) |
|---|---|
| Anaphylactic reaction to a vaccine contraindicates further doses of that vaccine. | Mild to moderate local reaction (soreness, redness, swelling) following a dose of an injectable antigen |
| Anaphylactic reaction to a vaccine constituent contraindicates the use of vaccines containing that substance | Mild acute illness with or without low-grade fever |
| | Current antimicrobial therapy |
| Moderate or severe illness with or without fever | Convalescent phase of illnesses |
| | Prematurity (same dosage and indications as for normal, full-term infants) |
| | Recent exposure to an infectious disease |
| | History of penicillin or other nonspecific allergies or fact that relatives have such allergies |

* This information is based on the recommendations of the Advisory Committee on Immunization Practices (ACIP) and those of the Committee on Infectious Diseases (Red Book Committee) of the American Academy of Pediatrics (AAP). Sometimes these recommendations vary from those contained in the manufacturers' package inserts. For more detailed information, providers should consult the published recommendations of ACIP, AAP, AAFP, and the manufacturers' package inserts.

From: National Vaccine Advisory Committee. *Standards for Pediatric Immunization Practices.* Atlanta, Ga: Centers for Disease Control and Prevention; 1993.

a permanent office log or file) contain the following information: date the vaccine was administered, the vaccine manufacturer, the vaccine lot number, and the name, address, and title of the person administering the vaccine. The Advisory Committee on Immunization Practices (ACIP) recommends that the above information be recorded for all vaccines and not only for those covered by the NCVIA.

Standard 16 states that clinicians should use patient-oriented and community-based approaches. The use of a patient- or parent-held record is one way to satisfy this standard. All states have official immunization cards for childhood immunizations, and immunization record forms are incorporated into several comprehensive health records for children, such as the *Child Health Guide* of the Put Prevention Into Practice campaign. Use of these records has been shown to be related to increased immunization rates for children in a broad range of socioeconomic groups in the United States.

## Ch. ii. Implementing Preventive Care — Overview

*Adult Immunizations*

The National Coalition for Adult Immunization has published standards for adult immunization practice (Table ii-5). Standards 2, 3, 4, 5, and 10 directly address the responsibilities of primary care clinicians. Standards 4 and 5 stress the important role that risk-factor assessment plays in adult immunization. A great many adults in special need of immunizations against influenza, pneumococcal disease, and hepatitis B do not receive them. High-risk adults have contacts with the health care system, such as during hospitalization, that should be better utilized as opportunities to provide needed immunizations. Proper record keeping, not only by providers but also by patients (Standards 3 and 10), is important for verifying the immunization status of adults and for developing recall systems as recommended in Standard 4.

### Table ii-5. National Coalition for Adult Immunization Standards for Adult Immunization Practices, 1990

The National Coalition for Adult Immunization (NCAI):

1. Encourages the promotion of appropriate vaccine use through information campaigns for health-care practitioners and trainees, employers, and the public about the benefits of immunizations; and
2. Encourages physicians and other health-care personnel (in practice and in training) to protect themselves and prevent transmission to patients by assuring that they themselves are completely immunized; and
3. Recommends that all health providers routinely determine the immunization status of their adult patients, offer vaccines to those for whom they are indicated, and maintain complete immunization records; and
4. Recommends that all health-care providers identify high-risk patients in need of influenza vaccine and develop a system to recall them for annual immunization each autumn; and
5. Recommends that all health-care providers and institutions identify high-risk adult patients in hospitals and other treatment centers and assure that appropriate vaccination is considered either prior to discharge or as part of discharge planning; and
6. Recommends that all licensing/accrediting agencies support the development by health-care institutions of comprehensive immunization programs for staff, trainees, volunteer workers, inpatients, and outpatients; and
7. Encourages states to establish pre-enrollment immunization requirements for colleges and other institutions of higher education; and
8. Recommends that institutions that train health-care professionals, deliver health-care, or provide laboratory or other medical support services require appropriate immunizations for persons at risk of contacting or transmitting vaccine-preventable illnesses; and
9. Encourages health-care benefit programs, third-party payers, and governmental health-care programs to provide coverage for adult immunization services; and
10. Encourages the adoption of a standard personal and institutional immunization record as a means of verifying the immunization status of patients and staff.

From: National Coalition for Adult Immunization. *Standards for Adult Immunization Practices.* Bethesda, Md: National Coalition for Adult Immunization; 1992.

## Ch. ii. Implementing Preventive Care — Overview

*Counseling*

1. The U.S. Preventive Services Task Force described 10 principles for patient education and counseling with which clinicians should be familiar (Table ii-6). Counseling should be culturally appropriate: information and services should be presented in a style and format that is sensitive to the culture, values, and traditions of the patient. Information and services should be provided at a level of comprehension consistent with the age and learning skills of the patient, using a dialect and terminology consistent with the patient's language and communication style.

2. Lack of time for counseling is often cited by busy clinicians as a key barrier to patient counseling. Poor reimbursement for counseling services is also frequently mentioned. Several measures may be taken to improve counseling efficiency:

    - The office or clinic environment can be tailored to promote preventive care. Using a variety of resources creates a milieu that reinforces healthy behaviors. Pamphlets, posters, and other materials should be conspicuously displayed and readily available. Patient education resources may be obtained from the sources listed in each chapter of this book.

    - Short patient questionnaires can quickly assess patient needs for counseling. Many such questionnaires are included in this book. Some are brief enough that they may be incorporated into patient intake questionnaires and history forms.

    - Patients' readiness to change their health-related behaviors should be assessed. This helps to focus the intervention. Research indicates that patients who are in the early stages of behavior change may benefit most from information, but probably not from more intensive interventions. Patients who are ready to change may benefit from more directive, task-oriented counseling and behavior modification. Finally, those who have successfully changed need support and follow-up.

    - Nursing and office/clinic staff and office systems can help perform and monitor counseling.

    - The clinician and staff should be familiar with community resources to which patients may be referred for types of counseling that cannot be provided in the practice.

    - Patient behavior changes, although difficult to achieve, may be more valuable for health than many of the screening tests and immunizations that patients receive. In general, patients value the advice of clinicians. Studies show that even brief interventions, such as simple advice to stop smoking, may have a beneficial effect. More counseling tends to be better counseling, but any counseling, no matter how brief, is better than none at all.

**Table ii-6. USPSTF Principles of Patient Education and Counseling**

1. Develop a therapeutic alliance
2. Counsel all patients
3. Ensure that patients understand the relationship between behavior and health
4. Work with patients to assess barriers to behavior change
5. Gain commitment from patients to change
6. Involve patients in selecting risk factors to change
7. Use a combination of strategies
8. Design a behavior modification plan
9. Monitor progress through follow-up contact
10. Involve office staff

From: From: U.S. Preventive Services Task Force. Recommendations for Patient Education and Counseling. In: *Guide to Clinical Preventive Services*. Baltimore, Md: Williams & Wilkins; 1989:chap. iv.

## Put Prevention Into Practice

The *Clinician's Handbook of Preventive Services* was designed to be used alone as a reference or textbook. It is also, however, a part of an integrated set of resources to improve the delivery of preventive services in clinical settings. These resources, which constitute the *Put Prevention Into Practice Education and Action Kit*, include minirecords for patients and parents and a collection of office materials to improve the tracking and prompting of preventive care. These materials, developed from research-proven prototypes, make preventive care delivery easier and more effective, improving both patient and clinician satisfaction. Information on ordering the *Put Prevention Into Practice Education and Action Kit* can be obtained from: Superintendent of Documents, Government Printing Office, Washington, DC 20402-9325; (202) 783-3238.

## Selected References

### *Establishing a Preventive Care Protocol*

Advisory Committee on Immunization Practices (ACIP). General recommendations on immunization. *MMWR*. In press.

American Academy of Family Physicians, Commission on Public Health and Scientific Affairs. *Age Charts for Periodic Health Examination*. Kansas City, Mo: American Academy of Family Physicians, 1993.

American Academy of Pediatrics, Committee on Infectious Diseases. *Report of the Committee on Infectious Diseases, 1991* ["*Red Book*"] 22nd ed. Elk Grove Village, Ill: American Academy of Pediatrics, 1991.

American Academy of Pediatrics. Committee on Practice and Ambulatory Care. Recommendations for preventive pediatric health care. *AAP News*. 1991;7:19.

American Cancer Society. *Summary of American Cancer Society Recommendations for the Early Detection of Cancer in Asymptomatic People*. Atlanta, Ga: American Cancer Society, 1992.

American College of Obstetricians and Gynecologists. *The Obstetrician-Gynecologist and Primary-Preventive Health Care.* Washington, DC: American College of Obstetricians and Gynecologists, 1993.

American College of Physicians Task Force on Adult Immunization and Infectious Diseases Society of America. *Guide for Adult Immunization* 2nd ed. Philadelphia, Pa: American College of Physicians, 1990.

American Medical Association. *Guidelines for Adolescent Preventive Services.* Chicago, Ill: American Medical Association, 1992.

Burack RC, Liang J. The early detection of cancer in the primary-care setting: factors associated with the acceptance and completion of recommended procedures. *Prev Med.* 1987;16:739-751.

Canadian Task Force on the Periodic Health Examination. The periodic health examination. *Can Med Assoc J.* 1979;121:1194-1254.

Davis K, Bialek R, Parkinson M, Smith J, Vellozzi C. Paying for prevention: moving the debate forward. *Am J Prev Med.* 1990;6(suppl):7-32.

Dietrich AJ, Goldberg H. Preventive content of adult primary care: do generalists and subspecialists differ? *Am J Public Health.* 1984;74:223-227.

Eddy DM, ed. *Common Screening Tests.* Philadelphia, Pa: American College of Physicians, 1991.

Frame PS. A critical review of adult health maintenance. *J Fam Pract.* 1986;22:341-346, 417-422, 511-520, and 23:29-39.

Frame PS, Carlson SJ. A critical review of periodic health screening using specific screening criteria. *J Fam Pract.* 1975;2:29-36.

Gemson DH, Elinson J. Prevention in primary care: variability in physician practice patterns in New York City. *Am J Prev Med.* 1986;2:226-234.

Hayward RSA, Steinberg EP, Ford DE, Roizen MF, Roach KW. Preventive care guidelines: 1991. *Ann Intern Med.* 1991;114:758-783.

McPhee SJ, Richard RJ, Solkowitz SN. Performance of cancer screening in a university internal medicine practice: comparison with the 1980 American Cancer Society guidelines. *J Gen Intern Med.* 1986;1:275-281.

Smart CR, Chu K, Conley V, Henson DE, Pommerenke F, Srivastova S. Cancer screening and early detection. In: Holland JF, Frei EF, Bast RC, Kufe DW, Morton DL, Weichselbaum RR, eds. *Cancer Medicine* 3rd ed. Vol 1. Philadelphia, Pa: Lea and Febiger, 1993:408-431.

US Preventive Services Task Force. *Guide to Clinical Preventive Services.* Baltimore, Md: Williams & Wilkins, 1989.

Williamson, PS, Driscoll CE, Dvorak, Garber KA, Shank JC. Health screening examinations: the patient's perspective. *J Fam Pract.* 1988;27:178-192.

Woo B, Woo B, Cook F, et al. Screening procedures in the asymptomatic adult: comparison of physicians' recommendations, patient desires, published guidelines, and actual practice. *JAMA.* 1985;254:1480-1484.

## *Implementing the Preventive Care Protocol in Practice*

Belcher DW, Berg AO, Inui TS. Practical approaches to providing better preventive care: are physicians a problem or a solution? *Am J Prev Med.* 1988;4(suppl):27-48.

Block L, Banspach SW, Gans K, et al. Impact of public education on physician attitudes and behavior concerning cholesterol. *Am J Prev Med.* 1988;4:255-260.

Carney P, Dietrich AJ, Keller A, Landgraf J, O'Connor GT. Tools, teamwork, and tenacity: elements of a cancer control office system for primary care. *J Fam Pract.* 1992;35:388-394.

Davidson RA, Fletcher SW, Retchin S, Duh S. A nurse-initiated reminder system for the periodic health examination. *Arch Intern Med.* 1984;144:2167-2170.

Dickey LL, Pettiti DB. A patient-held minirecord to promote adult preventive care. *J Fam Pract.* 1992;34:457-463.

Dietrich AJ, O'Connor GT, Keller A, Carney PA, Levy D, Whaley FS. Cancer: improving early detection and prevention. A community practice randomized trial. *Br Med J.* 1992;304:687-691.

Frame PS, Kowulich BA, Llewellyn AM. Improving physician compliance with a health maintenance protocol. *J Fam Pract.* 1984;19:340-344.

Harris RP, O'Malley MS, Fletcher SW, Knight BP. Prompting physicians for preventive procedures: a five-year study of manual and computer reminders. *Am J Prev Med.* 1990;6:145-152.

Larsen EB, Bergman J, Heidrich F, et al. Do postcard reminders improve influenza vaccination compliance? a prospective trial of different postcard cues. *Med Care.* 1982;20:639-648.

McCormick MC, Shapiro S, Starfield BH. The association of patient-held records and completion of immunizations. *Clin Pediatr (Phila).* 1981;20:270-274.

McDowell I, Newell C, Rosser W. Comparison of three methods of recalling patients for influenza vaccination. *Can Med Assoc J.* 1986;135:991-997.

McPhee SJ, Bird JA, Fordham D, Rodnick JE, Osborn EH. Promoting cancer prevention activities by primary care physicians. *JAMA.* 1991;266:538-544.

Ornstein SM, Garr DR, Jenkins RG, Rust PF, Arnon AA. Computer-generated physician and patient reminders: tools to improve population adherence to selected preventive services. *J Fam Pract.* 1991;32:82-90.

Pommerenke FA, Dietrich A. Improving and maintaining preventive services: I. applying the patient model. *J Fam Pract.* 1992;34:86-91.

Shank JC, Powell T, Llewelyn J. A five-year demonstration project associated with improvement in physician health maintenance behavior. *Fam Med.* 1989;21:273-278.

Turner RC, Wauvers LE, O'Brien KO. The effect of patient-carried reminder cards on the performance of health maintenance measures. *Arch Intern Med.* 1990;150:645-647.

## *Principles of Screening, Immunization, and Counseling*

Advisory Committee on Immunization Practices (ACIP). General recommendations on immunization. *MMWR.* In press.

Centers for Disease Control. National Childhood Vaccine Injury Act: requirements for permanent vaccination records and for reporting of selected events after vaccination. *MMWR.* 1988;37:197-200.

Centers for Disease Control. The public burden of vaccine preventable diseases among adults. *MMWR.* 1990;39:725-729.

Fedson DS, Harward MP, Reid RA, Kaiser DL. Hospital-based pneumococcal immunization: epidemiologic rationale from the Shenandoah study. *JAMA.* 1990;264:1117-1122.

Green LW. How physicians can improve patients' participation and maintenance in self-care. *West J Med.* 1987;147:346-349.

Greenfield S, Kaplan S, Ware JE. Expanding patient involvement in care: effects on patient outcomes. *Ann Intern Med.* 1985;102:520-528.

Kottke TE, Battista RN, DeFriese GH, Brekke ML. Attributes of successful smoking cessation interventions in medical practice: a meta-analysis of 39 controlled trials. *JAMA.* 1988;259:2882-2889.

Mullen PD, Green LW, Persinger G. Clinical trials of patient education for chronic conditions: a comparative analysis of intervention types. *Prev Med.* 1985;14:753-781.

National Coalition for Adult Immunization. *Standards for Adult Immunization Practices.* Bethesda, Md: National Coalition for Adult Immunization, 1992.

National Vaccine Advisory Committee. *Standards for Pediatric Immunization Practices.* Atlanta, Ga: Centers for Disease Control and Prevention, 1993. Also published in *MMWR.* 1993;42(RR-13):1-13.

Prochaska JO, DiClemente CC, Norcross JC. In search of how people change: applications to addictive behaviors. *Am Psychologist.* 1992;47:1102-1114.

Simons-Morton DG, Mullen PD, Mains DA, Tabak ER, Green LW. Characteristics of controlled studies of patient education and counseling for preventive health behaviors. *Pat Educ Couns.* 1992;19:175-204.

US Preventive Services Task Force. Methodology. In: *Guide to Clinical Preventive Services.* Baltimore, Md: Williams & Wilkins, 1989:xxvii-xxxviii.

US Preventive Services Task Force. Recommendations for patient education and counseling. In: *Guide to Clinical Preventive Services.* Baltimore, Md: Williams & Wilkins, 1989:lix-lxii.

Walsh DC, Hingson RW, Merrigan DM, et al. The impact of a physician warning on recovery after alcoholism treatment. *JAMA.* 1992;267:663-667.

Wells KB, Lewis CE, Leake B, Ware JE. Do physicians preach what they practice? a study of physicians' health habits and counseling practices. *JAMA.* 1984;252:2846-2848.

# Clinician's Handbook of Preventive Services

## Children/Adolescents

## Children/Adolescents — SCREENING

# 1. Anemia

Due to improved nutrition, anemia has diminished as a problem for children in the United States. Nonetheless, certain groups of children (particularly infants and adolescent girls) remain at significant risk of anemia. Among infants, the following characteristics confer special risk: low socioeconomic status, consumption of cow's milk starting before 6 months of age, consumption of formula not fortified with iron, and low birth weight. If untreated, anemia can lead to fatigue, apathy, impairment of growth and development, and decreased resistance to infection.

Iron deficiency is the most common cause of anemia for children and adolescents. Hemoglobinopathies, such as sickle cell disease and thalassemia, are also significant causes of anemia in children. See chapters 8 and 26 for information on screening for hemoglobinopathies in newborns and adults, respectively.

**Recommendations of Major Authorities**

- **American Academy of Family Physicians** and **U.S. Preventive Services Task Force** —All children should be screened for anemia once during infancy.

- **American Academy of Pediatrics**—Hemoglobin or hematocrit should be measured once during infancy (between 6 and 9 months), early childhood (between 1 and 5 years), late childhood (between 5 and 12 years), and adolescence (between 14 and 20 years).

- **Canadian Task Force on the Periodic Health Examination**—Hemoglobin concentration screening should be performed on children at high risk for iron-deficiency anemia: premature babies; babies born of a multiple pregnancy or an iron-deficient woman; and children in low socioeconomic conditions. This recommendation is currently under review.

**Basics of Anemia Screening**

1. Hemoglobin/hematocrit testing to screen for anemia can be accomplished by either of two basic methods: venipuncture with analysis by automated cell counter or capillary puncture with microhematocrit analysis by centrifuge. The latter method yields slightly higher values and is somewhat less sensitive than the former.

2. In general, screening should not be done if the child has experienced a fever or infection during the preceding 2 to 3 weeks.

3. If the microhematocrit method is used, the following principles of collection should be followed:

    - In infants, the best sites for collection are the medial and lateral aspects of the plantar surface of the heel. In older children, the best sites are the medial and lateral aspects

# Ch. 1. Anemia          Children/Adolescents — SCREENING

of the pulp of a finger; the puncture should be made perpendicular to the skin and across the dermal ridges.

- To increase blood flow, a warm (100° to 108°F), moist towel may be applied to the site.

- Before puncture, the site should be cleaned with an antiseptic and allowed to dry.

- Sterile, disposable lancets with tips less than 2.5 mm long should be used with infants 6 months of age or younger. Lancets with longer tips (up to 5 mm) may be used for older children.

- The first drop of blood, which contains tissue fluids, should be wiped away with a dry gauze.

- Massage of the collection site should be avoided if possible, as this may dilute the sample with tissue fluids.

4. Table 1-1 gives hemoglobin and hematocrit cut points for the diagnosis of anemia in children. It is derived from the Second National Health and Nutrition Examination Survey (NHANES II) conducted from 1976 through 1980. Although NHANES II did not provide data for children less than 1 year of age, by extrapolation the cut points for 6-month-old children can be determined to be essentially the same as (only a fraction of a unit less than) those for 1-year-old children.

Cut points for anemia should be adjusted upward for children who live at high altitudes and for children and adolescents who smoke (see Tables 26-1 and 26-2).

## Selected References

American Academy of Family Physicians, Commission on Public Health and Scientific Affairs. *Age Charts for Periodic Health Examination*. Kansas City, Mo: American Academy of Family Physicians; 1993.

American Academy of Pediatrics, Committee on Nutrition. *Pediatric Nutrition Handbook*. 3rd ed. Elk Grove Village, Ill: American Academy of Pediatrics; 1993.

American Academy of Pediatrics, Committee on Practice and Ambulatory Care. Recommendations for preventive pediatric health care. *AAP News*. 1991;7:19.

Centers for Disease Control. CDC criteria for anemia in children and childbearing-aged women. *MMWR*. 1989;38:400-404.

Dallman PR. Has routine screening of infants for anemia become obsolete in the United States? *Pediatrics*. 1987;80:439-441.

Dallman PR. New approaches to screening for iron deficiency. *J Pediatr*. 1977;90:678-681.

Dallman PR, Yip R, Johnson C. Prevalence and causes of anemia in the United States, 1976 to 1980. *Am J Clin Nutr*. 1984;39:437-445.

Lozoff B, Brittenham GM, Wolf AW, et al. Iron deficiency anemia and iron therapy effects on infant developmental test performance. *Pediatrics*. 1987;79:981-995.

Meites S, Levitt MJ. Skin-puncture and blood-collecting techniques for infants. *Clin Chem*. 1979;25:183-189.

**Table 1-1. Hemoglobin and Hematocrit Cutpoints for Anemia in Children 1 Year of Age or Older**

| Gender | Age, y | Hemoglobin, g/dL | Hematocrit, % |
|---|---|---|---|
| Both Genders | 1-1.9 | 11.0 | 33.0 |
| | 2-4.9 | 11.2 | 34.0 |
| | 5-7.9 | 11.4 | 34.5 |
| | 8-11.9 | 11.6 | 35.0 |
| Female | 12-14.9 | 11.8 | 35.5 |
| | 15-17.9 | 12.0 | 36.0 |
| | ≥18 | 12.0 | 36.0 |
| Male | 12-14.9 | 12.3 | 37.0 |
| | 15-17.9 | 12.6 | 38.0 |
| | ≥18 | 13.6 | 41.0 |

From: Centers for Disease Control. CDC criteria for anemia in children and childbearing-aged women. *MMWR.* 1989;38:400-404.

Randolph VS. Considerations for the clinical laboratory serving the pediatric patient. *Am J Med Technol.* 1982;48:7.

Reeves JD, Yip R, Kiley VA, Dallman PR. Iron deficiency in infants: the influence of mild antecedent infection. *J Pediatr.* 1984;105:874-879.

Thomas WJ, Collins TM. Comparison of venipuncture blood counts with microcapillary measurement in screening for anemia in one-year-old infants. *J Pediatr.* 1982;101:32-35.

US Preventive Services Task Force. Screening for anemia. In: *Guide to Clinical Preventive Services.* Baltimore, Md: Williams & Wilkins; 1989:chap 28.

Yip R, Binkin NJ, Fleshood L, Trowbridge FL. Declining prevalence of anemia among low-income children in the United States. *JAMA.* 1987;258:1619-1623.

Young PC, Hamill BH, Wasserman RC, Dickerman JD. Evaluation of the capillary microhematocrit as a screening test for anemia in pediatric office practice. *Pediatrics.* 1986;78:206-209.

# Children/Adolescents — SCREENING

## 2. Blood Pressure

Hypertension in children is defined as persistent blood pressure elevation that is at or above the blood pressure of 95% of children of the same age and sex on initial screening. If not recognized and treated, blood pressure may continue to rise and in some cases become life-threatening. For many children with hypertension who are less than 10 years of age, there is an identifiable cause. Older children and adolescents are more likely to suffer from essential hypertension. In adults, hypertension is a known risk factor for coronary artery disease, congestive heart failure, stroke, renal disease, and retinopathy. Early identification of children with elevated blood pressures may make it possible to halt the hypertensive process and the development of complications.

### Recommendations of Major Authorities

- **American Academy of Family Physicians** and **U.S. Preventive Services Task Force**—Measurement of blood pressure should be performed periodically beginning at 3 years of age.

- **American Academy of Pediatrics**—Blood pressure should be measured annually in children between 3 and 6 years of age, and every 2 years thereafter.

- **American Medical Association**—Blood pressure should be measured annually during adolescence.

- **National Heart, Lung, and Blood Institute Task Force on Blood Pressure Control in Children**—Blood pressure should be measured annually beginning at 3 years of age.

### Basics of Blood Pressure Screening

1. The patient should not have smoked (or otherwise used tobacco) or have ingested caffeine (including cola products) within 30 minutes prior to the measurement. This is especially important in screening adolescents.

2. The measurement should be performed in a quiet area, with the child sitting comfortably. The right arm should be fully exposed and supported at the level of the heart.

3. A mercury column or a calibrated aneroid gauge should be used. The inflatable bladder of the compression cuff should encircle 80% to 100% of the upper arm without impinging on the antecubital fossa. Use of a cuff that is too small will result in falsely elevated measurements, whereas a cuff that is too large will result in falsely low measurements.

4. The bell of the stethoscope should be placed lightly on the antecubital fossa over the brachial artery. Applying too much pressure may lead to inaccurate measurements. The cuff should be rapidly inflated to approximately 20 mm Hg above the point at which the pulse is no longer audible. The cuff should then be deflated at a rate of 2 to 3 mm Hg per

second. The onset of a tapping sound (the first Korotkoff phase) is used to determine systolic blood pressure. The fourth Korotkoff phase is identified by low-pitched muffled sounds. This is followed by the fifth phase, the disappearance of all sounds. The fifth phase may not be present in children. For this reason, the fourth Korotkoff phase should be used to determine diastolic blood pressure in children. In adolescents, the fifth phase is distinguishable and should be used to determine the diastolic blood pressure.

5. It may be helpful for future assessment to document the patient's position, limb used, cuff size, and whether the fourth or fifth Korotkoff phase was used.

6. The systolic and diastolic blood pressures corresponding to the 90th and 95th percentiles according to gender and age are given in Table 2-1. Blood pressures in the 90th through 94th percentiles should be considered high normal, whereas those at or greater than the 95th percentile should be considered elevated.

Table 2-1. 90th and 95th Percentile Blood Pressures (mm Hg) According to Gender and Age

| Age, y | Male Systolic 90% | Male Systolic 95% | Male Diastolic 90% | Male Diastolic 95% | Female Systolic 90% | Female Systolic 95% | Female Diastolic 90% | Female Diastolic 95% |
|---|---|---|---|---|---|---|---|---|
| 3  | 107 | 111 | 68 | 73 | 106 | 110 | 69 | 73 |
| 4  | 108 | 112 | 69 | 73 | 107 | 111 | 69 | 73 |
| 5  | 109 | 113 | 69 | 74 | 109 | 112 | 69 | 73 |
| 6  | 111 | 115 | 70 | 75 | 111 | 115 | 70 | 74 |
| 7  | 112 | 116 | 71 | 76 | 112 | 116 | 71 | 75 |
| 8  | 114 | 118 | 73 | 77 | 114 | 117 | 72 | 76 |
| 9  | 115 | 119 | 74 | 78 | 115 | 118 | 74 | 78 |
| 10 | 117 | 122 | 75 | 79 | 117 | 121 | 75 | 79 |
| 11 | 119 | 123 | 76 | 80 | 119 | 123 | 77 | 81 |
| 12 | 121 | 126 | 77 | 81 | 122 | 126 | 78 | 83 |
| 13 | 124 | 128 | 77 | 81 | 124 | 128 | 78 | 83 |
| 14 | 126 | 130 | 78 | 82 | 125 | 129 | 81 | 85 |
| 15 | 129 | 133 | 79 | 83 | 126 | 130 | 83 | 86 |
| 16 | 131 | 136 | 81 | 85 | 127 | 131 | 81 | 85 |
| 17 | 134 | 138 | 83 | 87 | 127 | 132 | 80 | 84 |
| 18 | 136 | 140 | 84 | 88 | 127 | 132 | 80 | 84 |

Adapted from: Task Force on Blood Pressure Control in Children. Report of the second task force on blood pressure control in children—1987. *Pediatrics.* 1987;79;1-25. Reproduced by permission of *Pediatrics*; copyright © 1987.

7. Elevated readings should be confirmed on at least two separate occasions and the average computed.

8. Fig 2-1 presents an algorithm for identifying children and adolescents with hypertension. It is important in assessing elevated blood pressure in children and adolescents to take into consideration the blood pressure-elevating effects of increased height and weight for age.

**Selected References**

American Academy of Family Physicians, Commission on Public Health and Scientific Affairs. *Age Charts for Periodic Health Examination*. Kansas City, Mo: American Academy of Family Physicians; 1993.

American Academy of Pediatrics, Committee on Practice and Ambulatory Care. Recommendations for preventive pediatric health care. *AAP News*. 1991;7:19.

American Medical Association. *Guidelines for Adolescent Preventive Services (GAPS)*. Chicago, Ill: American Medical Association; 1992.

Canadian Task Force on the Periodic Health Examination. The periodic health examination. *Can Med Assoc J*. 1979;121:1194-1254.

DeSwiet M, Dillon MJ. Hypertension in children. *Br Med J*. 1989;299(6697):469-470.

Fixler DE, Laird WP. Validity of mass blood pressure screening in children. *Pediatrics*. 1983;72:459-463.

Joint National Committee on Detection, Evaluation, and Treatment of High Blood Pressure. *The Fifth Report of the Joint National Committee on the Detection, Evaluation, and Treatment of High Blood Pressure*. Bethesda, Md: National Institutes of Health; 1993. US Dept of Health and Human Services publication NIH 93-1088. Also, *Arch Intern Med*. 1993;153:154-183.

Lauer RM, Burns TL, Clarke WR. Assessing children's blood pressure—considerations of age and body size: the Muscatine study. *Pediatrics*. 1985;75:1081-1090.

Mehta SK. Pediatric hypertension: a challenge for pediatricians. *AJDC*. 1987;141:893-894.

Sinaiko AR, Gomez-Marion O, Prineas RJ. Prevalence of "significant" hypertension in junior high school-aged children: the Children and Adolescent Blood Pressure Program. *J Pediatr*. 1989;114:664-669.

Task Force on Blood Pressure Control in Children. Report of the Second Task Force on Blood Pressure Control in Children—1987. *Pediatrics*. 1987;79:1-25.

US Preventive Services Task Force. Screening for hypertension. In: *Guide to Clinical Preventive Services*. Baltimore, Md: Williams & Wilkins; 1989:chap 3.

## Ch. 2. Blood Pressure — Children/Adolescents — SCREENING

**Figure 2-1. Algorithm for Identifying Children and Adolescents With Hypertension**

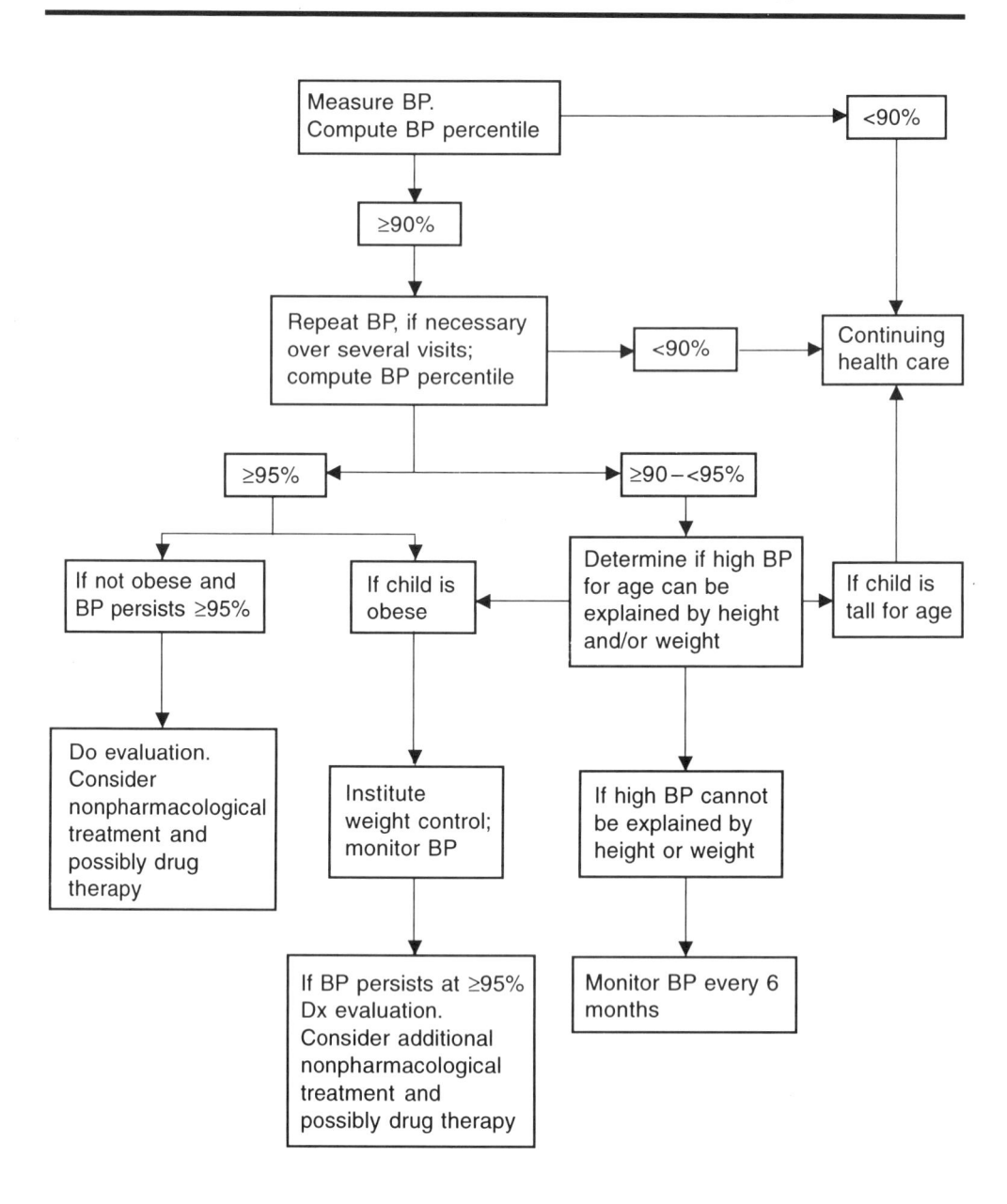

```
                  ┌──────────────────────┐
                  │ Measure BP.          │──────────────────────►  <90%
                  │ Compute BP percentile│                          │
                  └──────────┬───────────┘                          │
                             │ ≥90%                                 │
                             ▼                                      │
                  ┌──────────────────────┐                          │
                  │ Repeat BP, if        │                ┌─────────▼────────┐
                  │ necessary over       │──►  <90%  ──► │ Continuing       │
                  │ several visits;      │               │ health care      │
                  │ compute BP percentile│               └──────────────────┘
                  └──┬────────────────┬──┘                         ▲
                     │ ≥95%           │ ≥90–<95%                   │
                     ▼                ▼                            │
         ┌──────────┬──────────┐  ┌──────────────────┐   ┌────────────────┐
         │          │          │  │ Determine if high│──►│ If child is    │
         │ If not   │ If child │◄─│ BP for age can be│   │ tall for age   │
         │ obese and│ is obese │  │ explained by     │   └────────────────┘
         │ BP       │          │  │ height and/or    │
         │ persists │          │  │ weight           │
         │ ≥95%     │          │  └────────┬─────────┘
         └────┬─────┴────┬─────┘           │
              ▼          ▼                 ▼
     ┌──────────────┐ ┌────────────┐ ┌──────────────────┐
     │ Do evaluation│ │ Institute  │ │ If high BP cannot│
     │ Consider     │ │ weight     │ │ be explained by  │
     │ nonpharmaco- │ │ control;   │ │ height or weight │
     │ logical      │ │ monitor BP │ └─────────┬────────┘
     │ treatment and│ └──────┬─────┘           │
     │ possibly drug│        │                 ▼
     │ therapy      │        ▼         ┌──────────────────┐
     └──────────────┘ ┌──────────────┐ │ Monitor BP every │
                      │ If BP        │ │ 6 months         │
                      │ persists at  │ └──────────────────┘
                      │ ≥95% Dx      │
                      │ evaluation.  │
                      │ Consider     │
                      │ additional   │
                      │ nonpharmaco- │
                      │ logical      │
                      │ treatment and│
                      │ possibly drug│
                      │ therapy      │
                      └──────────────┘
```

Adapted from: NHLBI Task Force on Blood Pressure Control in Children. *Report of the Second Task Force on Blood Pressure Control in Children—1987*. Bethesda, MD: National Institutes of Health; 1987.

# Children/Adolescents — SCREENING

## 3. Body Measurement

Body measurement of infants and children serves to help identify significant childhood conditions, including growth retardation, malnutrition, obesity, and developmental abnormalities. Head circumference measurement can identify abnormal brain development, including hydrocephalus, in infants. In older children and adolescents, obesity and eating disorders are target conditions for screening. Obesity in children has been associated with the development of heart disease in adulthood.

### Recommendations of Major Authorities

- **American Academy of Family Physicians** and **U.S. Preventive Services Task Force**—Height and weight of children should be measured regularly throughout infancy and childhood. Neither authority has evaluated head circumference measurement.

- **American Academy of Pediatrics**—Height, weight, and head circumference should be measured at birth, at 2 to 4 weeks, and at 1, 2, 4, 6, 9, 12, 15, 18, and 24 months of age. Height and weight should also be measured at ages 3, 4, and 5 years, and every 2 years between ages 6 and 20 years.

- **American Medical Association**—All adolescents should be screened annually for eating disorders and obesity by measuring weight and stature and by asking about body image and dieting patterns.

- **Canadian Task Force on the Periodic Health Examination**—Height, weight, and head circumference should be measured at birth, at 2 to 4 weeks, at 2, 4, 6, 9, 12 to 15, and 18 months, and at 2 to 3, 4, 5 to 6, and 10 to 11 years of age to detect anomalies of physical growth. Height and weight should be measured periodically for children over the age of 12 years who are at high risk for malnutrition: adolescent girls, food "faddists," Native Americans, Inuits, and mothers who are nursing for unusually long periods. Evidence regarding screening for obesity in children is currently under review.

### Basics of Body Measurement

1. To ensure accurate measurements of infants and young children, it is helpful to have assistance. For accuracy, it may be necessary to take measurements more than once, particularly with young or uncooperative children.

2. Height should be obtained by measuring recumbent length of children less than 2 years of age and those aged 2 to 3 who cannot stand unassisted. A measuring board with a stationary headboard and a sliding vertical foot piece should be used if available. If unavailable, a stationary vertical surface, such as the side guard of the examining table, and a movable vertical surface, such as a heavy ruler, may be used along with a measuring tape. The general principles for taking the measurement are the same, regardless of apparatus: The child should lie flat against the center of the board or

examining table, the head should be held against the headboard and knees held so that the hips and legs are extended. The foot piece is then moved until it rests firmly against the child's heels. Measurements should be read to the nearest 1/8 inch (0.3 cm).

3. Standing height should be obtained on children beginning at 2 to 3 years of age. Measurements may be made accurately by using a graduated ruler or tape attached to a wall and a flat surface that is placed horizontally on top of the head. A stadiometer, an instrument specifically designed for height measurements, may also be used, if available. The child's feet should be bare or in socks only. The child should stand with head, shoulder blades, buttocks, and heels touching the wall. The knees should be straight and feet flat on the floor, and the child should be asked to look straight ahead. The flat surface (or movable headboard) should be lowered until it touches the crown of the head, compressing the hair. Height measuring rods attached to weight scales tend to become inaccurate with use; in general, they should not be used unless checked frequently for accuracy.

4. A balance-beam or electronic scale should be used to weigh infants and children. Spring-type scales are not sufficiently accurate for this use. The scale should be checked to make sure it is zeroed before each use. The infant or child should be weighed wearing only a dry diaper or light undergarments. Scales should be checked regularly for accuracy, and an effort should be made to use the same scale on subsequent visits.

5. Head circumference should be measured by extending a nonstretchable measuring tape (metal, fiberglass, and disposable paper tapes are better than cloth) around the most prominent part of the occiput to the middle of the forehead. The tape should be tightened to compress the hair.

6. Measurements should be plotted on age- and gender-specific National Center for Health Statistics (NCHS) growth charts for comparison with NCHS reference standards. Recording serial measurements over time provides an accurate record of growth, with large or sustained deviations signaling a potential problem. Measurements should be interpreted within the context of the individual child's family and growth history. For children whose measurements fall within the 10th through 25th percentile range or the 75th through 90th percentile range, past growth patterns and genetic and environmental factors should be assessed to help determine whether more in-depth follow-up is necessary. Measurements below the 5th percentile or above the 95th percentile should be re-checked. If these measurements are confirmed, detailed medical evaluations may be needed.

There is disagreement about the validity of using a single set of reference standards for all subpopulations of American children. Although measurements should be assessed within the context of genetic and environmental factors, most authorities support the use of the NCHS reference standards. Exceptions include children with genetic conditions such as Down, Turner's, Marfan's, and fragile X syndromes, achondroplasia, sickle cell disease, and neurofibromatosis. Separate growth charts have been developed for some of these conditions. Growth charts have also been developed for use with infants born prematurely (see Selected References).

7. During the first year of life, it is useful to take infant length into consideration when assessing head circumference. One formula developed for this purpose (Dine et al. 1981) defines the 5th and 95th percentile head circumferences as:

$$.5 \times \text{length} + 9.5 \text{ cm } [3.75 \text{ in}] \pm 2.5 \text{cm } [\pm 1 \text{ in}]$$

8. Some authorities, including the American Medical Association, recommend using body mass index (BMI) calculation to assess the weight of adolescents. See chapter 28 for information about the calculation and use of BMI.

**Family Resources**

*Child Health Guide*, part of the Put Prevention Into Practice campaign, contains growth charts and information about development and other important clinical preventive services needed by children. Superintendent of Documents, Government Printing Office, Washington, DC 20402-9325.

*Health Diary: Myself, My Baby* contains information about pregnancy and early childhood development. Superintendent of Documents, Government Printing Office, Washington, DC 20402-9325.

*The Child Health Record*, contains growth charts and other record forms; *Your Child's Growth: Developmental Milestones*, contains information on growth for children 3 months to 6 years of age. American Academy of Pediatrics, PO Box 927, Elk Grove Village, IL 60009-0927; 1-800 433-9016.

*Your Growing Baby*, includes information on growth. Ross Laboratories, Dept. L-1120, Columbus, OH 43260; 1-800 227-5767.

**Provider Resources**

*Growth charts*

Mead Johnson Nutritional Division; (812) 429-5000 for name and number of area representative.

Ross Laboratories, Dept. L-1120, Columbus, OH 43260; 1-800 227-5767.

**Selected References**

American Academy of Family Physicians, Commission on Public Health and Scientific Affairs. *Age Charts for Periodic Health Examination*. Kansas City, Mo: American Academy of Family Physicians; 1993.

Babson SG, Benda GI. Growth graphs for the clinical assessment of infants of varying gestational age. *J Pediatr.* 1976;89:814-820.

Canadian Task Force on the Periodic Health Examination. The periodic health examination. *Can Med Assoc J.* 1979;121:1194-1254.

Casey PH, Kraemer HC, Bernbaum J, et al. Growth Patterns of low birth weight preterm infants: an analysis of a large, varied sample. *J Pediatr.* 1990;117:289-307.

Chinn S, Price CE, Rona RJ. Need for new reference curves for height. *Arch Dis Child.* 1989;64:1545-1553.

Cronk C, Crocker AC, Pueschel SM, et al. Growth charts for children with Down syndrome: 1 month to 18 years of age. *Pediatrics.* 1988;81:102-110.

Dine MS, Gartside PS, Glueck CJ, et al. Relationship of head circumference to length in the first 400 days of life. *Pediatrics.* 1981;67:506-507.

Hamill PVV, Drizd TA, Johnson CL, et al. Physical growth: National Center for Health Statistics percentiles. *Am J Clin Nutr.* 1979;32:607-629.

Lohman TG, Roche AF, Martorell R. *Anthropometric Standardization Reference Manual.* Champaign, Ill: Human Kinetics Books; 1988.

Moore WM, Roche AF. *Pediatric Anthropometry.* Columbus, Ohio: Ross Laboratories: 1982.

Naeraa RW, Nielsen J. Standards for growth and final height in Turner's syndrome. *Acta Paediatr Scand.* 1990;79:182-190.

*Nutritional Screening of Children: A Manual for Screening and Followup.* Washington, DC: US Dept. of Health and Human Services, Public Health Service, Health Services Administration, Bureau of Community Health Services, Office of Maternal and Child Health; 1981. US DHHS publication HSA 81-5114.

National Center for Health Statistics Growth Charts. *Monthly Vital Statistics Report.* Hyattsville, Md: US Department of Health, Education, and Welfare; 1976; 25:1-22. US HEW publication HRA 76-1120.

US Preventive Services Task Force. Screening for obesity. In: *Guide to Clinical Preventive Services.* Baltimore, Md: Williams & Wilkins; 1989: chap 18.

Vaughn VC. On the utility of growth curves. *JAMA.* 1992;267:975-976.

Yip R, Scanlon K, Trowbridge F. Improving the growth status of Asian refugee children in the United States. *JAMA.* 1992;267:937-940.

# Children/Adolescents — SCREENING

## 4. Cholesterol

Of the leading risk factors for coronary heart disease, hyperlipidemia is the most prevalent in children. Twenty-five percent of children have total cholesterol levels above 170 mg/dL. Autopsy studies have found the presence of aortic fatty streaks in children to be correlated with total cholesterol and low-density lipoprotein levels. Children with high cholesterol levels are at increased risk of having high cholesterol levels as adults. Nonetheless, many children with high cholesterol do not go on to have high cholesterol levels as adults, and the safety and effectiveness of treating high cholesterol in childhood as a means of preventing coronary artery disease in adulthood has not been established.

### Recommendations of Major Authorities

- **Expert Panel on Blood Cholesterol Levels in Children and Adolescents of the National Heart, Lung, and Blood Institute's National Cholesterol Education Program, American Academy of Family Physicians, American Academy of Pediatrics,** and **American Medical Association**—Universal screening of children for cholesterol levels is not recommended. Children older than 2 years of age who have a parent with a total cholesterol level of 240 mg/dL or greater should be screened for total cholesterol. Children above the age of 2 years with a family history of premature cardiovascular disease—i.e., a parent or grandparent who, at the age of 55 years or younger, suffered a documented myocardial infarction, angina pectoris, peripheral vascular disease, cerebrovascular disease, or sudden cardiac death, or underwent diagnostic coronary arteriography and was found to have atherosclerosis, or underwent coronary artery bypass surgery or angioplasty—should be screened for lipoprotein levels. Screening of other children may be indicated if the family history is unobtainable, especially if risk factors for coronary artery disease (high blood pressure, smoking, overweight, or excessive consumption of saturated fat and cholesterol) are present.

- **Canadian Task Force on the Periodic Health Examination**—There is insufficient evidence to recommend routine cholesterol screening for children and adolescents. Individual clinical judgment should be exercised to determine the need for screening.

### Basics of Cholesterol Screening

1. The child may eat a normal diet before total cholesterol screening. Children undergoing lipoprotein analysis should fast, taking nothing but water for 12 hours before the blood sample is taken.

2. Children should not be screened when acutely ill, including with infectious diseases. Pregnant adolescents should not be screened.

3. A venous sample obtained in the sitting position yields the most accurate results (recumbency lowers lipid levels). For screening purposes, however, finger-stick capillary technique is adequate and position is not important.

4. The clinician should take into account the cholesterol-raising effect of certain medications, including corticosteroids, isotretinoin, thiazides, anticonvulsants, beta blockers, and certain anabolic steroids. If a patient meeting screening criteria is on one of these drugs, it is probably simplest to do the test and, if the result is elevated, to consider the magnitude of the elevation and the ease and safety of suspending medication for retesting in the absence of drugs.

5. The laboratory used for analysis should be a participant in a program of external standardization to ensure compliance with standards of precision and accuracy. The National Cholesterol Education Program's Laboratory Standardization Panel has recommended that bias not exceed ±3% from the true value and that the intralaboratory coefficient of variation not exceed ±3%.

6. The National Cholesterol Education Program has recommended protocols for assessing cholesterol levels in screening of children (Figs 4-1 and 4-2).

**Figure 4-1. Assessment and Follow-up of Total Cholesterol Measurements**

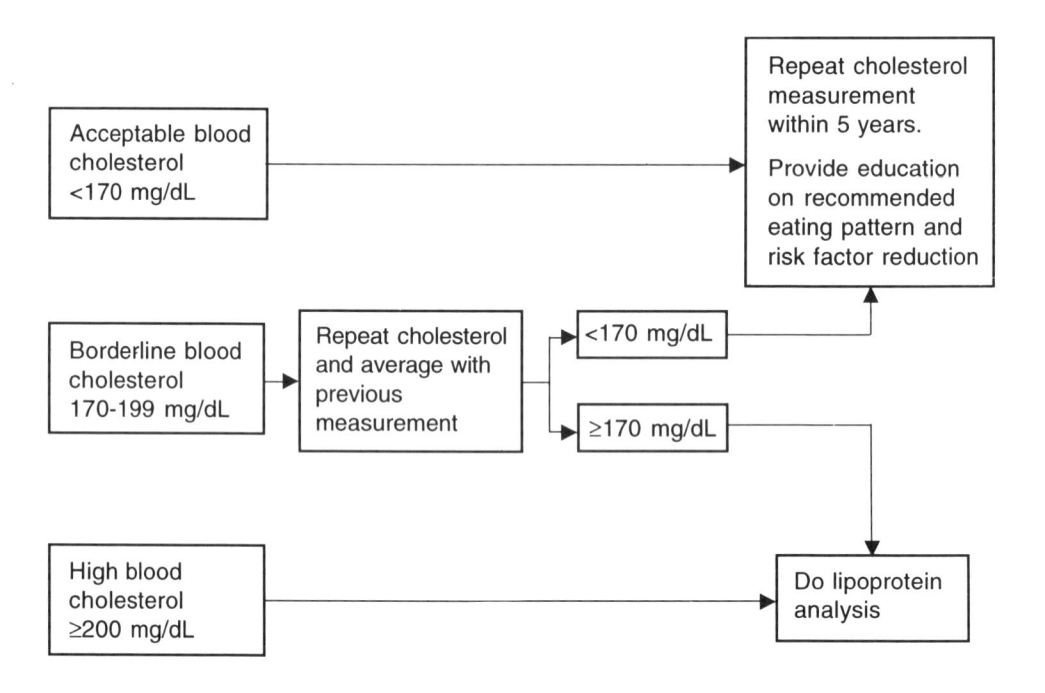

```
Acceptable blood               ─────────────►  Repeat cholesterol
cholesterol                                    measurement
<170 mg/dL                                     within 5 years.
                                               Provide education
                                               on recommended
                                               eating pattern and
                                               risk factor reduction

Borderline blood  ──►  Repeat cholesterol  ──► <170 mg/dL
cholesterol            and average with
170-199 mg/dL          previous
                       measurement          ──► ≥170 mg/dL

High blood                     ─────────────►  Do lipoprotein
cholesterol                                    analysis
≥200 mg/dL
```

From: National Cholesterol Education Program. *Report of the Expert Panel on Blood Cholesterol Levels in Children and Adolescents*. Bethesda, MD: National Institutes of Health, National Heart, Lung, and Blood Institute; 1991. USDHHS publication no. NIH 91-2732.

## Ch. 4. Cholesterol — Children/Adolescents — SCREENING

**Figure 4-2. Assessment and Follow-up of Lipoprotein Analysis**

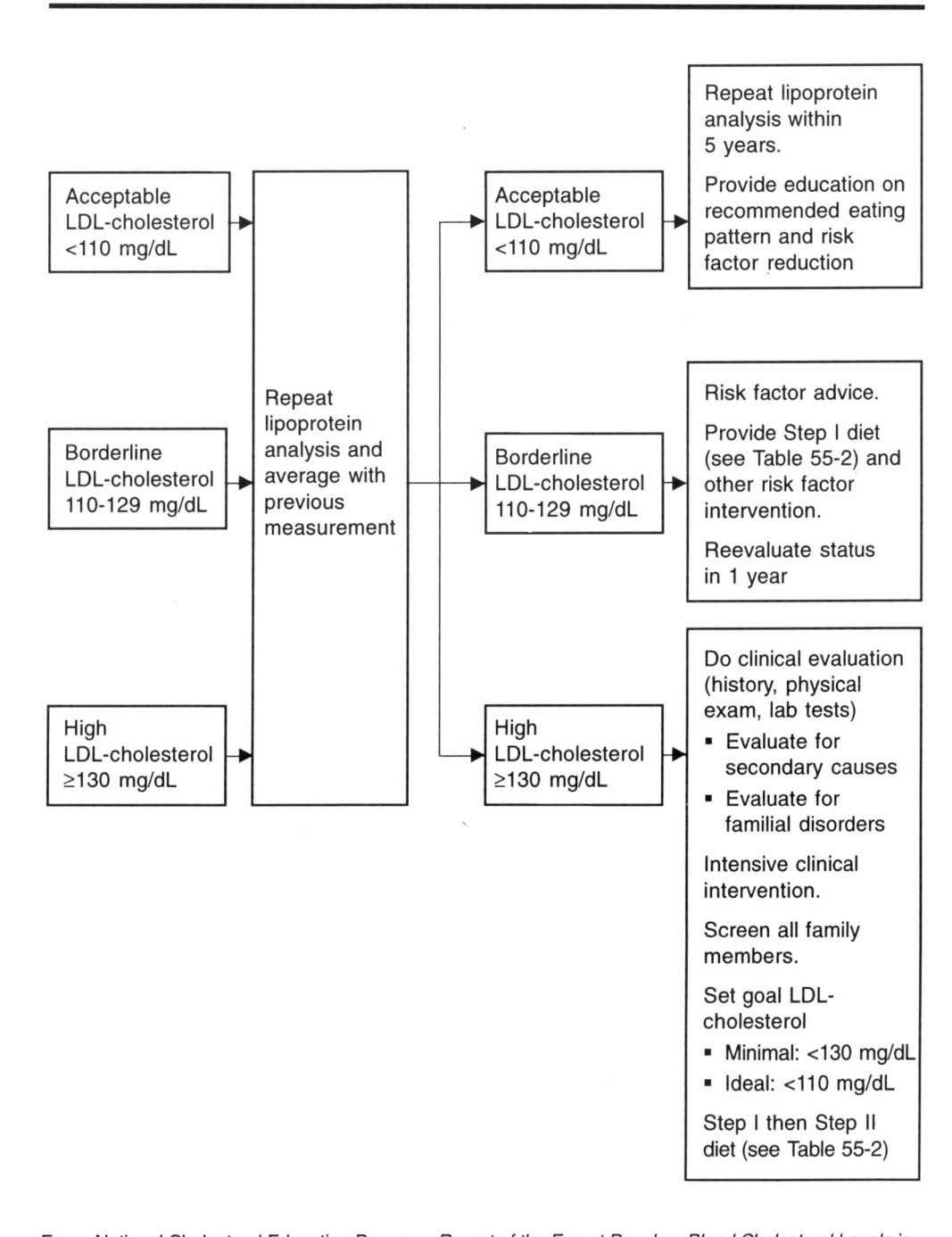

```
Acceptable                                    Acceptable                Repeat lipoprotein
LDL-cholesterol ──┐                      ┌─▶  LDL-cholesterol  ──▶      analysis within 5 years.
<110 mg/dL        │                      │    <110 mg/dL                Provide education on
                  │                      │                              recommended eating
                  │                      │                              pattern and risk
                  │                      │                              factor reduction
                  │   Repeat             │
                  │   lipoprotein        │                              Risk factor advice.
Borderline        │   analysis and       │    Borderline                Provide Step I diet
LDL-cholesterol ──┼─▶ average with    ───┼─▶  LDL-cholesterol  ──▶      (see Table 55-2) and
110-129 mg/dL     │   previous           │    110-129 mg/dL             other risk factor
                  │   measurement        │                              intervention.
                  │                      │                              Reevaluate status
                  │                      │                              in 1 year
                  │                      │
                  │                      │                              Do clinical evaluation
                  │                      │                              (history, physical
                  │                      │                              exam, lab tests)
High              │                      │    High                       ▪ Evaluate for
LDL-cholesterol ──┘                      └─▶  LDL-cholesterol  ──▶         secondary causes
≥130 mg/dL                                    ≥130 mg/dL                  ▪ Evaluate for
                                                                           familial disorders
                                                                        Intensive clinical
                                                                        intervention.
                                                                        Screen all family
                                                                        members.
                                                                        Set goal LDL-
                                                                        cholesterol
                                                                          ▪ Minimal: <130 mg/dL
                                                                          ▪ Ideal: <110 mg/dL
                                                                        Step I then Step II
                                                                        diet (see Table 55-2)
```

From: National Cholesterol Education Program. *Report of the Expert Panel on Blood Cholesterol Levels in Children and Adolescents*. Bethesda, MD: National Institutes of Health, National Heart, Lung, and Blood Institute; 1991. USDHHS publication no. NIH 91-2732.

## Family Resources

*Growing up Healthy: Fat, Cholesterol and More*. American Academy of Pediatrics, Division of Publications, PO Box 927, Elk Grove Village, IL 60009-0927; 1-800 433-9016.

*Eating With Your Heart in Mind* (ages 7 to 10 years); *Healthy Heart Habits* (ages 15 to 19 years); *Heart Health—Your Choice* (ages 11 to 14 years); *Parents Guide: Cholesterol in Children—Healthy Eating is a Family Affair*. National Heart, Lung, and Blood Institute Information Center, PO Box 30105, Bethesda, MD 20824-0105; (301) 251-1222.

## Selected References

American Academy of Family Physicians, Commission on Public Health and Scientific Affairs. *Age Charts for Periodic Health Examination*. Kansas City, Mo: American Academy of Family Physicians; 1993.

American Academy of Pediatrics. Prudent life-style for children: dietary fat and cholesterol. *Pediatrics*. 1986;78:521-525.

American Academy of Pediatrics. *Pediatric Nutrition Handbook*. 3rd ed. Elk Grove Village, Ill: American Academy of Pediatrics; 1993.

American Academy of Pediatrics, Committee on Nutrition. Statement on cholesterol. *Pediatrics*. 1992;90:469-473.

American Medical Association. *Guidelines for Adolescent Preventive Services (GAPS)*. Chicago, Ill: American Medical Association; 1992.

Canadian Task Force on the Periodic Health Examination. Periodic health examination, 1993 update: 2. Lowering the blood total cholesterol level to prevent coronary heart disease. *Can Med Assoc J*. 1993;148:521-535.

Garcia RE, Moodie DS. Routine cholesterol surveillance in childhood. *Pediatrics*. 1989;84:751-755.

Kuehl KS. Cholesterol screening in childhood. Targeted versus universal approaches. *Ann N Y Acad Sci*. 1991;623:193-199.

National Cholesterol Education Program. *Recommendations for Improving Cholesterol Measurement*. Bethesda, Md: National Institutes of Health, National Heart, Lung, and Blood Institute; 1990. US Department of Health and Human Services, Public Health Service, publication NIH 90-2964.

National Cholesterol Education Program, Expert Panel on Blood Cholesterol Levels in Children and Adolescents. *Report of the Expert Panel on Blood Cholesterol Levels in Children and Adolescents*. Bethesda, Md: National Institutes of Health, National Heart, Lung, and Blood Institute; 1991. US Department of Health and Human Services, Public Health Service, publication NIH 91-2732.

Newman WP, Wattigney W, Berenson G. Autopsy studies in United States children and adolescents. Relationship of risk factors to atherosclerotic lesions. *Ann N Y Acad Sci*. 1991;623:17-25.

Newman TB, Browner W, Hulley SB. The case against childhood cholesterol screening. *JAMA*. 1990;264:3039-3043.

Resnicow K, Berenson G, Shea S, Srinivasan S, et al. The case against the "case against childhood cholesterol screening." *JAMA*. 1991;265:3003-3005.

Resnicow K, Morley-Kotchen J, Wynder E. Plasma cholesterol levels of 6585 children in the United States; results of the know your body screening in five states. *Pediatrics*. 1989;84:969-976.

## Children/Adolescents — SCREENING

# 5. Depression and Suicide

Depression in childhood and adolescence is a significant health problem in the United States. It is a condition that is often overlooked and misdiagnosed in primary care. Major depressive disorders have prevalence rates of approximately 1.8% in prepubertal children and 4.7% in adolescents. Risk factors for depression in children and adolescents include a history of verbal, physical, or sexual abuse; frequent separation from or loss of a loved one; a family history of depression (particularly parental); incarceration; pregnancy; lower socioeconomic status; homosexuality; mental retardation; attention deficit disorder; hyperactivity; and chronic illness. The complications of depression in childhood and adolescence include poor school performance, poor peer relations, alcohol and drug abuse, promiscuity, teenage pregnancy, other psychiatric illnesses, and suicide.

Suicide now ranks as the third leading cause of death among individuals between 15 and 24 years old in the United States and sixth among children 5 to 14 years old. Suicide rates for children 5 to 14 years old more than doubled between 1970 and 1988. Risk factors for adolescent suicide, in addition to those listed above for depression, include a strong family history of psychiatric disorders (especially depression or suicidal behavior), previous suicide attempts, serious medical illness, family violence, alcohol and other drug abuse, and the availability and accessibility of firearms in the home. Primary care clinicians often have an opportunity to intervene, as many suicide attempters have been seen by a clinician shortly before committing the act.

### Recommendations of Major Authorities

- **American Academy of Family Physicians**, **Canadian Task Force on the Periodic Health Examination,** and **U.S. Preventive Services Task Force**—Routine screening for depression and suicide is not recommended; nonetheless, clinicians should remain alert for symptoms of depression and suicide risk factors.

- **American Academy of Pediatrics**—Behavioral assessment should be a routine part of health supervision throughout childhood and adolescence. Adolescents and their parents should be asked about suicidal thoughts or threats, or both.

- **American Medical Association**—All adolescents should be asked annually about behaviors or emotions that indicate recurrent or severe depression or risk of suicide. Parents or other adult caregivers of adolescents with suicidal intent should be counseled to remove weapons and potentially lethal medications from the home.

### Basics of Screening for Depression and Suicide

*Depression*

1. Clinicians should be familiar with the risk factors (see above) and symptoms (see Table 5-1) of depression.

**Table 5-1. Symptoms of Major Depression**

| |
|---|
| Depressed mood (or can be irritable mood in children and adolescents) |
| Markedly diminished interest or pleasure in activities |
| Significant weight loss or gain when not dieting, or decrease or increase in appetite (in children, consider failure to make expected weight gains) |
| Insomnia or hypersomnia |
| Psychomotor agitation or retardation |
| Fatigue or loss of energy |
| Feelings of worthlessness or excessive or inappropriate guilt |
| Diminished ability to think or concentrate, or indecisiveness |
| Recurrent thoughts of death, recurrent suicidal ideation |

From: American Psychiatric Association, Committee on Nomenclature. *Diagnostic and Statistical Manual of Mental Disorders, Third Edition, Revised.* Washington, DC: American Psychiatric Association; 1987. Reproduced by permission of the publisher; copyright © 1987.

2. The presence of any risk factors or symptoms should alert the clinician to the need for in-depth evaluation.

3. Early referral to a mental health professional should be considered for evaluation and treatment.

## *Suicide*

1. Clinicians should be familiar with the risk factors for suicide (see above).

2. Patients should be asked in a direct, straightforward manner about suicidal thoughts.

3. Patients with suicidal thoughts should be questioned regarding the extent and specificity of plans for suicide. Immediate referral to a mental health professional is advisable, especially for those patients with serious intent.

4. Parents should be counseled about the importance of restricting the access of children and adolescents to dangerous prescription drugs and firearms in the home.

## Family Resources

*Facts for Families: The Depressed Child; Teen Suicide; Children and Grief; Manic Depressive Illness in Teens.* American Academy of Child and Adolescent Psychiatry, 3615 Wisconsin Ave. NW, Washington, DC 20016; (202) 966-7300.

*Surviving: Coping with Adolescent Depression and Suicide; Caring for Your Adolescent: Age 12 to 21.* American Academy of Pediatrics, P.O. Box 927, Elk Grove Village, IL 60000-0927; 1-800 443-9016.

## Selected References

American Academy of Family Physicians, Commission on Public Health and Scientific Affairs. *Age Charts for Periodic Health Examination*. Kansas City, Mo: American Academy of Family Physicians; 1993.

American Academy of Pediatrics, Committee on Adolescence. Suicide and suicide attempts in adolescents and young adults. *Pediatrics*. 1988;81:322-324.

American Academy of Pediatrics, Committee on Psychosocial Aspects of Child and Family Health. *Guidelines for Health Supervision*. Elk Grove Village, Ill: American Academy of Pediatrics; 1988.

American Medical Association. *Guidelines for Adolescent Preventive Services (GAPS)*. Chicago, Ill: American Medical Association; 1992.

American Psychiatric Association, Committee on Nomenclature. *Diagnostic and Statistical Manual*. 3rd ed., rev. Washington, DC: American Psychiatric Association; 1987.

Brent DA, Perper JA, Goldstein CE, et al. Risk factors for adolescent suicide. *Arch Gen Psychiatry*. 1988;45:581-587.

Canadian Task Force on the Periodic Health Examination. Periodic health examination, 1990 update: 2. Early detection of depression and prevention of suicide. *Can Med Assoc J*. 1990;142:1233-1238.

Chang G, Warner V, Weissman MM. Physicians' recognition of psychiatric disorders in children and adolescents. *AJDC*. 1988;142:736-739.

Costello EJ, Angold A. Scales to assess child and adolescent depression: checklists, screens, and nets. *J Am Acad Child Adolesc Psychiatry*. 1988;27:726-737.

Grayson P, Carlson G. The utility of a DSM-III-R-based checklist in screening child psychiatric patients. *J Am Acad Child Adolesc Psychiatry*. 1991;30:669-673.

Kashani J, Sherman D. Childhood depression: epidemiology, etiological models, and treatment implications. *Integr Psychiatry*. 1988;6:1-21.

Roberts N, Vargo B, Ferguson HB. Measurement of anxiety and depression in children and adolescents. *Psychiatr Clin North Am*. 1989;12:837-860.

Slap G, Vorters D, Khalid N, Margulies S, Forke C. Adolescent suicide attempters: do physicians recognize them? *J Adolesc Health*. 1992;13:286-292.

US Preventive Services Task Force. Screening for depression. In: *Guide to Clinical Preventive Services*. Baltimore, Md: Williams & Wilkins; 1989:chap 44.

US Preventive Services Task Force. Screening for suicidal intent. In: *Guide to Clinical Preventive Services*. Baltimore, Md: Williams & Wilkins; 1989:chap 45.

# Children/Adolescents — SCREENING

## 6. Hearing

Hearing impairment occurs in an estimated 1% to 2% of infants and children in the United States. Approximately half of these cases are congenital or acquired during infancy. The incidence of severe or profound hearing loss is 1 in every 750 live births. Approximately 5% of infants in neonatal intensive care units have evidence of significant hearing loss. Temporary hearing loss is also common among school-age children, usually as a complication of otitis media with middle ear effusion. Approximately 8 million school-age children suffer from temporary hearing impairment.

Hearing is necessary for normal development of speech and language and is also important for acquiring psychosocial skills during infancy and childhood. Because most speech and language development occurs between birth and age 3 years, early detection of hearing impairment in infants and children and the initiation of medical and educational interventions are critical.

**Recommendations of Major Authorities**

*Normal-Risk Children*

- **American Academy of Family Physicians, Canadian Task Force on the Periodic Health Examination (CTFPHE),** and **U.S. Preventive Services Task Force (USPSTF)**—There is insufficient evidence to recommend routine hearing screening (pure-tone audiometry) for children. The **USPSTF** recommendation is under review. **CTFPHE** has recommended repeated examination of hearing for young children, especially during the first year of life. Suggested guidelines for this examination include checking the startle or turning response to a novel noise produced outside the infant's field of vision at birth and 6 months of age and checking for the absence of babbling at 6 months of age.

- **American Academy of Pediatrics**—Pure-tone audiometry should be performed at 4, 5, 12, and 18 years of age. Subjective assessment of hearing should be performed at other ages.

- **American Speech-Language-Hearing Association**—Annual pure-tone audiometry should be performed for children functioning at a developmental level of age 3 years to grade 3 and for any high-risk children, including those above grade 3. A recommendation for universal screening of neonates is under consideration.

- **National Institutes of Health Consensus Development Conference on Hearing Impairment in Infants and Young Children**—Universal newborn hearing screening within the first 3 months of life and preferably before hospital discharge, using otoacoustic emission techniques, is recommended.

*High-Risk Children*

- **Joint Committee on Infant Hearing (American Speech-Language-Hearing Association, American Academy of Pediatrics, American Academy of Otolaryngology-Head and Neck

**Surgery,** and **Council for Education of the Deaf)**—Neonates (birth to 28 days of age) with one or more of the neonatal risk criteria should have audiology screening, preferably prior to hospital discharge but no later than 3 months of age. A recommendation for universal screening of neonates is under consideration.

*Neonatal Risk Criteria*: Family history of congenital early onset or delayed onset childhood sensorineural or conductive hearing loss, or both; birth weight of less than 1500 g; presence of a syndrome known to include sensorineural hearing loss; presence of craniofacial anomalies; congenital infection with toxoplasmosis, syphilis, rubella, cytomegalovirus, or herpes; bacterial meningitis; hyperbilirubinemia requiring exchange transfusion; ototoxic medications used for more than 5 days; loop diuretic used with aminoglycoside; severe depression at birth, including Apgar scores of 0 to 3 at 5 minutes, failure to have spontaneous respiration by 10 minutes, or hypotonia lasting more than 2 hours; mechanical ventilation for cardiopulmonary disease for 48 hours or longer; and neonatal intracranial hemorrhage.

Infants and children less than 2 years of age with one or more of the following risk criteria should have audiology screening as soon as possible, but no later than 3 months after the child has been identified as high risk.

*Risk Criteria under 2 Years of Age*: Parent or other care-giver concern regarding hearing, speech, language, or developmental delay; infection with bacterial meningitis; head trauma with temporal bone fracture; stigmata or other findings; ototoxic medications used for more than 5 days; loop diuretic used with aminoglycoside; neonatal risk factors that may be associated with delayed onset or progressive sensorineural hearing loss; infectious diseases known to be associated with sensorineural hearing loss (mumps, measles); a neurodegenerative disorder associated with hearing loss.

- **American Academy of Family Physicians** and **U.S. Preventive Services Task Force**—Screening for hearing impairment should be performed on all high-risk neonates. See neonatal risk criteria listed above. If not tested at birth, high-risk children should be screened before 3 years of age. Adolescents regularly exposed to excessive noise in recreational or other settings should receive hearing screening. The optimal interval for screening is left to clinical discretion. This recommendation is under review.

- **American Academy of Pediatrics** and **American Speech-Language-Hearing Association (ASHA)**—Children with frequently recurring otitis media or middle ear effusion, or both, should have audiology screening and monitoring of communication skills development. **ASHA** has recommended annual pure-tone audiometry testing for all children at high risk for hearing impairment.

## Basics of Hearing Screening

1. The family and medical history of every child should be assessed for risk factors for hearing impairment.

2. Parents should be asked about the auditory responsiveness and speech and language development of young children. Any parental reports of impairment should be seriously evaluated.

3. In infants, assessment of hearing by observational techniques is very imprecise. Clinicians should consider referring all infants and young children with suspected hearing difficulties to an audiologist for evaluation.

4. When performing physical examinations, clinicians should remain alert for structural defects of the ear, head, and neck. They should also remain alert for abnormalities of the ear canal (inflammation, cerumen impaction, tumors, or foreign bodies) and the eardrum (perforation, retraction, or evidence of effusion).

5. Children as young as 3 years of age, depending on how cooperative they are, may be screened by pure-tone audiometry. The test should be performed in a quiet environment using earphones, since ambient noise can significantly affect test performance, particularly at the lower frequencies (i.e., 500 and 1000 Hz). Hand-held audiometers are of unproven effectiveness in screening children. Each ear should be tested at 500, 1000, 2000, and 4000 Hz. Air-conduction hearing threshold levels of greater than 20 dB at any of these frequencies indicate possible impairment. If possible, the ears should be examined before pure-tone audiometry screening is performed.

6. Audiometric evidence of hearing impairment should be substantiated by repeat screening. Earphones should be removed and repositioned and instructions carefully repeated to the child to assure proper understanding and attention to the test. Referral to a qualified specialist (ie., audiologist, otolaryngologist) is recommended for confirmation and work-up of hearing impairment.

7. The audiometer should be calibrated yearly; the operator should listen to it each day of use to detect gross abnormalities.

## Family Resources

*Is My Baby's Hearing Normal?* American Academy of Otolaryngology-Head and Neck Surgery, Order Department, 1 Prince St., Alexandria, VA 22314; (703) 836-4444.

*ASHA Answers Questions About Otitis Media, Hearing, and Language Development; How Does Your Child Hear and Talk?; Recognizing Communication Disorders.* American Speech-Language-Hearing Association, 10801 Rockville Pike, Rockville, MD 20852; 1-800 638-8255; (301) 897-5700.

## Selected References

American Academy of Family Physicians, Commission on Public Health and Scientific Affairs. *Age Charts for Periodic Health Examination.* Kansas City, Mo: American Academy of Family Physicians; 1993.

American Academy of Otolaryngology-Head and Neck Surgery, Joint Committee on Infant Hearing. 1990 position statement. *American Academy of Otolaryngology-Head and Neck Surgery Bulletin.* March 1991:15-18.

American Academy of Pediatrics. Joint Committee on Infant Hearing position statement 1982. In: *Policy Reference Guide: A Comprehensive Guide to AAP Policy Statements through December 1991.* Elk Grove, Ill: American Academy of Pediatrics; 1991;333-334.

American Academy of Pediatrics. Middle ear disease and language development. In: *Policy Reference Guide: A Comprehensive Guide to AAP Policy Statements through December 1991.* Elk Grove, Ill: American Academy of Pediatrics; 1991;418.

American Academy of Pediatrics, Committee on Practice and Ambulatory Medicine. Recommendations for pediatric preventive health care. *AAP News.* 1991;7:19.

American Speech-Language-Hearing Association. Guidelines for the audiologic assessment of children from birth through 36 months of age. *Asha.* 1991;33(suppl.5):37-43.

American Speech-Language-Hearing Association. Guidelines for audiologic screening of newborn infants who are at risk for hearing impairment. *Asha.* 1989;31(3):89-92.

American Speech-Language-Hearing Association. Guidelines for Identification Audiometry. *Asha.* 1985;May:49-53.

American Speech-Language-Hearing Association. Guidelines for screening for hearing impairment and middle-ear disorders. *Asha.* 1990;32(suppl.2):17-24.

American Speech-Language-Hearing Association. *Preferred Practice Patterns for the Professions of Speech-Language Pathology and Audiology.* Rockville, Md: *Asha.* In press.

American Speech-Language-Hearing Association. The prevention of communication disorders tutorial. *Asha.* 1991;33(suppl.6):15-41.

Canadian Task Force on the Periodic Health Examination. The periodic health examination. *Can Med Assoc J.* 1979;121:1194-1254.

Canadian Task Force on the Periodic Health Examination. The periodic health examination: 2. 1984 update. *Can Med Assoc J.* 1984;130:1278-1285.

Canadian Task Force on the Periodic Health Examination. Periodic health examination, 1989 update: 3. Preschool examination for developmental, visual and hearing problems. *Can Med Assoc J.* 1989;141:1136-1140.

Canadian Task Force on the Periodic Health Examination. Periodic health examination, 1990 update: 4. Well-baby care in the first 2 years of life. *Can Med Assoc J.* 1990;143:867-872.

National Institutes of Health. *Early Identification of Hearing Impairment in Infants and Young Children.* Bethesda, Md: National Institutes of Health. In press.

Thompson MD, Thompson G. Early identification of hearing loss: listen to parents. *Clin Pediatr* (Philadelphia, Pa.). 1991;30:77-80.

US Preventive Services Task Force. Screening for Hearing Impairment. In: *Guide to Clinical Preventive Services.* Baltimore, Md: Williams & Wilkins; 1989:chap 33.

Watkin PM, Baldwin M, Laoide S. Parental suspicion and identification of hearing impairment. *Arch Dis Child.* 1990;65:846-850.

# Children/Adolescents — SCREENING

## 7. Lead

Lead poisoning is one of the most common and preventable childhood environmental health problems in the United States. Although low-income, inner-city children have higher rates of lead poisoning, no socioeconomic group, geographic area, or racial or ethnic population is spared. In 1990, up to 3 million children under 6 years of age, 15% of all children in this age group, had blood lead levels greater than 10 µg/dL. Studies have shown associations between diminished intelligence, impaired neurobehavioral development, decreased hearing acuity, and growth inhibition and lead levels as low as 10 to 15 µg/dL. A recent study (Ruff et al. 1993) demonstrated in a cohort of children with moderate lead poisoning (25 to 55 µg/dL), most of whom received residential lead abatement, that decreases in blood lead levels were associated with improvements in cognitive functioning. Higher levels can cause severe damage to the central nervous, renal, and hematopoietic systems and can be fatal.

### Recommendations of Major Authorities

- **American Academy of Family Physicians**—Until 6 years of age, children should be assessed for risk of lead exposure, using a structured questionnaire (see Table 7-1). Children with an increased risk for lead exposure should have whole blood lead level testing.

- **American Academy of Pediatrics**—Pediatric-care providers should increase their efforts to screen children for lead exposure. Blood lead screening should be a part of routine health supervision for children and can best be addressed by increasing children's access to health care. Because lead is ubiquitous in the U.S. environment, this screening should occur at about 9 to 12 months of age and, if possible, again at about 24 months of age. The Centers for Disease Control and Prevention has raised the possibility that there may be low-risk communities that do not require screening, but no explicit guidance has been developed for determining a community's risk. As more data are collected, it may become evident that there are locales where selective screening of children is more appropriate than routine screening. Currently no adequate laboratory capacity exists nationwide to screen each child, but the requirement to phase in screening should generate those resources.

- **Centers for Disease Control and Prevention (CDC)**—All children should have routine blood lead-level testing, except in communities where large numbers or percentages of children have been screened and found not to have elevated levels. A structured questionnaire (see Table 7-1) should be used to assess risk. A child for whom an answer to any of the questions is "yes" should be considered at high risk. Infants at low risk of lead poisoning should be screened at 12 months of age and, if the initial test result is <10 µg/dL and resources allow, at 24 months of age. Infants at high risk should be screened initially at 6 months of age and, if the initial test result is <10 µg/dL, every 6 months. After two consecutive measurements are <10 µg/dL, or three are <15 µg/dL, the child should be retested in one year. High-risk children ≥36 and <72 months of age without previous testing should have blood lead testing. Re-screening should occur any time history suggests exposure has increased. In general, screening may stop at 6 years of age, unless indicated (for example, in a developmentally delayed child with pica). See Table 7-2 for CDC's recommendations for interpretation and follow-up of blood lead measurement results.

- **U.S. Preventive Services Task Force**—Recommendation currently under review.

## Basics of Lead Screening

1. Risk assessment and counseling should begin during prenatal visits and continue after birth during regular office visits until at least the age of 6 years.

2. Each child's risk of lead toxicity should be evaluated. For this purpose, a structured set of questions such as that developed by CDC (Table 7-1) can be very helpful. If the answer to any of these questions is positive, the child is considered at high risk for exposure.

3. Screening by measurement of the blood lead level is more sensitive and specific than measurement of the erythrocyte protoporphyrin (EP) level. Blood lead levels <25 µg/dL cannot be reliably detected by EP testing. Elevated EP levels (≥35 µg/dL) require confirmation with blood lead testing.

4. Because of possible contamination of capillary specimens from environmental sources, venous blood samples are preferable to capillary sampling for blood lead levels. If capillary samples must be used, the precautions listed in Table 7-3 should be followed to minimize the chance of contamination. Elevated blood lead results (≥15 µg/dL) obtained on capillary specimens must be confirmed using venous blood. A child with a capillary lead level ≥70 µg/dL should be considered a medical emergency and retested with a venous sample immediately.

5. Blood lead test results can be interpreted and managed according to the CDC recommendations listed in Table 7-2.

6. Laboratories where blood is tested for lead levels should participate in a blood-lead proficiency testing program, such as the collaborative program between the Health Resources and Services Administration and CDC. Information on this program is available by calling (404) 488-7330.

7. Because iron deficiency can enhance lead absorption and toxicity, all children with blood lead levels ≥20 µg/dL should be tested for iron deficiency.

8. In addition to screening, it is important to provide guidance to parents about creating an environment safe from lead exposure for their children. Counseling should include advice on eliminating peeling or chipping paint, decreasing the lead content of water, preventing contact via hobbies or contaminated work clothing, remaining alert for pica behavior, and assuring good hygiene. See Family Resources for publications to aid in counseling.

## Family Resources

*Getting the Lead Out.* Food and Drug Administration. Superintendent of Documents, Consumer Information Center-3C, PO Box 100, Pueblo, CO 81002.

*Home Buyer's Guide to Environmental Hazards.* Environmental Protection Agency. Superintendent of Documents, Consumer Information Center-3C, PO Box 100, Pueblo, CO 81002.

### Table 7-1. Recommended Questions for Assessing Exposure Risk

| |
|---|
| Does your child live in or regularly visit a house with peeling or chipping paint built before 1960? (This includes day care centers, preschools, homes of baby-sitters or relatives, etc.) |
| Does your child live in or regularly visit a house built before 1960 with recent, ongoing, or planned renovation or remodeling? |
| Does your child have a brother or sister, housemate or playmate being followed or treated for lead poisoning (blood lead level ≥15 µg/dL)? |
| Does your child live with an adult whose job or hobby involves exposure to lead? (Such hobbies include ceramics, furniture refinishing, and stained glass work.) |
| Does your child live near an active lead smelter, battery recycling plant, or other industry likely to release lead? |

Adapted from: Centers for Disease Control. *Preventing Lead Poisoning in Young Children: A Statement by the Centers for Disease Control.* Atlanta, GA: Centers for Disease Control; 1991.

*Important Facts About Childhood Lead Poisoning Prevention.* Centers for Disease Control and Prevention, Lead Poisoning Prevention Program, 1600 Clifton Rd., Atlanta, GA 30333; (404) 488-4880.

*What Everyone Should Know About Lead Poisoning.* Alliance to End Childhood Lead Poisoning, 600 Pennsylvania Ave. SE, Suite 100, Washington, DC 20003 (individual copies); Channing L. Bete Co., Inc., 200 State Rd., South Deerfield, MA 01373; 1-800 628-7733 (bulk copies).

*What You Should Know About Lead-Based Paint in Your Home.* U.S. Consumer Product Safety Commission, Washington, DC 20207; 1-800 638-2666.

**Provider Resources**

*Case Studies in Environmental Medicine: Lead Toxicity.* Agency for Toxic Substances and Disease Registry, Division of Health Education, Mailstop E33, 1600 Clifton Rd., Atlanta, GA 30333; (404) 639-6205.

*Preventing Lead Poisoning in Young Children: A Statement by the Centers for Disease Control.* Centers for Disease Control and Prevention, Lead Poisoning Prevention Program, 1600 Clifton Rd., Atlanta, GA 30333; (404) 488-4880.

*Blood-Lead Proficiency Testing Program*; Centers for Disease Control and Prevention. (404) 488-4880.

**Table 7-2. CDC Recommendations for Follow-up of Blood Lead Measurements**

| Class | Blood Lead Concentration (µg/dL) | Action | |
|---|---|---|---|
| I | ≤9 | Low risk: | 6-35 months of age—Retest at 24 months of age (when blood levels peak), if resources allow.<br>≥36 and <72 months of age—Retesting not necessary unless history suggests exposure has increased. |
| | | High risk: | 6-35 months of age—Retest every 6 months. After two subsequent consecutive measurements are <10 µg/dL, or three are <15 µg/dL, retest once a year.<br>≥36 to 72 months of age—Retest once a year until sixth birthday. |
| IIA | 10-14 | Low risk: | 6-35 months of age—Retest every 3-4 months. After two consecutive measurements are <10 µg/dL or three are <15 µg/dL, retest once a year.<br>≥36 and <72 months of age—Retesting not necessary if all previous test results are <15 µg/dL, unless history suggests exposure has increased. |
| | | High risk: | 6-35 months of age—Retest every 3-4 months. After two consecutive measurements are <10 µg/dL or three are <15 µg/dL, retest once a year.<br>≥36 and <72 months of age—Retest once a year until sixth birthday. |
| IIB | 15-19 | | Retest every 3-4 months. The family should be given education and nutritional counseling and a detailed environmental history should be taken to identify any obvious sources or pathways of lead exposure. If venous blood level is in this range in two consecutive tests 3-4 months apart, environmental investigation and abatement should be conducted, if resources permit. |
| III | 20-44* | | Retest every 3-4 months. Conduct a complete medical evaluation, including iron deficiency testing. Environmental lead sources should be identified and eliminated. Pharmacologic treatment may be necessary. |
| IV | 45-69* | | Begin medical treatment and environmental assessment and remediation within 48 hours. |
| V | ≥70* | | Begin medical treatment and environmental assessment and remediation immediately. |

*Based on confirmatory blood lead level.

Adapted from: Centers for Disease Control. *Preventing Lead Poisoning in Young Children: A Statement by the Centers for Disease Control.* Atlanta, GA: Centers for Disease Control; 1991.

**Table 7-3. Recommendations for Minimizing the Contamination of Capillary Blood Samples Obtained by Finger Stick**

| |
|---|
| Personnel who collect specimens should be well-trained in and completely familiar with the collection procedure. |
| Puncturing the fingers of infants less than 1 year of age is not recommended. The heel is a more suitable site for these children. |
| If examination gloves are coated with powder, they should be rinsed with tap water. |
| The child's hands should be thoroughly washed with soap and water, and then dried with a clean, low-lint towel. |
| Once washed, the finger or heel to be punctured should be cleansed with alcohol and not allowed to come into contact with any surface, including the child's other fingers. |
| Although its effectiveness in reducing contamination is under study, silicone spray can be used to form a protective layer between the skin and blood droplets. |
| The first droplet of blood, which contains tissue fluids, should be wiped off with sterile gauze or a cotton ball. |
| Do not collect blood that has run down the finger or onto the fingernail. |
| Contact between the skin and the collection container should be avoided. |

Adapted from: Centers for Disease Control. *Preventing Lead Poisoning in Young Children: A Statement by the Centers for Disease Control.* Atlanta, GA: Centers for Disease Control; 1991.

## Selected References

American Academy of Family Physicians, Commission on Public Health and Scientific Affairs. *Age Charts for Periodic Health Examination.* Kansas City, Mo: American Academy of Family Physicians; 1993.

American Academy of Pediatrics. Lead poisoning: from screening to primary prevention. *AAP News.* 1993;9:9.

American Academy of Pediatrics, Committee on Environmental Hazards, Committee on Accident and Poison Prevention. Statement on childhood lead poisoning. *Pediatrics.* 1987;79:457-464.

Centers for Disease Control. *Preventing Lead Poisoning in Young Children: A Statement by the Centers for Disease Control.* Atlanta, Ga: Centers for Disease Control; 1991. US Dept of Health and Human Services.

Centers for Disease Control. Childhood lead poisoning—United States: report to the Congress by the Agency for Toxic Substances and Disease Registry. *MMWR.* 1988;37:481-485.

Crocetti AF, Mushak P, Schwartz J. Determination of numbers of lead-exposed US children by areas of the United States: an integrated summary of a report to the US Congress on childhood lead poisoning. *Environ Health Perspect.* 1990;89:109-120.

DeBaun MR, Sox HC. Setting the optimal erythrocyte protoporphyrin screening decision threshold for lead poisoning: a decision analytic approach. *Pediatrics.* 1991;88:121-131.

Mahaffey KR, Annest JL, Roberts J, Murphy RS. National estimates of blood lead levels: United States, 1976-1980. *N Engl J Med.* 1982;307:573-579.

Needleman HL. The persistent threat of lead: a singular opportunity. *Am J Public Health.* 1989;79:643-645.

Needleman HL, Schell A, Bellinger D, Leviton A, Allred EN. The long-term effects of exposure to low doses of lead in childhood: an 11-year follow-up report. *N Engl J Med.* 1990;322:83-88.

Ratcliffe SD, Lee J, Lutz LJ, Woolley FR, et al. Lead toxicity and iron deficiency in Utah migrant children. *Am J Public Health*. 1989;79:631-633.

Ruff HA, Bijur PE, Markowitz M, Yeou-Cheng M, Rosen JF. Declining blood lead levels and cognitive changes in moderately lead-poisoned children. *JAMA*. 1993;269:1641-1654.

US Preventive Services Task Force. Screening for lead toxicity. In: *Guide to Clinical Preventive Services*. Baltimore, Md: Williams & Wilkins; 1989: chap 30.

# Children/Adolescents — SCREENING

## 8. Newborn Screening

Newborn screening for congenital hypothyroidism and phenylketonuria (PKU) is required in virtually all states. Testing for galactosemia and hemoglobinopathies is required in a majority of the states. Other conditions for which some states require newborn screening are maple syrup urine disease, homocystinuria, biotinidase deficiency, tyrosinemia, congenital adrenal hyperplasia, cystic fibrosis, and toxoplasmosis. Screening for some conditions is voluntary in some states. See Table 8-1 for a state-by-state listing of newborn screening policies.

### *Hypothyroidism*

Most children with congenital hypothyroidism who are not identified and treated promptly suffer the irreversible mental retardation and varying degrees of growth failure, deafness, and neurologic abnormalities comprising the syndrome of cretinism. Incidence is 1 per 3600 to 1 per 5000 live births. Infants who receive adequate treatment with thyroxine within the first weeks of life have normal or near-normal intellectual performance when tested at 4 to 7 years of age.

### *Phenylketonuria (PKU)*

This autosomal recessive aminoacidopathy leads to severe, irreversible mental retardation (IQ below 50) when untreated during infancy. Incidence is 1 per 10,000 to 1 per 25,000 live births. With early screening, diagnosis, and optimal treatment with a dietary restriction of phenylalanine, most children are in the normal range of intelligence.

### *Galactosemia*

This disease causes failure to thrive, vomiting, liver disease, cataracts, and irreversible mental retardation. Death often results from *Escherichia coli* septicemia. The incidence is 1 per 60,000 to 1 per 80,000 live births. Removal from the diet of galactose-containing foods, especially milk, leads to a dramatic improvement in the patient, and all clinical features except mental retardation may improve or disappear.

### *Hemoglobinopathies*

Sickle cell disease and other hemoglobinopathies, such as thalassemia and hemoglobin E, are most common in individuals of African, Mediterranean, Asian, Caribbean, and South and Central American ancestry. Affected individuals may have overwhelming sepsis, chronic hemolytic anemia, episodic vascular occlusive crises, hyposplenism, periodic splenic sequestration, and bone marrow aplasia. Carriers (genetic heterozygotes) do not suffer significant morbidity. In newborns with sickle cell disease, early detection allows prevention of septicemia with prophylactic penicillin and prompt clinical intervention for infection and sequestration crises.

## Recommendations of Major Authorities

- **American Academy of Pediatrics**—Newborn screening should be performed according to each state's regulations.

National authorities have made recommendations for the following specific conditions:

### Hypothyroidism

- **American Academy of Family Physicians, American Thyroid Association, Canadian Task Force on the Periodic Health Examination**, and **U.S. Preventive Services Task Force**—All neonates should be screened for congenital hypothyroidism prior to discharge from the hospital nursery but not later than day 6 of life. Infants at risk for not being screened include those who are born at home, ill at birth, or transferred between hospitals early in life.

### Phenylketonuria (PKU)

- **American Academy of Family Physicians** and **U.S. Preventive Services Task Force**—All infants should be screened for PKU at time of nursery discharge or transfer regardless of age, but no later than 7 days of age. Infants screened earlier than 24 hours after birth should be screened again before the third week of life.

- **Canadian Task Force on the Periodic Health Examination (CTFPHE)**—CTFPHE has made a similar recommendation, stating that since screening of newborns under 4 days of age may result in under-referral, a second test is justifiable.

### Hemoglobinopathies

- **Sickle Cell Disease Guideline Panel of the Agency for Health Care Policy and Research, U.S. Public Health Service**—Universal screening for sickle cell disease should be conducted on all newborns. This recommendation has been endorsed by the **American Academy of Pediatrics**, **American Nurses Association**, and **National Medical Association**.

- **American Academy of Family Physicians, Canadian Task Force on the Periodic Health Examination**, and **U.S. Preventive Services Task Force**—Screening for hemoglobinopathies should be done for those in high-risk ethnic groups.

## Basics of Newborn Screening

### Schedule

1. A blood spot on filter paper should be obtained from every neonate before discharge or transfer from the nursery, regardless of the nature or status of the infant's feeding or age.

2. For the full-term, well neonate, the specimen should be obtained as close as possible to the time of discharge from the nursery, and in no case later than 7 days of age. If the initial specimen is obtained earlier than 24 hours after birth, a second specimen should be obtained at 1 or 2 weeks of age to decrease the probability that PKU and other disorders with metabolite accumulation will be missed as a consequence of testing on the first day of life.

3. Any premature infant, any infant receiving parenteral feeding, or any neonate being treated for illness should have a specimen obtained for screening at or near the 7th day of life if a specimen has not been obtained before that time, regardless of feeding status. If an infant requires transfusion or dialysis prior to the routine time for obtaining the specimen and if the clinical status of the neonate permits, it is optimal to obtain the sample for screening prior to transfusion or dialysis. If a sample cannot be obtained beforehand, the clinician should ensure that an adequate specimen is obtained at a time when the plasma or red blood cells, or both, will again reflect the child's own metabolic processes or phenotype.

Adapted from: American Academy of Pediatrics, Committee on Genetics. Issues in newborn screening. *Pediatrics*. 1992;89:345-349. Reproduced by permission of *Pediatrics*; copyright © 1992.

## *Collection Technique*

1. The same standards and techniques for the collection of blood specimens for neonatal screening programs should be applied for all of the congenital diseases. State screening agencies hold individual hospitals accountable for instituting policies that assure the correct collection of filter-paper blood samples.

2. The required information should be entered on the specimen collection kit with a ballpoint pen, not a soft-tip pen or typewriter.

3. *Universal precautions*: All appropriate precautions, including wearing gloves, should be taken for handling blood and disposing of used lancets in a biohazard container for sharp objects.

4. *Site Selection*: The source of blood must be the most lateral surface of the plantar aspect (walking surface) of the infant's heel. Skin punctures to obtain blood specimens **must not be performed** on the central area of the newborn's foot (area of the arch) or on the fingers of newborns. Puncturing the heel on the posterior curvature will permit blood to flow away from the puncture, making proper spotting difficult. A previous puncture site should not be lanced.

5. *Site Preparation*: Warming the puncture site can increase blood flow. A warm, moist towel at a temperature no higher than 42°C (108°F) should be placed on the site for 3 minutes. Also, holding the infant's leg in a position lower than the heart will increase venous pressure.

6. *Cleaning the Site*: The infant's heel should be cleaned with 70% isopropyl alcohol (rubbing alcohol). Excess alcohol should be wiped away with a dry sterile gauze or cotton ball and the heel allowed to air dry thoroughly. Failure to wipe off alcohol residue may dilute the specimen and adversely affect test results.

7. *Puncture*: To ensure that sufficient flow of blood is obtained, the plantar surface of the infant's heel should be punctured with a sterile lancet to a depth of 2.0 to

2.4 mm or with an automated lancet device. The first drop of blood should be wiped away with sterile gauze. In small premature infants, the heel bone may be no more than 2.4 mm beneath the plantar heel skin surface and half this distance at the posterior curvature of the heel. Puncturing deeper may risk bone damage. The puncture site should not be milked or squeezed, as this may cause hemolysis and admixture of tissue fluids with the specimen.

8. *Filter Paper Handling and Application*: Care should be taken to avoid touching the area within the printed circle on the filter paper before collection. The filter paper should be touched gently against a large drop of blood and, in one step, a sufficient quantity of blood allowed to soak through to fill completely the circle on the filter paper. The paper must not be pressed against the puncture site on the heel. Blood should be applied to only one side of the filter paper. Both sides of the filter paper should be examined to assure that the blood has penetrated and saturated the paper. Successive drops of blood should not be layered within the circle. If blood flow diminishes so that the circle is incompletely filled, the sampling steps must be repeated at a different site. The blood sample should not be touched after collection, and water, feeding formulas, antiseptic solutions, or any other contaminant should not be allowed to come into contact with the sample. The sample should be allowed to dry thoroughly before insertion into the envelope. Insufficient drying can adversely affect test results.

9. *Hemostasis:* After blood has been collected from the heel of the newborn, the foot should be elevated above the body and a sterile gauze pad or cotton ball pressed against the puncture site until the bleeding stops. It is not advisable to apply adhesive bandages over skin puncture sites in newborns.

Adapted from: National Committee for Clinical Laboratory Standards. *Blood Collection on Filter Paper for Neonatal Screening Programs—Second Edition; Approved Standard*. Villanova, Pa: National Committee for Clinical Laboratory Standards; 1992. Permission to use portions of NCCLS document LA4-A2 has been granted by the National Committee for Clinical Laboratory Standards; copyright © 1992.

## *Documentation*

Clinicians should ensure that children have received proper newborn screening and that test results have been received and evaluated. Clinicians should be aware of those patients at increased risk for not being screened. These include sick or premature neonates, neonates undergoing adoption or being transferred within or between hospitals, infants born at home, children of transient or homeless families, and infants born outside the United States and Canada. Newborn screening results should be documented in an easily accessible part of the patient record for future reference.

## *Follow-up*

All abnormal results require confirmatory testing. With certain rare exceptions (eg., galactosemia and maple syrup urine disease) treatment should not be instituted until a confirmatory test has been obtained. Prompt physical examination of patients with abnormal results is important. All patients with sickle cell disease should be started on penicillin prophylaxis as soon as the diagnosis is confirmed.

## *Counseling*

Appropriate counseling should be provided to all parents of children with abnormal results. This counseling should provide information about the significance of the results and need for retesting, implications for the child's health, treatment regimens, symptoms to be alert for, and genetic issues for future childbearing.

## Family Resources

*Sickle Cell Disease: Guide for Parents*. Agency for Health Care Policy and Research Publications Clearinghouse, PO Box 8547, Silver Spring, MD 20907; 1-800 358-9295.

*Understanding PKU*. PKU Clinic, Children's Hospital Medical Center, 300 Longwood Ave., Boston, MA 02115; (617) 735-6650.

Most state health departments have their own pamphlets on newborn screenings for parents that can be ordered by clinicians.

## Provider Resources

*Blood Collection on Filter Paper for Neonatal Screening Programs—Second Edition; Approved Standard*. National Committee for Clinical Laboratory Standards (NCCLS), 771 E. Lancaster Ave., Villanova, PA 19085; (215) 525-2435. An educational videotape depicting the LA4-A2 collection procedure is also available from NCCLS.

*Sickle Cell Disease: Clinical Practice Guideline*; *Sickle Cell Disease: Guideline Report*; *Sickle Cell Disease: Quick Reference Guide*. Agency for Health Care Policy and Research Publications Clearinghouse, PO Box 8547, Silver Spring, MD 20907; 1-800 358-9295.

## Selected References

American Academy of Family Physicians, Commission on Public Health and Scientific Affairs. *Age Charts for Periodic Health Examination*. Kansas City, Mo: American Academy of Family Physicians; 1993.
American Academy of Pediatrics, Committee on Genetics. Issues in newborn screening. *Pediatrics*. 1992;89:345-349.
American Academy of Pediatrics, Committee on Genetics. Newborn screening fact sheets. *Pediatrics*. 1989;83:449-464.
Canadian Task Force on the Periodic Health Examination. The periodic health examination. *Can Med Assoc J*. 1979;121:1193-1254.
Council of Regional Networks for Genetic Services (CORN). *Newborn Screening Report: 1990, Final Report*. New York, NY: Council on Regional Networks for Genetic Screening; 1993.
Donnell G, ed. *Galactosemia: New Frontiers in Research*. Bethesda, Md: National Institutes of Health, National Institute of Child Health and Development; 1992.

Illinois Department of Public Health. *Newborn Screening: An Overview of Newborn Screening Programs in the United States and Canada.* Springfield, Ill: Illinois Department of Public Health; 1990.

National Committee for Clinical Laboratory Standards. *Blood Collection on Filter Paper for Neonatal Screening Programs—Second Edition; Approved Standard.* Villanova, Pa: National Committee for Clinical Laboratory Standards; 1992.

National Institutes of Health. Newborn Screening for Sickle Cell Disease and Other Hemoglobinopathies. *National Institutes of Health Consensus Development Conference Statement.* 1987;6(9):1-22.

National Screening Status Report. *Infant Screening.* 1993;16(1):7.

Sickle Cell Disease Guideline Panel, Agency for Health Care Policy and Research. *Sickle Cell Disease: Screening, Diagnosis, Management, and Counseling in Newborns and Infants.* Clinical Practice Guideline No. 6. Rockville, Md: US Dept of Health and Human Services; April 1993. DHHS publication no. AHCPR 93-0562.

US Preventive Services Task Force. Screening for phenylketonuria. In: *Guide to Clinical Preventive Services.* Baltimore, Md: Williams & Wilkins; 1989:chap 19.

US Preventive Services Task Force. Screening for thyroid disease. In: *Guide to Clinical Preventive Services.* Baltimore, Md: Williams & Wilkins; 1989:chap 17.

## Ch. 8. Newborn Screening

### Table 8-1. Newborn Screening by State

| State | PKU | HYP | GAL | BIO | CAH | HEMO | MSUD | HOMO | TYRO | CF | TOXO |
|---|---|---|---|---|---|---|---|---|---|---|---|
| Alabama | x[1] | x[1] | x[1] | | | x | | | | | |
| Alaska | x[2] | x[2] | x[2] | x[2] | x[1] | | x[2,3] | x[2] | x[1] | | |
| Arizona | x[2] | x | x | x | | x | x | x | | | |
| Arkansas | x | x | | | | x | | | | | |
| California | x | x | x | | | x | | | | | |
| Colorado | x[1] | x | x | x | | x | x | x | | x | |
| Connecticut | x[1] | x | x | x | | x | x | x | | | |
| Delaware | x | x | x | x | | x[3] | x | x | x | | |
| Dist. Columbia | x[2] | x[2] | x | | | x | x[2] | x[2] | | | |
| Florida | x | x | x | | | x | | | | | |
| Georgia | x | x | x | | x | x[3,4] | x | x | x | | |
| Hawaii | x | x | | | | | | | | | |
| Idaho | x[2] | x[2] | x[2] | x[2] | | | x[2] | x[2] | x[1] | | |
| Illinois | x | x | x | x | x | x | | | | | |
| Indiana | x[2] | x[2] | x[2] | | | x | x[2] | x[2] | | | |
| Iowa | x | x | x | | x | x | x | | | | |
| Kansas | x | x | x | | | x | | | | | |
| Kentucky | x | x | x | | | x[4] | | | | | |
| Louisiana | x | x | | | | x | | | | | |
| Maine | x | x | x | | | x[3,4] | x | x | | | |
| Maryland | x[2] | x[2] | x[2] | x[2] | | x | x[2] | x[2] | x | | |
| Massachusetts | x | x | x | | x | x | x | x | | | x |
| Michigan | x[2] | x[2] | x[2] | x[2] | x | x | x | | | | |
| Minnesota | x | x | x | | x | x | | | | | |
| Mississippi | x | x | x | | | x | | | | | |
| Missouri | x[2] | x[2] | x[2] | | | x[3] | | | | | |
| Montana | x | x | x | | | | | | | | |
| Nebraska | x | x | | x | | | | | | | |
| Nevada | x[1] | x[1] | x[1] | x[1] | | x | x[1] | x[1] | x[1] | | |
| New Hampshire | x | x | x | | | x[3,4] | x | x | | | x |
| New Jersey | x | x | x | | | x | | | | | |
| New Mexico | x[1] | x | x | | | x[3,4] | | | | | |
| New York | x | x | x | x | | x | x | x | | | |

*(Continued)*

## Ch. 8. Newborn Screening Children/Adolescents — SCREENING

Table 8-1. Newborn Screening by State—Continued

| State | Conditions Screened |||||||||||
|---|---|---|---|---|---|---|---|---|---|---|
| | PKU | HYP | GAL | BIO | CAH | HEMO | MSUD | HOMO | TYRO | CF | TOXO |
| North Carolina | $x^3$ | $x^3$ | $x^3$ | | x | $x^4$ | | | | | |
| North Dakota | $x^1$ | $x^1$ | x | | x | | x | | | | |
| Ohio | x | x | x | | | x | | $x^1$ | | | |
| Oklahoma | x | x | x | | | x | | | | | |
| Oregon | $x^1$ | $x^1$ | $x^1$ | $x^1$ | | | $x^1$ | $x^1$ | $x^1$ | | |
| Pennsylvania | x | x | | | | x | x | | | | |
| Rhode Island | x | x | x | | | x | x | x | | | |
| South Carolina | x | x | x | | x | x | | | | | |
| South Dakota | x | x | | | | | | | | | |
| Tennessee | x | x | x | | | x | | | | | |
| Texas | $x^1$ | $x^1$ | $x^1$ | | $x^1$ | $x^1$ | | | | | |
| Utah | $x^1$ | x | x | | | | | | | | |
| Vermont | $x^3$ | $x^3$ | $x^3$ | | | $x^{3,4}$ | x | $x^3$ | | | |
| Virginia | x | x | x | x | | x | x | x | | | |
| Washington | $x^1$ | $x^1$ | | | $x^1$ | x | | | | | |
| West Virginia | x | x | x | | | $x^{3,4}$ | | | | | |
| Wisconsin | x | x | x | x | x | x | x | x | | $x^3$ | |
| Wyoming | $x^2$ | x | x | x | | x | x | x | | | x |

### Key

| | | | |
|---|---|---|---|
| PKU | Phenylketonuria | x | Screening required by state law |
| HYP | Congenital Hypothyroidism | $x^1$ | Repeat screening required |
| GAL | Galactosemia | $x^2$ | Repeat screening required only on a |
| BIO | Biotinidase Deficiency | | discretionary basis (i.e., for early |
| CAH | Congenital Adrenal Hyperplasia | | discharges) |
| HEMO | Hemoglobinopathies | $x^3$ | Screening voluntary |
| MSUD | Maple Syrup Urine Disease | $x^4$ | Screening targeted (i.e., African, Middle |
| HOMO | Homocystinuria | | Eastern descent) |
| TYRO | Tyrosinemia | | |
| CF | Cystic Fibrosis | | |
| TOXO | Toxoplasmosis | | |

Adapted from: Council of Regional Networks for Genetic Services (CORN). *Newborn Screening Report: 1990, Final Report.* New York, NY: Council of Regional Networks for Genetic Screening; 1993; and National Screening Status Report. *Infant Screening.* 1993;16(1):7. Reproduced by permission of the publisher; copyright © 1993.

## Children/Adolescents — SCREENING

# 9. Tuberculosis
## (Including Prophylaxis and BCG Vaccination)

Tuberculosis (TB) is an increasing public health problem in the United States. In 1990, the number of reported TB cases increased 9.4% compared with 1989 and 15.5% compared with 1984. There were 1596 cases of TB reported in children younger than 15 years old in 1990, and 86% of those cases were in racial and ethnic minorities. Factors contributing to the increase in TB cases include adverse social and economic conditions, the HIV epidemic, immigration of individuals with TB infection, and clinician and patient noncompliance with recommended screening and treatment regimens. The recent emergence of multiple-drug resistant strains of *Mycobacterium tuberculosis* has added urgency to the need for improved preventive efforts to combat the disease.

Populations at high risk include: 1) medically underserved, low-income populations, including those of African-American, Hispanic, Asian, Native American, and Alaskan Native heritage; 2) foreign-born individuals from high-prevalence countries (e.g., Asia, Africa, and Latin America); 3) children in close contact with infectious TB cases (sharing accommodations as well as playing or working in the same enclosed area); 4) individuals with medical conditions known to substantially increase the risk of TB (see Table 9-1); 5) alcoholics and injection drug users; 6) residents of high-risk environments, including long-term care facilities, correctional institutions, and mental institutions.

Prophylaxis with isoniazid has been shown to be very effective in preventing the onset of clinical disease. When taken for 12 months, isoniazid reduces the incidence of clinical TB infection by 54% to 88%. Efficacy is directly related to the length of prophylaxis and the extent of patient compliance with the prophylaxis regimen. The effectiveness of *bacille Calmett-Guérin* (BCG) vaccination is considerably less certain, with effectiveness rates that vary from 0% to 82% in major trials.

See chapter 42 for information on TB screening and prophylaxis and BCG vaccination in adults.

**Recommendations of Major Authorities**

*Screening*

- **American Academy of Family Physicians, American Medical Association, American Thoracic Society (ATS), Centers for Disease Control and Prevention (CDC), and U.S. Preventive Service Task Force**—Tuberculin testing should be performed on children and adolescents at high risk of disease. **ATS** and **CDC** have recommended that the frequency of testing be determined by the likelihood of exposure to infectious TB. Annual TB testing is recommended for children in high-risk populations, such as those born abroad and those in medically underserved, low-income groups.

- **American Academy of Pediatrics (AAP)** —All children should receive tuberculin testing at 1, 4, and 14 years of age. All high-risk children should receive annual tuberculin testing.

- **Canadian Task Force on the Periodic Health Examination**—Tuberculin testing of children at high risk for disease should be performed at 5 to 6 years of age and after 16 years of age at a frequency determined by clinical judgment. This recommendation is currently under review.

## Prophylaxis

- **AAP** and **CDC**—Children with a positive Mantoux test and without active disease should receive prophylaxis with isoniazid. Certain children with a negative Mantoux test should be considered for isoniazid prophylaxis: 1) newborn infants whose mothers have active TB; 2) patients who are anergic and from populations where the prevalence of TB is greater than 10%, such as injection drug users, homeless individuals, migrant laborers, and individuals born in Asia, Africa, or Latin America; 3) patients with close contact within the last 3 months with an infectious TB case.

## BCG Vaccination

- **AAP**—BCG vaccination should be considered for children, particularly infants, who 1) are tuberculin-test negative and have repeated household contacts with an individual who has sputum-positive TB and who is persistently untreated or inadequately treated; and 2) live in a group with an excessive rate of new infection for which the usual methods of surveillance and treatment have failed.

- **ATS** and **CDC**—Infants and children should be considered for BCG vaccination if their TB skin test is negative and they fall into any of the following categories: 1) those who have continuous, unavoidable exposure to individuals with active disease and who cannot be placed on isoniazid preventive therapy; 2) those with continuous exposure to patients infected with organisms resistant to isoniazid and rifampin; 3) those belonging to groups with new infection rates greater than 1% and who do not participate in usual surveillance and treatment programs.

**Table 9-1. Medical Conditions That Increase the Risk of Tuberculosis Infection**

| |
|---|
| HIV infection |
| Silicosis |
| Gastrectomy |
| Jejunoileal bypass |
| Weight 10% or more below ideal weight |
| Chronic renal failure |
| Diabetes mellitus |
| Conditions requiring prolonged high-dose corticosteroid therapy or other immunosuppressive therapy |
| Some hematologic disorders (e.g., leukemia and lymphomas) |
| Other malignancies |

From: Centers for Disease Control. Screening for tuberculosis and tuberculous infection in high-risk populations; Recommendations of the Advisory Committee for Elimination of Tuberculosis. *MMWR.* 1990;39:1-7.

## Basics of Tuberculosis Screening and Prophylaxis and BCG Vaccination

*Screening*

1. The Mantoux test should be used if possible. Multiple-puncture tests have inadequate specificity and sensitivity. A reaction to any multiple-puncture test should be confirmed by the standard Mantoux test unless vesiculation occurs, in which case the reaction should be considered positive.

2. For the Mantoux test, 0.1 mL of purified protein derivative (PPD) containing 5 tuberculin units should be used. PPD should be administered using a disposable tuberculin syringe to give an intradermal injection on the volar or dorsal surface of the forearm. The bevel of the needle should be facing upward and a pale, discrete elevation of the skin (weal) 6 to 10 mm in diameter should be produced.

3. The test should be read 48 to 72 hours after the injection by measuring the diameter of induration (not erythema) transverse to the long axis of the forearm. A ballpoint pen may be helpful to delineate the margin of induration.

4. The criteria for a "positive" Mantoux test differ somewhat between AAP and CDC.

   - AAP considers a reaction to be positive if the diameter is:

     *5 mm or greater* and any of the following apply: the child is a known contact of a sputum- or smear-positive adult; lives in an area that is not endemic for nontuberculous mycobacterial infection; is HIV-seropositive; or is immunosuppressed for any reason.

     *10 mm or greater:* all children and adolescents.

   - CDC considers a reaction to be positive if the diameter is:

     *5 mm or greater* and has any of the following: close contact with a patient with infectious TB; known or suspected HIV infection; a chest radiograph with a fibrotic lesion likely to represent old, healed TB.

     *10 mm or greater* and any of the following apply: less than 4 years of age; born in an area with high prevalence (Asia, Africa, and Latin America); member of a medically underserved, low-income population (including high-risk minorities, especially African Americans, Hispanics, Native Americans, and other populations identified locally as at high risk); injection drug user; resident of a long-term care facility; has medical conditions that substantially increase the risk of TB infection (see Table 9-1; note that for HIV infection, diameters of 5 mm or greater are considered positive).

     *15 mm or greater:* all children and adolescents.

BCG vaccination can cause false-positive Mantoux reactions, but these decrease with time and rarely cause reactions of 15 mm or greater. In general, BCG-vaccinated individuals with positive Mantoux tests should be considered to have true infection with *M. tuberculosis* and given appropriate follow-up care.

5. Adverse reactions to TB skin testing are very uncommon. Reactions described include pain, fever, vesiculation, and regional adenopathy.

6. Children with HIV infection should have PPD testing in conjunction with anergy testing with at least two delayed-type hypersensitivity skin tests (i.e., Candida, mumps, or tetanus toxoid). Anergy testing should also be considered for children in other groups who have an increased risk of TB infection.

7. Patients who have a documented history of a positive Mantoux test should not be retested, because such testing has no diagnostic utility and may lead to adverse reactions.

8. Live-virus vaccines, such as MMR and OPV, may interfere with response to a tuberculin test. Tuberculin testing, if otherwise indicated, may be administered either on the same day as live-virus vaccines or postponed until 4 to 6 weeks afterward.

*Prophylaxis*

1. *Indications:* A child with a positive Mantoux test and without active disease should be considered for isoniazid prophylaxis. Certain children should be considered for isoniazid prophylaxis without documentation of a positive Mantoux test: newborn infants whose mothers have active disease (even if noncontagious) at delivery; children who are anergic and from populations where the prevalence of TB is greater than 10% (such as injection drug users, homeless individuals, migrant laborers, and individuals from Asia, Africa, or Latin America); and children with close contact within the last 3 months with an infectious TB case.

2. *Dosage and Administration:* The recommended dosage of isoniazid is 10 mg/kg (up to a maximum of 300 mg) given orally once daily. For noncompliant patients, 20-40 mg/kg (to a maximum of 900 mg) may be given twice weekly under the direct observation of a health professional.

3. *Duration*: Isoniazid prophylaxis should be continued for 6 to 12 months. AAP, ATS, and CDC recommend a minimum of 9 months of prophylaxis. CDC recommends that newborn prophylaxis be discontinued at 3 months of age if a Mantoux test at that age is negative; all known adult contacts have negative sputum samples and are compliant with anti-TB medications; and a repeat Mantoux test is performed at 6 months of age. AAP recommends maintaining isoniazid prophylaxis until a negative PPD test is obtained at 6 months of age. In general, patients who are HIV-positive or who have evidence of prior TB on chest radiograph should receive isoniazid prophylaxis for 12 months.

4. *Precautions:* Patients must be monitored monthly while on isoniazid for signs and symptoms of hepatotoxicity. These include loss of appetite, nausea, vomiting, persistent dark urine, jaundice, fever, and abdominal tenderness (especially in the right upper quadrant). The incidence of hepatitis during isoniazid therapy is low enough in otherwise healthy children that liver function testing is not required. Peripheral neuritis and convulsions due to inhibition of pyridoxine metabolism by isoniazid have rarely occurred. Pyridoxine supplementation may be considered on an individual basis for breast-feeding children, children with deficient diets (particularly if low in meat and milk), and pregnant women.

## *BCG Vaccination*

1. *Indications:* Recommendations differ slightly among authorities. See Recommendations of Major Authorities.

2. *Vaccine Types:* There is one BCG vaccine (Tice®) available in North America.

3. *Dosage and Administration:* 0.2 to 0.3 mL of the vaccine is dropped on the cleansed surface of the skin. It is administered percutaneously with the application of a multiple-puncture disc through the vaccine. After vaccination, the vaccine should flow into the puncture wounds and dry. A dressing is not required, but the patient should be advised to keep the site dry for 24 hours. Infants less than 30 days old should receive half the usual dose. If the indications for vaccination persist, infants should also receive a full dose at 1 year of age.

4. *Precautions:* BCG vaccine should not be given to individuals who are immunocompromised or immunosuppressed, including those with HIV infection.

5. *Adverse reactions:* Side effects occur in 1% to 10% of vaccinated individuals and may include severe or prolonged ulceration at the vaccination site, lymphadenitis, and lupus vulgaris.

6. *Interactions:* BCG vaccination can cause false-positive Mantoux reactions, but this decreases with time and rarely causes reactions of 15 mm or greater. In general, BCG-vaccinated individuals with positive Mantoux tests should be considered to have true infection with *M. tuberculosis* and given appropriate follow-up care.

## Family Resources

*Facts About the TB Skin Test; Facts About Tuberculosis.* American Lung Association, 1740 Broadway, New York, NY 10019-4374; (212) 315-8700.

*TB: Get the Facts; Tuberculosis: Connection between TB and HIV.* Centers for Disease Control and Prevention, Attn: Information Systems Office, 1600 Clifton Rd. NE, Atlanta, GA 30333; (404) 639-1819.

## Provider Resources

*Core Curriculum on Tuberculosis.* American Thoracic Society/Centers for Disease Control; 1991. Tuberculosis Elimination, National Center for Prevention Services, Centers for Disease Control and Prevention, 1600 Clifton Rd. NE, Mailstop E-10, Atlanta, GA 30333; (404) 639-2508.

*Initial Therapy for TB in the Era of Multiple Drug Resistance; Mantoux Tuberculin Skin Testing* (videotape). Centers for Disease Control and Prevention, Attn: Information Services Office, 1600 Clifton Rd., NE, Atlanta, GA 30333; (404) 639-1819.

## Selected References

American Academy of Family Physicians, Commission on Public Health and Scientific Affairs. *Age Charts for Periodic Health Examination.* Kansas City, Mo: American Academy of Family Physicians; 1993.

American Academy of Pediatrics, Committee on Infectious Diseases. *Report of the Committee on Infectious Diseases.* Elk Grove Village, Ill: American Academy of Pediatrics; 1991.

American Thoracic Society. Control of tuberculosis in the United States. *Am Rev Respir Dis.* 1992;146:1623-1633.

American Thoracic Society/Centers for Disease Control. Diagnostic standards and classification of tuberculosis. *Am Rev Respir Dis.* 1990;142:725-735.

Centers for Disease Control. Guidelines for preventing the transmission of tuberculosis in health-care settings, with special focus on HIV-related issues. *MMWR.* 1990;39:1-29.

Centers for Disease Control. Prevention and control of tuberculosis in US communities with at-risk minority populations and prevention and control of tuberculosis among homeless persons. *MMWR.* 1992;4:1-23.

Centers for Disease Control. Purified protein derivative (PPD) tuberculin anergy and HIV infection: guidelines for anergy testing and management of anergic persons at risk of tuberculosis. *MMWR.* 1991:40(RR-5):27-33.

Centers for Disease Control. Screening for tuberculosis and tuberculous infection in high-risk populations: Recommendations of the Advisory Committee for Elimination of Tuberculosis. *MMWR.* 1990;39:1-7.

Centers for Disease Control. Use of BCG vaccines in the control of tuberculosis: a joint statement by the ACIP and the Advisory Committee for Elimination of Tuberculosis. *MMWR.* 1988;37:1-5.

*Physicians' Desk Reference.* Oradell, NJ: Medical Economics Company; 1993. Pp 898-899; 1689-1692.

Pust, RE. Tuberculosis in the 1990's: resurgence, regimens, and resources. *South Med J.* 1992;85:584-593.

US Preventive Services Task Force. Screening for tuberculosis. In: *Guide to Clinical Preventive Services.* Baltimore, Md: Williams & Wilkins; 1989:chap 21.

## Children/Adolescents — SCREENING

# 10. Urinalysis

Screening urinalysis can detect many types of abnormalities in the urine, including the presence of glucose, protein, red and white blood cells, bacteria, and bacterial breakdown products. In asymptomatic children, screening for red blood cells and protein is generally not very productive because of the transient and benign nature of the disorders causing them. Screening for glucosuria is also of questionable utility because of varying renal thresholds for glucose spillage and the short interval between the onset of glucosuria and onset of the symptoms of diabetes mellitus. Screening for indicators of occult infection, such as white blood cells and bacteria, may be beneficial as a means of promoting early treatment.

During infancy, the prevalence of asymptomatic bacteriuria is higher in boys (2.5%) than in girls (0.9%). This is partly due to the higher incidence of structural abnormalities of the urinary tract in boys. After infancy, the prevalence of asymptomatic bacteriuria is much higher in girls (1% to 2%) than in boys (less than 0.1%). Asymptomatic bacteriuria develops into symptomatic urinary tract infections in less than 10% of cases. These infections can lead to renal scarring and permanent renal damage. Most such damage occurs, however, in children before 2 to 3 years of age, when screening is difficult because of problems of specimen collection. Treatment of asymptomatic bacteriuria with antibiotics may alter the composition of body's flora and lead to infections with resistant bacteria.

Asymptomatic sexually transmitted diseases, particularly infection with *Chlamydia trachomatis*, are common in adolescents and young adults. The prevalence of asymptomatic chlamydial urethral infection in young males ranges from 6% to 11%. These infections can be passed to female partners, resulting in pelvic inflammatory disease, ectopic pregnancy, and infertility. Recently, dipstick urinalysis has been advocated as a noninvasive initial screening technique for detecting such occult infections in sexually active young males. Such testing is of moderate sensitivity but low specificity—necessitating further follow-up testing of positives. For *Chlamydia trachomatis* infection, the leukocyte esterase dipstick test has a sensitivity of 70% to 80% and a specificity of 70% to 85%.

**Recommendations of Major Authorities**

- **American Academy of Family Physicians** and **U.S. Preventive Services Task Force**—It may be clinically prudent to perform urinalysis to detect bacteriuria in preschool children. The optimal frequency for urine testing has not been determined and is left to clinical discretion. This recommendation is under review.

- **American Academy of Pediatrics**—Urinalysis should be performed at 6 months and at 2, 8, and 18 years of age, although current medical evidence suggests the need for reevaluation of the frequency and timing of urinalyses. This recommendation is currently being reevaluated.

- **American Medical Association**—Sexually active adolescent males should be screened yearly for gonorrhea and chlamydia by urinalysis with a dipstick leukocyte esterase test. If this test is positive, tests to make a definitive diagnosis should be performed.

- **Canadian Task Force on the Periodic Health Examination**—Urinalysis should not be included in the periodic health examination because of the low yield in detecting occult infection and the frequent recurrence of infection after treatment.

## Basics of Urinalysis

1. Obtaining urine to screen infants and young children for bacteriuria requires use of a plastic urine bag applied to the perineum. This method has a relatively high rate of false-positive results (up to 30%), due to contamination. Positive results for bacteriuria obtained by bag collection should be confirmed by catheterization or suprapubic aspiration.

2. In screening children and adolescents for bacteriuria, it is best to obtain specimens using midstream "clean catch" techniques. This permits follow-up culture testing of dipstick-positive specimens. The vulva of girls and the glans of boys should be cleansed well with a mild soap solution. Antiseptic solutions should not be used because of the potential of suppressing bacterial growth in the sample. During urination, the labia of girls should be held open to avoid impinging on the flow of urine. This may be accomplished without manual holding by having the girl sit backward with legs astride a toilet seat. The foreskin of uncircumcised boys should be retracted to avoid impinging on the flow of urine.

3. The sensitivity of screening for bacteriuria may be improved by obtaining a specimen from the first void of the day. This void tends to be more concentrated and contain higher amounts of bacteria and bacterial breakdown products than subsequent voids. Specimen collection from later voids is acceptable and may be more practical.

4. The specimen is most efficiently screened for bacteriuria by using a dipstick leukocyte esterase test. The sensitivity and specificity (each approximately 80%) of the leukocyte esterase test (compared with culture) is roughly equivalent to that obtained by more labor-intensive microscopic analysis. The nitrite test is also available on many dipsticks; if used alone, however, it is inadequate for screening purposes because of low sensitivity (approximately 30%). A positive nitrite test, however, has high specificity (approximately 99%) for significant bacteriuria.

5. In screening males for sexually transmitted diseases, urine samples should be collected from the first 15-20 mL of a void. The unspun sample is then tested with a leukocyte esterase dipstick. Because of the poor specificity of the test and the cost and the potential morbidity associated with treatment, positive tests should be confirmed with more specific techniques, such as enzyme immunoassay or culture.

## Selected References

American Academy of Family Physicians, Commission on Public Health and Scientific Affairs. *Age Charts for Periodic Health Examination.* Kansas City, Mo: American Academy of Family Physicians; 1993.

American Academy of Pediatrics, Committee on Practice and Ambulatory Care. Recommendations for preventive pediatric health care. *AAP News.* 1991;7:19.

American Academy of Pediatrics, Section on Urology. Screening school children for urologic disease. *Pediatrics.* 1977;60:239-243.

American Medical Association. *Guidelines for Adolescent Preventive Services (GAPS).* Chicago, Ill: American Medical Association; 1992.

Aronson MD, Phillips RS. Screening young men for *Chlamydia* infection. *JAMA.* 1993;270:2097-2098.

Boehm JJ, Haynes JL. Bacteriology of "midstream catch" urines. *Am J Dis Child.* 1966;111:366-369.

Canadian Task Force on the Periodic Health Examination. The periodic health examination 1979. *Can Med Assoc J.* 1979;121:1193-1254.

Dodge WF. Cost effectiveness of renal disease screening. *Am J Dis Child.* 1977;131:1274-1280.

Edelman CM, Ogwo JE, Fine BP, Martinez AB. The prevalence of bacteriuria in full-term and premature newborn infants. *J Pediatr.* 1973;82:125-132.

Genc M, Ruusuvaara, Mardh PA. An economic evaluation of screening for *Chlamydia trachomatis* in adolescent males. *JAMA.* 1993;270:2057-2064.

Goldsmith BM, Campos JM. Comparison of urine dipstick, microscopy, and culture for the detection of bacteriuria in children. *Clin Pediatr.* 1990;29:214-218.

Lindberg U. Asymptomatic bacteriuria in school girls: V. The clinical course and response to treatment. *Acta Paediatr Scand.* 1975;64:718-724.

Lohr JA, Donowitz LG, Dudley SM. Bacterial contamination rates for non-clean-catch and clean-catch midstream urine collections in boys. *J Pediatr.* 1986;109:659-660.

Lohr JA, Donowitz LG, Dudley SM. Bacterial contamination rates in voided urine collections in girls. *J Pediatr.* 1989;114:91-93.

Kemper KJ, Avner ED. The case against screening urinalyses for asymptomatic bacteriuria in children. *Am J Dis Child.* 1992;146:343-346.

Kunin CM. *Detection, Prevention and Management of Urinary Tract Infections.* 4th ed. Philadelphia, Pa: Lea & Febiger, 1987.

Mitchell N, Stapleton FB. Routine admission urinalysis examination in pediatric patients: a poor value. *Pediatrics.* 1990;86:345-349.

Savage DCL, Howie G, Adler K, Wilson MI. Controlled trial of therapy in covert bacteriuria of childhood. *Lancet.* 1975;1:358-361.

Schlager TA, Dunn ML, Dudley SM, Lohr JA. Bacterial contamination rate of urine collected in a urine bag from healthy non-toilet-trained male infants. *J Pediatr.* 1990;116:738-739.

Shafer M, Schachter J, Moncada J, et al. Evaluation of urine-based screening strategies to detect *Chlamydia trachomatis* among sexually active asymptomatic young males. *JAMA.* 1993;270:2065-2070.

US Preventive Services Task Force. Screening for asymptomatic bacteriuria, hematuria, and proteinuria. In: *Guide to Clinical Preventive Services.* Baltimore, Md: Williams & Wilkins; 1989:chap 27.

Zhanel GG, Harding GKM, Guay DRP. Asymptomatic bacteriuria. Which patients should be treated? *Arch Intern Med.* 1990;150:1389-1396.

# Children/Adolescents — SCREENING

## 11. Vision

Refractive errors are the most common vision disorders of children, occurring in 20% by 16 years of age. Amblyopia ("lazy eye") develops in 2% to 4% of children. The risk of developing amblyopia is greatest during the first 2 to 3 years of life, but the potential for its development exists until visual development is complete at 9 years of age. Left untreated, amblyopia may lead to irreversible visual deficits. Strabismus occurs in 2% of children and is one of the primary causes of amblyopia. Other eye diseases occurring during infancy and childhood include cataracts (1 per 1000 live births), congenital glaucoma (1 per 10,000 live births), retinoblastoma (1 per 20,000 live births), and retinopathy of prematurity. More than 100,000 eye injuries occur annually in the general population, an estimated 90% of which are preventable.

Through careful history, examination, vision testing, and appropriate referral, amblyopia and other ophthalmologic disorders can be detected and visual impairment lessened or averted. Early detection and prompt intervention are essential.

### Recommendations of Major Authorities

*Normal-Risk Children*

- **American Academy of Family Physicians** and **U.S. Preventive Services Task Force**—All children should have testing for amblyopia and strabismus once before entering school, preferably at 3 to 4 years of age. Stereotesting is more effective than visual acuity testing for this purpose. Routine visual acuity testing is not recommended for asymptomatic school-age children. Clinicians should be alert for signs of ocular misalignment in examining all infants and children.

- **American Academy of Ophthalmology (AAO), American Academy of Pediatrics (AAP), American Association for Pediatric Ophthalmology and Strabismus (AAPOS),** and **American Optometric Association (AOA)**—Eye and vision screening should be performed at birth and at approximately 6 months, 3 years, and 5 years of age. **AAO** has published recommendations regarding screening methods and indications for referral to be used by primary care clinicians in screening preschool children (see Table 11-1). **AAP** recommends that clinicians perform objective vision screening on school-aged children at 3, 4, 5, 6, 8, 12, and 18 years of age. **AAO** and **AAPOS** recommend that screening after 5 years of age be carried out at routine school checks or after the appearance of symptoms. **AOA** recommends that color vision screening be included in the routine screening of boys prior to school entry.

- **Canadian Task Force on the Periodic Health Examination**—Eye examination and the cover/uncover test should be performed on children during the first week of life and at 2 to 4 weeks, 2 months, and 2 to 3 and 5 to 6 years of age. Visual acuity testing with a wall chart should be performed at 2 to 3 and 5 to 6 years of age. Visual acuity testing is discretionary for children at 10 to 11 years of age.

*High-Risk Children*

- **American Academy of Ophthalmology**—Asymptomatic children should have a comprehensive examination by an ophthalmologist if they are at high risk due to: health and developmental problems that make screening by the primary care clinician difficult or inaccurate (e.g., retinopathy of prematurity or diagnostic evaluation of a complex disease with ophthalmic manifestations); a family history of conditions that cause or are associated with eye or vision problems (e.g., retinoblastoma, significant hyperopia, strabismus [particularly accommodative esotropia], amblyopia, congenital cataract, or glaucoma); multiple health problems, systemic disease, or use of medications that are known to be associated with eye disease and vision abnormalities (e.g., neurodegenerative disease, juvenile rheumatoid arthritis, systemic steroid therapy, systemic syndromes with ocular manifestations, or developmental delay with visual system manifestations).

- **American Optometric Association**—The primary care clinician should remain alert for visual/ocular abnormalities associated with the following high-risk groups: babies who are premature, have been on oxygen therapy, or are of low birth weight; infants with a family history of retinoblastoma, congenital cataracts, or metabolic or genetic disease; infants whose mothers have had rubella, venereal disease, or AIDS-related infections during pregnancy. All infants weighing less than 1500 grams or less than 34 weeks gestation should be screened for retinopathy of prematurity with an ophthalmoscopic fundus evaluation through dilated pupils before the 6th week of life and at least every 6 months for the first 2 years of life.

**Basics of Vision Screening**

1. *History:* Gathering information in the following areas is important in screening for present or potential visual disorders:

   - Family history of vision or eye problems.

   - History of maternal, intrapartum, or neonatal conditions that may place the child at high risk for visual disorders (see Recommendations for High-Risk Children).

   - Parental concerns about a child's visual functioning—It is important to listen carefully to parents who note that their child has a problem with his or her eyes or vision. Parental observations are often correct.

   - School performance—Worsening grades and other school difficulties may be signs of vision problems.

2. *Physical Examination:* A comprehensive examination of the eye includes the lids, lashes, tear ducts, orbit, conjunctiva, sclera, cornea, iris, pupillary responsiveness, range of motion, anterior chamber, lens, vitreous, retina, and optic nerve and vessels. It can be difficult to gain cooperation of young children with an ophthalmoscopic examination. It may be helpful to demonstrate the examination procedure on the parent beforehand and to have the child sit on the parent's lap.

## Ch. 11. Vision — Children/Adolescents — SCREENING

**Table 11-1. Eye and Vision Examination Recommendations for Primary Care Physicians**

| Age | Screening Method | Indicators Requiring Further Evaluation |
|---|---|---|
| Newborn to 3 months old | Red reflex | Abnormal or asymmetric |
| | Corneal light reflex | Asymmetric |
| | Inspection | Structural abnormality |
| 6 months to 1 year old | Red reflex | Abnormal or asymmetric |
| | Corneal light reflex | Asymmetric |
| | Differential occlusion | Failure to object equally to covering each eye |
| | Fix and follow with each eye | Failure to fix and follow |
| | Inspection | Structural abnormality |
| 3 years old (approximately) | Visual acuity[a] | 20/50 or worse or difference of 2 lines between eyes |
| | Red reflex | Abnormal or asymmetric |
| | Corneal light reflex/cover-uncover | Asymmetric/ocular refixation movements |
| | Stereoacuity[b] | Failure to appreciate random dot or Titmus Stereogram |
| | Inspection | Structural abnormality |
| 5 years old (approximately) | Visual acuity[a] | 20/30 or worse |
| | Red reflex | Abnormal or asymmetric |
| | Corneal light reflex/cover-uncover | Asymmetric/ocular refixation movements |
| | Stereoacuity[b] | Failure to appreciate random dot or Titmus Stereogram |
| | Inspection | Structural abnormality |

[a] Allen figures, HOTV, Tumbling E, or Snellen

[b] Optional, sometimes advocated in lieu of visual acuity; Random Dot E Game (RDE), Titmus Stereograms, Randot Stereograms

From: American Academy of Ophthalmology, Quality of Care Committee, Pediatric Ophthalmology Panel. *Comprehensive Pediatric Eye Evaluation.* San Francisco, CA: American Academy of Ophthalmology; 1992. Reproduced by permission of the publisher; copyright © 1992.

3. *Testing Procedures:*

- *Red Reflex:* The red reflex exam may be performed with an ophthalmoscope or other light source. In a darkened room, the light source should be held at arm's length from the infant and the infant's attention drawn to look directly at the light. Both retinal reflexes should be red or red-orange and of equal intensity.

- *Corneal Light Reflex:* The corneal light reflex test, for detection of strabismus, is also performed with an ophthalmoscope or other light source. Corneal light reflections should fall symmetrically on corresponding points of the patient's eyes. Improper alignment will appear as asymmetry of reflections.

- *Differential Occlusion:* The test for differential occlusion is performed by gently covering the infant's eyes, one at a time. Aversion to the occlusion is normal. However, this test may give a false-positive result and is generally less accurate than the corneal light reflex test for detecting strabismus.

- *Fixation:* In examining for fixation, a light or a small object is held in front of the infant. In a normal exam, the infant's eyes will be aligned in the same direction, without deviation.

- *Cover/Uncover:* The cover/uncover test is performed by having the child focus on a stationary target. While placing a hand or cover in front of one eye, the examiner observes the other eye. Movement of the observed eye is abnormal and demonstrates the presence of strabismus. As the covered eye is uncovered, the examiner observes it for movement. Movement is abnormal and indicates the presence of heterophoria.

- *Stereotesting:* Stereopsis (binocular depth perception) can be tested using a stereotesting technique, such as the Random Dot E stereogram. While wearing polarized glasses, the child views test cards that contain fields of random dots. If stereopsis is present, the child will see a form stand out from the background of the cards.

- *Visual Acuity*: Several eye charts are available to test visual acuity in children. In order of decreasing cognitive difficulty, these are: Snellen Letters, Snellen Numbers, Tumbling E, HOTV, Allen Figures, and LH (Leah Hyvarinen) Test. The test with the highest level of difficulty that the child is capable of performing should be used. In general, the Snellen tests are too advanced for use by preschool children. Visual acuity may be tested at 10, 15, or 20 feet (using the appropriate chart). For young children, a distance of 10 feet may result in better compliance due to closer interaction with the examiner. Care should be taken to make sure the child does not "peek" with the eye not being tested. This may require that the examiner hold the occluder or that an adhesive occluder be used. A passing score should be given for a line on which the child gives more than 50% correct responses. Recommended criteria for referral to an ophthalmologist or optometrist vary slightly. In general, referral should be made for any child with a difference in scores of two or more lines between eyes; children younger than 5 years of age scoring 20/40 or worse in either eye; and children 5 years of age or older scoring 20/30 or worse in either eye.

4. *Safety Counseling:* Parents and children should be counseled about eye safety and the appropriate use of protective equipment. Children who participate in school shop or science labs or in certain sports (i.e., racquetball, squash) should wear safety lenses and safety frames approved by the American National Standards Institute. Children with good vision in only one eye should wear safety lenses and safety frames to protect the good eye, even if they do not otherwise need to wear glasses.

## Family Resources

*Amblyopia: Is it Affecting Your Child's Sight?*; *Cataracts in Children: Eye Safety and Children*; *Eyeglasses for Infants and Children*; *Home Eye Test for Children and Adults*; *Strabismus.* American Academy of Ophthalmology, PO Box 7424, San Francisco, CA 94120; (415) 561-8500.

*Answers to Your Questions About: Lazy Eye, Nearsightedness, Astigmatism, Eye Coordination, Color Deficiency, Crossed-Eyes*; *Signs of a Child's Vision Problems*; *Toys, Games and Your Child's Vision*; *Your Child's Eyes*; *Your Preschool Child's Eyes*; *Your School-Aged Child's Eyes.* American Optometric Association, 243 N. Lindbergh Blvd., St. Louis, MO 63141; (314) 991-4100.

## Provider Resources

*Comprehensive Pediatric Eye Evaluation.* American Academy of Ophthalmology, PO Box 7424, San Francisco, CA 94120; (415) 561-8500,

*Guidelines for Preventive Eye Care.* American Optometric Association, 243 N. Lindbergh Blvd., St. Louis, MO 63141; (314) 991-4100.

## Selected References

American Academy of Family Physicians, Commission on Public Health and Scientific Affairs. *Age Charts for Periodic Health Examination.* Kansas City, Mo: American Academy of Family Physicians; 1993.
American Academy of Ophthalmology, Quality of Care Committee, Pediatric Ophthalmology Panel. *Comprehensive Pediatric Eye Evaluation.* San Francisco, Ca: American Academy of Ophthalmology; 1992.
American Academy of Ophthalmology. *Infant and Children's Vision Screening: Policy Statement.* San Francisco, Ca: American Academy of Ophthalmology; 1991.
American Academy of Pediatrics, Committee on Practice and Ambulatory Medicine. Vision screening and eye examination in children. *Pediatrics.* 1986;77:918-919.
American Optometric Association. *Guidelines for Preventive Eye Care.* St. Louis, Mo: American Optometric Association; 1993.
Canadian Task Force on the Periodic Health Examination. The periodic health examination. *Can Med Assoc J.* 1979;121:1194-1254.

Canadian Task Force on the Periodic Health Examination. Periodic health examination: 2; 1989 update. *Can Med Assoc J.* 1989;141:4-24.

Gaynon, MW. Retinopathy of Prematurity. *Pediatrician.* 1990;17:127-133.

Hope C. Random dot stereogram E in vision screening of children. *Austr N Zea J Ophthalmol.* 1990;18;319-324.

Romano PE. Advances in vision and eye screening: screening at six months of age. *Pediatrician.* 1990;17:134-141.

Romano PE. Vision/eye screening: Test twice and refer once. *Pediatr Annals.* 1990;19:359-367.

US Preventive Services Task Force. Screening for diminished visual acuity. In: *Guide to Clinical Preventive Services.* Baltimore, Md: Williams & Wilkins; 1989:chap 31.

Children/Adolescents — IMMUNIZATION/PROPHYLAXIS

# 12. Diphtheria, Tetanus, and Pertussis

Over the past decade, 1 to 5 cases of diphtheria and approximately 50 to 100 cases of tetanus have been reported each year in the United States. Due to the successful immunization of children, the majority of these cases occurred in nonimmunized or partially immunized adults. Small epidemics of pertussis persist in this country. Of the 11,446 reported cases during 1989 to 1991, the highest incidence was among children less than 1 year of age. Of the cases of pertussis reported in children aged 7 months to 4 years, about two-thirds occurred in children inadequately immunized.

See chapter 51 for information on tetanus and diphtheria immunization and prophylaxis in adults.

### Recommendations of Major Authorities

- All major authorities, including **Advisory Committee on Immunization Practices (ACIP), American Academy of Family Physicians, American Academy of Pediatrics (AAP), Canadian Task Force on the Periodic Health Examination**, and **U.S. Preventive Services Task Force**—All children should receive immunization against diphtheria, tetanus, and pertussis with completion of a primary series of vaccinations by approximately 18 months of age. A booster dose should be received at 4 to 6 years of age. Booster vaccinations against tetanus and diphtheria should be received every 10 years thereafter. See below for details of schedule.

### Basics of Diphtheria, Tetanus, and Pertussis Immunization and Tetanus Prophylaxis

*Immunization*

1. *Vaccine Types:* The standard vaccine for the first three vaccinations during infancy is DTP, which is a preparation of diphtheria and tetanus toxoids combined with inactivated pertussis bacilli. A combined DTP-HbOC vaccine (TETRAMUNE®) has recently been licensed for single-injection vaccination of children against diphtheria, tetanus, pertussis, and *Haemophilus influenzae* type b (Hib). DTaP, in which the pertussis portion of the vaccine is acellular, has fewer side effects and is the vaccine of choice for the fourth and fifth vaccinations. The efficacy of DTaP in infants is unknown, and DTaP should not be used for the first three vaccinations. If DTaP is unavailable, DTP may be used for all five vaccinations. DT and Td contain only the diphtheria and tetanus toxoids, with Td containing fewer flocculating units of diphtheria toxoid dose per dose than DT. If a child under 7 years of age has a contraindication to pertussis vaccine, DT should replace DTP or DTaP in the immunization schedule. Only Td should be used to immunize children 7 years of age and older.

2. *Schedule*: ACIP currently recommends routine immunization with DTP at 2, 4, and 6 months of age. The first vaccination may be given as early as 6 weeks of age, and the

first three vaccinations may be given a minimum of 4 weeks apart. The fourth vaccination (with DTaP or DTP) is recommended at 15 months of age. (AAP has recommended this dose at 15-18 months of age). If DTP is used and at least 6 months have passed since the third vaccination, the fourth vaccination may be given as early as 12 months of age. DTaP is not currently recommended for use at less than 15 months of age. The fifth vaccination with DTaP or DTP should be given at 4 to 6 years of age. The fifth vaccination is not necessary if the fourth vaccination was given at 4 years of age or older.

For a partially immunized child, the immunization schedule should continue without repetition to complete the primary series. If a nonimmunized child is 7 years of age or older, three doses of Td should be given. The second dose should be given 4 to 8 weeks after the first dose. The third dose should be given 6 to 12 months after the second dose.

Booster immunizations with diphtheria and tetanus toxoid in the form of Td should be given every 10 years; for children immunized according to the recommended schedule, the first booster will be needed at 14 to 16 years of age.

3. *Dosage and Administration*: The recommended dosage of DTP, DTaP, DTP-HbOC, DT, Td, and the single-antigen absorbed preparations is 0.5 mL, given intramuscularly. In infants less than 12 months of age, the preferred site of administration is the anterolateral thigh. The thigh muscle should be bunched, using the free hand, and the needle (22-25 gauge, $7/8$ to 1 inch in length) directed inferiorly at an angle to reach the muscle but avoid contact with neurovascular structures or bone. In toddlers and older children, the vaccination may be given in the deltoid (if muscle mass appears adequate), using a 22-25 gauge needle that is $5/8$ to $1 1/4$ inches in length. DTP and DTaP may be given simultaneously with other childhood vaccinations. It is preferable to avoid giving other vaccinations in the same limb with DTP or DTaP.

The Food and Drug Administration has approved reconstituting lyophilized PRP-T *Haemophilus Influenzae* type b vaccine with DTP vaccine produced by Connaught Laboratories. These are currently the only two vaccines licensed to be mixed by the person administering the vaccine and given in the same syringe.

4. *Precautions:* See Table ii-4 for a listing of appropriate and inappropriate contraindications and precautions for giving childhood immunizations. Table 12-1 lists appropriate and inappropriate contraindications specific to DTP/DTaP vaccination.

5. *Adverse Reactions:* Local side effects (redness, swelling, or pain) and mild systemic reactions (fever >38°C/100.4°F, drowsiness, fretfulness, vomiting, or anorexia) are fairly common. These side effects occur somewhat less frequently with the use of the acellular DTaP vaccine than with the DTP vaccine. The following moderate-to-severe systemic events have rarely occurred after DTP and DTaP vaccination:

- Severe allergic hypersensitivity.

- Fever ≥40.5°C (104.9°F) within 48 hours.

- Collapse or shocklike state (hypotonic-hyporesponsive episode) within 48 hours.

- Persistent, inconsolable crying for 3 hours or more, or an unusual, high-pitched cry within 48 hours.

More severe neurologic events, such as convulsions and encephalopathy, have also been rarely reported. It is anticipated, but not proven, that moderate and severe side effects will also be less common with DTaP use.

By law, the following adverse events after DTP vaccination must be reported to the Vaccine Adverse Event Reporting System (VAERS): anaphylaxis or anaphylactic shock within 24 hours; encephalopathy or encephalitis within 7 days; shock-collapse or hypotonic-hyporesponsive collapse within 7 days; residual seizure disorder (fever less than 102°F, first seizure within 3 days and two seizures within 1 year); any acute complication or sequela (including death) of the preceding (without time limit); and events described in the manufacturer's package insert as contraindications to additional doses of vaccine. Providers are encouraged to report adverse reactions of all kinds, particularly if serious or unusual, to VAERS. VAERS forms and instructions are available in the *FDA Drug Bulletin* (Food and Drug Administration) and the *Physicians' Drug Reference*, or by calling the 24-hour VAERS information recording at 1-800 822-7967.

Acetaminophen, given in a dose of 15 mg/kg at the time of DTP or DTaP vaccination and 4 hours later, may help prevent or relieve minor side effects (e.g., fever, pain) of the vaccine.

6. *Patient Education:* Effective April 15, 1992, as mandated by the National Childhood Vaccine Injury Act, every patient who receives a DTP immunization must receive written information about the nature of the diseases immunized against; manifestations of adverse reactions; precautionary measures that should be taken to reduce the risk for major adverse reactions; contraindications to, and the basis for delay of, administration of the vaccine; and notice of the availability of the National Vaccine Injury Compensation Program. The U.S. Department of Health and Human Services has developed a pamphlet for this purpose (see Family Resources). Clinicians may choose to use other patient educational materials, as long as they provide the information required by the National Childhood Vaccine Injury Act. For additional information about this requirement, contact the Training Coordinator, National Immunization Program, Centers for Disease Control and Prevention; (404) 639-8226.

7. *Vaccine Storage and Handling:* Vaccine should be stored at 2° to 8°C (36° to 46°F), but not frozen. Vaccine that has been frozen should not be used. Handle all vaccine preparations according to manufacturers' instructions.

**Table 12-1. Contraindications and Precautions for DTP/DTaP Vaccination**

| True Contraindications and Precautions | NOT Contraindiactions (vaccine may be given) |
|---|---|
| Encephalopathy within 7 days of administration of previous dose of DTP/DTaP | Temperature <40.5°C (104.9°F) following a previous dose of DTP/DTaP |
| *Fever ≥40.5°C (104.9°F) within 48 hours after vaccination with a previous dose of DTP/DTaP | Family history of convulsions** |
| *Collapse or shock-like state (hypotonic-hyporesponsive episode) within 48 hours of receiving a previous dose of DTP/DTaP | Family history of sudden infant death syndrome |
|  | Family history of an adverse event following DTP administration |
| *Seizures within 3 days of receiving a previous dose of DTP/DTaP |  |
| *Persistent, inconsolable crying lasting ≥3 hours within 48 hours of receiving a previous dose of DTP/DTaP |  |

*Precautions, although not contraindications, should be carefully reviewed. The benefits and risks of administering a specific vaccine to an individual under the circumstances should be considered. If the risks are believed to outweigh the benefits, the immunization should be withheld; if the benefits are believed to outweigh the risks (for example, during an outbreak or foreign travel), it should be given. Whether and when to administer DTP/DTaP to children with proven or suspected underlying neurologic disorders should be decided on an individual basis. Children in the first year of life with a neurologic disorder that prevents the use of the pertussis vaccine also should not receive diphtheria or tetanus vaccine. After the first birthday, the child may receive DT vaccine if the contraindication to pertussis vaccine persists.

**Acetaminophen (15 mg/kg per dose) given prior to administering DTP or DTaP and thereafter every 4 hours for 24 hours should be considered for children with a personal or a family history of convulsions.

Adapted from: National Vaccine Advisory Committee. *Standards for Pediatric Immunization Practices.* Atlanta, GA: Centers for Disease Control and Prevention; 1993.

## Tetanus Prophylaxis

1. *Indications:* Patients who may have been exposed to tetanus because of wounds may need immediate passive immunization with tetanus immune globulin (TIG) or active immunization with tetanus toxoid, or both. See Table 51-1 for guidelines on passive and active immunization according to the nature of the wound and the patient's immunization status.

2. *Dosage and Administration:* The recommended dosage of TIG is 250 units. This should be given intramuscularly, in a different site and with a different syringe than used for concurrent DTP, DTaP, or Td immunization. If active immunization is not completed at the time of wound management, it should be completed subsequently according to the usual schedule.

3. *Adverse Reactions:* The side effects of TIG are relatively minor (site soreness and mild temperature elevation), but a few cases of more serious side effects (anaphylaxis, angioneurotic edema, and nephrotic syndrome) have been reported.

## Family Resources

*Childhood Vaccines: What They Are and Why Your Child Needs Them.* American Academy of Family Physicians, 8880 Ward Parkway, Kansas City, MO 64114-2797; 1-800 944-0000.

*Diphtheria, Tetanus, and Pertussis: What You Need To Know.* U.S. Dept. of Health and Human Services. Available from state and local health departments; American Academy of Family Physicians, 8880 Ward Parkway, Kansas City, MO 64114-2797; 1-800 944-0000; or American Academy of Pediatrics, Division of Publications, PO Box 927, Elk Grove Village, IL 60009-0927; 1-800 433-9016.

*DTP Vaccine Info Sheet* ; *Protecting Your Child Against Diphtheria, Tetanus, and Pertussis*; *Immunization Protects Children.* American Academy of Pediatrics, Division of Publications, 141 Northwest Point Blvd., PO Box 927, Elk Grove Village, IL 60009-0927; 1-800 433-9016.

*Parents Guide to Childhood Immunization.* U.S. Dept. of Health and Human Services. Copies available from state and local health departments.

## Selected References

Advisory Committee on Immunization Practices (ACIP). General recommendations on immunization. *MMWR*. In press.

Advisory Committee on Immunization Practices (ACIP). Diphtheria, tetanus, and pertussis: guidelines for vaccine prophylaxis and other preventive measures. *MMWR*. 1985;34:405-426.

Advisory Committee on Immunization Practices (ACIP). Diphtheria, tetanus, and pertussis: recommendations for vaccine use and other preventive measures. *MMWR*. 1991;40(RR-10):1-28.

Advisory Committee on Immunization Practices (ACIP). New recommended schedule for active immunization of normal infants and children. *MMWR*. 1986;35:577-579.

Advisory Committee on Immunization Practices (ACIP). Pertussis vaccination: acellular pertussis vaccine for reinforcing and booster use—supplementary ACIP statement. *MMWR*. 1992;41(RR-1):1-10.

Advisory Committee on Immunization Practices (ACIP). Pertussis immunizations; family history of convulsions and use of antipyretics—supplementary ACIP statement. *MMWR*. 1987;36:281-282.

American Academy of Family Physicians, Commission on Public Health and Scientific Affairs. *Age Charts for Periodic Health Examination*. Kansas City, Mo: American Academy of Family Physicians; 1993.

American Academy of Pediatrics, Committee on Infectious Diseases. Acellular pertussis vaccine: Recommendations for use as the fourth and fifth doses. *Pediatrics*. 1992;90:121-123.

American Academy of Pediatrics, Committee on Infectious Diseases. Haemophilus influenzae type b conjugate vaccines: Recommendations for immunization with recently and previously licensed vaccines. *AAP News*. 1993;9:17-19.

American Academy of Pediatrics, Committee on Infectious Disease. *1991 Report*. Elk Grove Village, Ill: American Academy of Pediatrics; 1991.

Canadian Task Force on the Periodic Health Examination. The periodic health examination. *Can Med Assoc J*. 1979;121:1193-1254.

Centers for Disease Control and Prevention. FDA approval of use of a new Haemophilus b conjugate vaccine and a combined diphtheria-tetanus-pertussis and Haemophilus b conjugate vaccine for infants and children. *MMWR*. 1993;42:296-298.

Centers for Disease Control. Summary of notifiable diseases, United States, 1989. *MMWR*. 1990; 38:51-59.

Centers for Disease Control. Tetanus surveillance—United States, 1989-1990. *MMWR*. 1992;41:1-9.

Centers for Disease Control. Vaccine Adverse Event Reporting System—United States. *MMWR*. 1990;39:730-733.

Edwards KM, Karzon DT. Pertussis Vaccines. *Pediatr Clin North Am*. 1990;37:549-563.

Farizo KM, Cochi SL, Zell ER, Brink EW, Wassilak SG, Patriarca PA. Epidemiological features of pertussis in the United States, 1980-89. *Clin Infect Dis*. 1992;14:708-719.

McAuliffe JSM, Wadland WC. Pertussis vaccination. *Am Fam Physician*. 1988;37(3):231-235.

National Vaccine Advisory Committee. *Standards for Pediatric Immunization Practices*. Atlanta, Ga: Centers for Disease Control and Prevention, 1993.

U.S. Preventive Services Task Force. Childhood immunizations. In: *Guide to Clinical Preventive Services*. Baltimore, Md: Williams and Wilkins; 1989:chap 56.

# Children/Adolescents — IMMUNIZATION/PROPHYLAXIS

## 13. Haemophilus influenzae Type b

*Haemophilus influenzae* type b (Hib) is one of the leading causes of invasive bacterial disease in children under 5 years of age, and it is the leading cause of meningitis in this age group. Even with the use of antibiotics, the mortality rate from meningitis is approximately 5%. Among survivors, 20% to 30% suffer permanent neurologic sequelae. The peak incidence of Hib infection occurs between 6 and 12 months of age, and 75% of all illness occurs in children younger than 24 months of age. African Americans, Hispanics, and Native Americans are at increased risk for infection. Other risk factors include attendance at day-care centers, exposure to a family member of elementary school age, asplenia, sickle cell disease, and antibody-deficiency syndromes. Hib conjugate vaccines given as a primary series in infancy have high efficacy (in some studies over 90%) in preventing disease; recent studies have shown a significant decline in invasive disease since the introduction of this vaccination. The efficacy of Hib vaccination in older children with chronic conditions associated with increased risk of Hib disease is unknown. Studies suggest, however, good immunogenicity in patients with sickle cell disease, leukemia, splenectomy, and HIV infection.

Rifampin chemoprophylaxis eradicates Hib carriage in 95% or more of contacts of primary cases, and it reduces the risk of secondary invasive disease in exposed household contacts. The efficacy of rifampin chemoprophylaxis in day-care settings is not well defined.

**Recommendations of Major Authorities**

*Immunization*

- **Advisory Committee on Immunization Practices, American Academy of Family Physicians, American Academy of Pediatrics,** and **U.S. Preventive Services Task Force**— All children should receive a primary series of one of the conjugate vaccines licensed for infant use beginning at 2 months of age. See below for details of schedule.

*Prophylaxis*

- **Advisory Committee on Immunization Practices** and **American Academy of Pediatrics**— Rifampin prophylaxis should be given to all household contacts of persons with invasive disease, irrespective of age, in households with at least one contact younger than 48 months of age. A contact is defined as an individual residing with the index patient or a nonresident who spent 4 or more hours with the index patient for at least 5 of the 7 days preceding the day of hospital admission of the index patient. Prophylaxis is not necessary if all members of the household are fully immunized. Immunization, in this case, is defined as at least one dose of conjugate vaccine at 15 months of age or older, or two doses at 12 to 14 months, or two or more doses when younger than 12 months of age with a booster dose at 12 months of age or older. All members of a household with a child younger than 12 months of age (e.g., a child who has not yet received the booster dose) should receive rifampin prophylaxis. Members of households with a fully vaccinated immunocompromised child should receive rifampin because it is possible that the vaccination may have been ineffective. Rifampin prophylaxis should be employed in day-care homes resembling

# Ch. 13. Hib      Children/Adolescents — IMMUNIZATION/PROPHYLAXIS

households, such as those with children less than 2 years of age in which contact is 25 hours per week or more. Prophylaxis is unnecessary in day-care facilities where all contacts are older than 2 years of age.

## Basics of *Haemophilus influenzae* Type b Immunization and Prophylaxis

### *Immunization*

1. *Vaccine Types:* There are currently four types of conjugate vaccines licensed for use in the United States: HbOC (HibTITER® made by Lederle-Praxis), PRP-OMP (Pedvax HIB® made by Merck Sharp & Dohme), PRP-D (ProHIBIT® made by Connaught Laboratories), and PRP-T (ActHIB® distributed by Connaught Laboratories). A combined DTP and Hib (HbOC) vaccine (TETRAMUNE® distributed by Lederle-Praxis) was recently licensed for use in children aged 2 months to 5 years when indications for vaccination with DTP vaccine and Hib conjugate vaccine coincide. PRP-D is not licensed for use in primary immunization of children less than 15 months of age; it may, however, be used as a booster beginning at 12 months of age. Ideally, the same type of conjugate vaccine should be given throughout the entire primary vaccination series. To facilitate this, the vaccine type should be noted on the parent-held record and in the patient chart. If the type of vaccine used in previous immunizations is not known, the provider should ensure that the 2- to 6-month-old patient receives a total of at least three doses of conjugate vaccine. It is acceptable to use any type of conjugate Hib vaccine for booster doses irrespective of the type used for the primary series.

2. *Schedule:* If HbOC or PRP-T is used, a primary series should be given to previously unvaccinated infants at 2, 4, and 6 months of age. If PRP-OMP is used, a primary series of 2 vaccinations at 2 and 4 months of age is recommended. The first vaccination in a primary series may be given as early at 6 weeks of age. For children who start the primary series at 4-6 months of age or who are more than 1 month behind, an accelerated schedule can be used with intervals of at least 1 month between primary vaccinations. Children who start the primary series at 7-11 months of age should receive a primary series of 2 doses of HbOC, PRP-T, or PRP-OMP. Children beginning the primary series at 12-14 months of age should receive a primary series of 1 dose of HbOC, PRP-T, or PRP-OMP. Combined DTP-HbOC vaccine (TETRAMUNE®) should be given in compliance with recommendations for use of both HbOC and DTP.

    According to ACIP, a booster dose of any conjugate Hib vaccine should be given at 12-15 months of age and preferably at least 2 months after the previous dose, although an interval of 1 month is acceptable if necessary.

    Children beginning the Hib vaccine series at 15-59 months of age should receive one dose only of any licensed conjugate Hib vaccine. In general, Hib vaccine should not be given after the fifth birthday, except in certain special circumstances (such as asplenia or sickle cell anemia) that may make a child particularly vulnerable to Hib infection.

3. *Dosage and Administration:* The recommended dosage of Hib vaccines (including DTP-HbOC) is 0.5 mL, given intramuscularly. In infants less than 12 months of age, the

preferred site is the anterolateral thigh (although, if necessary, the deltoid also may be used). The thigh muscle should be bunched, using the free hand, and the needle (22-25 gauge, 7/8 to 1 inch in length) directed inferiorly at an angle to reach the muscle but avoid contact with neurovascular structures or bone. In toddlers and older children, the vaccination may be given in the deltoid (if muscle mass appears adequate), using a 22-25 gauge needle that is 5/8 to 1 1/4 inches in length. Hib vaccines may be given simultaneously with other childhood vaccinations at different sites.

The Food and Drug Administration has approved reconstituting lyophilized PRP-T *Haemophilus Influenzae* type b vaccine with DTP vaccine produced by Connaught Laboratories. These are currently the only two vaccines licensed to be mixed by the person administering the vaccine and given in the same syringe.

4. *Precautions:* There are no known specific contraindications to the Hib vaccination. See Table ii-4 for a listing of appropriate and inappropriate contraindications and precautions for giving childhood immunizations.

5. *Adverse Reactions:* The side effects from Hib vaccination are minor and limited to mild fever and redness and/or swelling at the injection site. Providers are encouraged to report adverse reactions of all kinds, particularly if serious or unusual, to the Vaccine Adverse Event Reporting System (VAERS). VAERS forms and instructions are available in the *FDA Drug Bulletin* (Food and Drug Administration) and the *Physicians' Drug Reference*, or by calling the 24-hour VAERS information recording at 1-800-822-7967.

6. *Patient Education:* Patient information statements about Hib vaccination developed by the Centers for Disease Control and Prevention (see Family Resources below) must be employed in settings where federally-purchased vaccines are used. Their use in other settings is encouraged.

7. *Vaccine Storage and Handling:* Vaccine should be stored at 2° to 8°C (36° to 46°F), but not frozen. Vaccine that has been frozen should not be used. Handle all vaccine preparations according to manufacturers' instructions.

## *Prophylaxis*

1. *Schedule:* Rifampin chemoprophylaxis should be instituted as soon as possible, since most cases of secondary disease occur within the first week after occurrence of the index case. Chemoprophylaxis is of questionable efficacy 2 weeks after occurrence of the index case.

2. *Dosage and Administration:* The recommended dosage of rifampin for chemoprophylaxis is 20 mg/kg (maximum of 600 mg), given orally once daily for 4 days. The recommended dosage for infants younger than 1 month is not established, although some experts recommend reducing the dosage to 10 mg/kg. For children unable to swallow capsules, rifampin powder may be mixed with several teaspoons of applesauce or a suspension may be prepared by a pharmacist.

3. *Precautions:* Rifampin should not be used by pregnant women.

4. *Adverse Reactions:* Side effects of rifampin chemoprophylaxis include orange discoloration of urine and other bodily fluids, discoloration of soft contact lenses, decreased effectiveness of oral contraceptives, nausea, vomiting, diarrhea, headache, and dizziness.

## Family Resources

*Childhood Vaccines: What They Are and Why Your Child Needs Them.* American Academy of Family Physicians, 8880 Ward Parkway, Kansas City, MO 64114-2797; 1-800 944-0000.

*Immunization Protects Children.* American Academy of Pediatrics, PO Box 927, Elk Grove Village, IL 60009-0927; 1-800 433-9016.

*Important Information About* Haemophilus Influenzae *Type b Disease and* Haemophilus b *Conjugate Vaccine*; *Parents Guide to Childhood Immunization.* Centers for Disease Control and Prevention. Available from state and local health departments.

## Selected References

American Academy of Family Physicians, Commission on Public Health and Scientific Affairs. AAFP recommendations: new *Haemophilus influenzae* type b immunization schedule. *Am Fam Physician.* 1991;43(4):1473-1474.

Adams WG, Deaver KA, Cochi, et al. Decline of childhood *Haemophilus influenzae* type b (Hib) disease in the Hib vaccine era. *JAMA.* 1993;269:221-226.

Advisory Committee on Immunization Practices (ACIP). General recommendations on immunization. *MMWR.* In press.

Advisory Committee on Immunization Practices (ACIP). *Haemophilus* b conjugate vaccines for prevention of *Haemophilus influenzae* disease among infants and children two months of age and older. *MMWR.* 1991; 40(RR-1):1-7.

Advisory Committee on Immunization Practices (ACIP). Update: prevention of *Haemophilus influenzae* type b disease. *MMWR.* 1986;35:170-174, 179-180.

American Academy of Pediatrics, Committee on Infectious Diseases. *Haemophilus influenzae* type b conjugate vaccines: recommendations for immunization of infants and children 2 months of age and older: update. *Pediatrics.* 1991;88:169-172.

American Academy of Pediatrics, Committee on Infectious Diseases. *Haemophilus influenzae* type b conjugate vaccines: recommendations for immunization with recently and previously licensed vaccines. *AAP News.* 1993;9:17-19.

American Academy of Pediatrics, Committee on Infectious Diseases. *1991 Report.* Elk Grove Village, Ill: American Academy of Pediatrics; 1991.

Centers for Disease Control and Prevention. FDA approval of use of a new *Haemophilus* b conjugate vaccine and a combined diphtheria-tetanus-pertussis and *Haemophilus* b conjugate vaccine for infants and children. *MMWR.* 1993;42:296-298.

Pomeroy SL, Holmes SJ, Dodge PR, Feigin RD. Seizures and other neurologic sequelae of bacterial meningitis in children. *N Engl J Med.* 1990;323:1651-1657.

Wilfert CM. Epidemiology of *Haemophilus influenzae* type b infections. *Pediatrics.* 1990;85(suppl 4):631-635.

Children/Adolescents — IMMUNIZATION/PROPHYLAXIS

# 14. Hepatitis B

Infection with the hepatitis B virus (HBV) is a major, growing health problem in the United States. The reported incidence of acute HBV infection increased by 37% from 1979 to 1989, and an estimated 250,000 to 300,000 new infections occurred annually during that period. Approximately 4000 to 5000 people die every year from chronic liver disease due to HBV infection. People with chronic infection are also at increased risk of death from hepatocellular cancer. See Table 14-1 for a list of groups at high risk for HBV infection.

In the United States, most HBV infections are acquired in adolescence or adulthood, largely as a result of injection drug use, sexual contact, or occupational or household exposure. Certain populations, including Alaska Natives, Pacific Islanders, and immigrants from HBV-endemic areas (particularly East Asia and Africa), have high rates of infection. Efforts to control HBV infection through vaccination and education of high-risk individuals, testing of pregnant women, and vaccination of the offspring of carrier women have been only partially successful. Children of HBV-infected mothers are at high risk for developing infection during the perinatal period and the first 5 years of life. Perinatal infection leads to a 90% risk of chronic infection and a 25% risk of death from chronic liver disease as an adult.

**Table 14-1. Groups at High Risk for Hepatitis B Infections**

| |
|---|
| Health care workers and others at occupational risk |
| Clients and staff of institutions for the developmentally disabled—including nonresidential day-care programs if attended by known HBV carriers |
| Hemophiliacs and other recipients of certain blood products |
| Hemodialysis patients |
| Household contacts and sex partners of HBsAg-positive persons |
| Household contacts of adoptees from HBV-endemic, high-risk countries who are HBsAg-positive |
| International travelers who spend more than 6 months in areas with high HBV infection rates and have close contact with the local population; also short-term travelers who have contact with blood, or sexual contact with residents in high- or intermediate-risk areas |
| Injection drug users |
| Sexually active homosexual or bisexual males |
| Heterosexual individuals who have had more than one sex partner in the previous 6 months and/or those with a recent episode of a sexually transmitted disease |
| Inmates of long-term correctional institutions |

Adapted from: Advisory Committee on Immunization Practices (ACIP). Hepatitis B virus: a comprehensive strategy for eliminating transmission in the United States through universal childhood vaccination. *MMWR*. 1991;40 (RR-13):1-25.

Vaccination is highly effective (up to 95%) in preventing HBV infection in susceptible patients. Due to its relatively recent development, HBV vaccine is known to be effective for only 10 years, but much longer lasting immunity is likely. The combination of vaccination with the use of HBV immune globulin (HBIG) is 80% to 95% effective at preventing perinatal HBV infection after acute exposure.

See chapter 47 for information on hepatitis immunization and prophylaxis for adults.

## Recommendations of Major Authorities

### Immunization

- **Advisory Committee on Immunization Practices (ACIP)**, **American Academy of Family Physicians (AAFP)**, and **American Academy of Pediatrics(AAP)**—All children should receive a complete series of hepatitis B immunizations during the first 18 months of life. Infants born to HBsAg-positive mothers should begin receiving these immunizations at birth. Immunization of adolescents should be carried out in areas with increased rates of injection drug use, teenage pregnancy, or sexually transmitted diseases. All older children and adolescents at high risk for HBV infection should receive a complete series of immunizations. See Table 14-1 for a listing of those at high risk. In addition to recommending HBV immunization for high-risk adolescents, the **American Medical Association** encourages widespread immunization for all adolescents.

- **Canadian Task Force on the Periodic Health Examination** and **U.S. Preventive Services Task Force**—Infants born to HBsAg-positive mothers, individuals exposed to HBV, and individuals at high risk for HBV infection should receive immunization. See Table 14-1 for a listing of those at high risk. This recommendation is under review by both groups.

### Prophylaxis

- **All major authorities**—HBIG should be used for prophylaxis of nonimmunized or inadequately immunized individuals exposed to active HBV infection. Prophylactic treatment may be needed in the following situations: percutaneous or mucosal exposure to HBsAg-positive blood, sexual exposure to an HBsAg-positive person, perinatal exposure of an infant to an HBsAg-positive mother, or household exposure of an infant less than 12 months of age to a primary care-giver who has acute HBV infection.

## Basics of Hepatitis B Immunization and Prophylaxis

### Immunization

1. *Vaccine Types:* There are currently two licensed HBV vaccines produced in the United States: Engerix-B® and Recombivax HB® (available in three preparations for different age groups). Both are produced by recombinant DNA technology. These vaccines may be used interchangeably at any point in the vaccination schedule, although the dosage may vary. A plasma-derived vaccine, (Heptavax®) is also licensed, but it is no longer produced in the United States.

2. *Schedule:* According to ACIP, the schedule for administering HBV vaccine to infants of HBsAg-negative mothers should be flexible and integrated into the routine childhood immunization schedule. Two alternative schedules are recommended: at birth (before

hospital discharge), 1 to 2 months, and 6 to 18 months of age (AAP prefers this schedule); or at 1 to 2 months, 4 months, and 6 to 18 months of age. For children not immunized according to these schedules, three immunizations should be given by 18 months of age, with a minimum of 1 month between the first two doses, and a minimum of 2 (but preferably 4) months between the second and third doses. Because of possible decreased seroconversion rates, premature infants of HBsAg-negative mothers with birth weights less than 2000 g should receive the first dose at the time of hospital discharge if the infant then weighs at least 2000 g, or when the routine childhood immunizations are initiated (at 2 months of age).

For infants (even if premature) born to HBsAg-positive mothers, immunization should be initiated within 12 hours of birth. Subsequent doses should be received at 1 and 6 months after the first dose. A four-dose schedule (birth, 1, 2, and 12 months) for post-exposure immunization has been licensed for Engerix-B®. This schedule may increase slightly the likelihood of development of immunity, but it has not been demonstrated to offer clinical advantage over the three-dose regimens. For information on immunization for post-exposure prophylaxis, see Table 47-1.

High-risk children and adolescents not immunized as infants should receive a series of three immunizations, with the second and third doses administered 1 and 6 months, respectively, after the first dose.

Long-term studies of healthy adults and children indicate that immunologic memory remains intact for at least 10 years, although antibody levels may become low or undetectable. Therefore, for children and adults whose immune status is normal, booster doses of vaccine are not recommended, and serologic testing to assess antibody levels is not necessary. The possible need for booster doses will be assessed as additional information becomes available.

3. *Dosage and Administration:* The recommended dosage of HBV vaccine varies according to the vaccine type and the age of the child (see Table 14-2). HBV vaccine should be administered as an intramuscular injection. In infants less than 12 months of age, the preferred site is the anterolateral thigh (although, if necessary, the deltoid also may be used). The thigh muscle should be bunched, using the free hand, and the needle (22-25 gauge, $7/8$ to 1 inch in length) directed inferiorly at an angle to reach the muscle but avoid contact with neurovascular structures or bone. In toddlers and older children, the vaccination may be given in the deltoid (if muscle mass appears adequate), using a 22-25 gauge needle that is $5/8$ to $1 1/4$ inches in length. HBV vaccines may be given simultaneously with other childhood vaccinations at different sites.

4. *Precautions:* History of an anaphylactic reaction to common baker's yeast is a contraindication to HBV vaccination. The only other contraindication to HBV vaccination is known serious adverse reaction to the vaccine. Pregnancy and lactation are not contraindications.

**Table 14-2. Recommended Dosages for Children of Currently Licensed Recombinant Hepatitis B Vaccines**

| | Vaccines | | | |
|---|---|---|---|---|
| | Recombivax HB®* | | Engerix-B® | |
| Group | µg | mL | µg | mL |
| Infants of HBsAg-negative mothers and children <11 years of age | 2.5 | 0.25 | 10 | 0.5 |
| Infants of HBsAg-positive mothers; prevention of perinatal infection | 5 | 0.5 | 10 | 0.5 |
| Children and adolescents 11-19 years of age | 5 | 0.5 | 20 | 1.0 |
| Dialysis patients and other immunocompromised individuals | 40 | 1.0** | 40 | 2.0*** |

*Licensure is expected shortly for a child formulation of Recombivax HB®. This formulation will have a lower concentration (5 µg/mL), allowing a dosage of 0.5 mL for infants of HBsAg-negative mothers and children less than age 11.

**Special formulation

***Two 1.0-mL doses administered at one site, in a four-dose schedule at birth, 1, 2, and 6 months.

Adapted from: Advisory Committee on Immunization Practices (ACIP). Hepatitis B virus: a comprehensive strategy for eliminating transmission in the United States through universal childhood vaccination. *MMWR.* 1991;40(RR-13):1-25.

5. *Adverse Reactions:* The side effects of HBV vaccination are relatively minor in children. These include pain at the injection site (3% to 29%) and temperature greater than 38°C (100.4°F) (0.5% in infants and 1% to 6% in other children). Based on surveillance for adverse reactions in adults in the United States, a possible association has been shown between Guillain-Barré syndrome (GBS) and receipt of plasma-derived HBV vaccine; however, available data do not indicate an association between receipt of recombinant HBV vaccine and GBS. Although systematic surveillance for adverse events following administration of recombinant HBV vaccine to infants and children has been limited, no association has been found between vaccination and the occurrence of severe adverse events, including seizures and GBS. Providers are encouraged to report adverse reactions of all kinds, particularly if serious or unusual, to the Vaccine Adverse Event Reporting System (VAERS). VAERS forms and instructions are available in the *FDA Drug Bulletin* (Food and Drug Administration) and the *Physicians' Drug Reference,* or by calling the 24-hour VAERS information recording at 1-800 822-7967.

6. *Patient Education:* Patient information statements about HBV vaccination developed by the Centers for Disease Control and Prevention (see Family Resources below) must be employed in settings where federally purchased vaccines are used. Their use in other settings is encouraged.

**Ch. 14. HBV**          Children/Adolescents — IMMUNIZATION/PROPHYLAXIS

7. *Vaccine Storage and Handling:* Vaccine should be stored at 2° to 8°C (36° to 46°F), but not frozen, which would destroy the potency of the vaccine. Vaccine that has been frozen should not be used. Handle all vaccine preparations according to manufacturers' instructions.

## Postexposure Prophylaxis

1. *Schedule:* See Table 14-3 for the recommended schedule of HBV immunoprophylaxis to prevent perinatal transmission. See Table 47-1 for the recommended schedule of HBV immunoprophylaxis for percutaneous and mucosal exposure in children and adults.

2. *Dosage and Administration:* The recommended dose of HBIG for infants 12 months of age or younger is 0.5 mL. The dose for children over 12 months of age is 0.06 mL/kg. HBIG should be administered as an intramuscular injection. The recommended site is the anterolateral thigh muscle for infants and the deltoid muscle for children and adolescents. HBIG may be given at the same time as HBV vaccine, but at a different site. The recommended dosage of HBV vaccine for perinatal exposure varies according to vaccine type. See Table 14-3.

3. *Precautions:* The only contraindication to HBIG injection is a history of hypersensitivity to HBIG.

4. *Adverse Reactions:* The main side effects of HBIG injection are pain and swelling at the injection site. Urticaria, angioedema, and very rarely, anaphylaxis can occur. HIV is not known to be transmitted by HBIG injection.

## Family Resources

*Childhood Vaccines: What They Are and Why Your Child Needs Them.* American Academy of Family Physicians, 8880 Ward Parkway, Kansas City, MO 64114-2797; 1-800 944-0000.

*Immunization Protects Children.* American Academy of Pediatrics, PO Box 927, Elk Grove Village, IL 60009-0927; 1-800 433-9016.

*Hepatitis B Virus Infection—From Mother to Child: A Cycle of Tragedy* (videotape); *Hepatitis B Prevention*; *Hepatitis Screening: What Does It Mean for You and Your Baby?* (videotape); *Important Information about Hepatitis B and Hepatitis B Vaccine*; *Why Does My Baby Need Hepatitis B Vaccine?* Centers for Disease Control and Prevention. Available from state and local health departments.

## Provider Resources

*Hepatitis B Vaccination for Infants: A "Universal" Message for Physicians* (audiotape). Centers for Disease Control and Prevention. Available from state and local health departments.

**Table 14-3. Recommended Schedule of Hepatitis B Immunoprophylaxis To Prevent Perinatal Transmission**

| Infant Born to Mother Known To Be HBsAg-Positive ||
|---|---|
| **Vaccine/HBIG Schedule** | **Age of Infant** |
| First HBV | Birth (within 12 hours) |
| HBIG | Birth (within 12 hours) |
| Second HBV | 1 month |
| Third HBV | 6 months* |
| **Infant Born to Mother Not Screened for HBsAg** ||
| **Vaccine/HBIG Schedule** | **Age of Infant** |
| First HBV | Birth (within 12 hours) |
| HBIG | If mother is found to be HBsAg-positive, administer a dose to infant as soon as possible, but not later than 1 week after birth |
| Second HBV | 1-2 months** |
| Third HBV | 6 months* |

*If the four-dose schedule (Engerix-B®) is used, the third dose is administered at 2 months of age and the fourth dose at 12-18 months of age.

**Infants of women who are HBsAg-negative may be vaccinated at 2 months of age.

Adapted from: Advisory Committee on Immunization Practices (ACIP). Hepatitis B virus: a comprehensive strategy for eliminating transmission in the United States through universal childhood vaccination. *MMWR.* 1991;40; 1-25. (RR-13)

## Selected References

Advisory Committee on Immunization Practices(ACIP). General recommendations on immunization. *MMWR.* In press.

Advisory Committee on Immunization Practices (ACIP). Hepatitis B virus: a comprehensive strategy for eliminating transmission in the United States through universal childhood vaccination. *MMWR.* 1991;40(RR-13):1-25.

Advisory Committee on Immunization Practices (ACIP). Protection against viral hepatitis. *MMWR.* 1990;39(RR-2):1-26.

American Academy of Family Physicians. *Recommendations for Hepatitis B Preexposure Vaccination and Postexposure Prophylaxis.* Kansas City, Mo: American Academy of Family Physicians; 1992.

American Academy of Pediatrics. Universal hepatitis B immunization. *AAP News.* February 1992:13-15, 22.

American Academy of Pediatrics, Committee on Infectious Diseases. *1991 Report.* Elk Grove Village, Ill: American Academy of Pediatrics; 1991.

Canadian Task Force on the Periodic Health Examination. The periodic health examination: 2. 1984 update. *Can Med Assoc J.* 1984;130:1278-1285.

National Vaccine Advisory Committee. *Standards for Pediatric Immunization Practices.* Atlanta, Ga: Centers for Disease Control and Prevention; 1993.

US Preventive Services Task Force. Adult immunizations. In: *Guide to Clinical Preventive Services*. Baltimore, Md: Williams & Wilkins; 1989:chap 57.

# Children/Adolescents — IMMUNIZATION/PROPHYLAXIS

## 15. Measles, Mumps, and Rubella

Measles (rubeola) remains a significant health problem in the United States. In the period 1989 to 1990, the incidence of measles increased sharply, reaching a peak in 1990 of over 27,000 cases. In 1992, after concerted national efforts to increase immunization, the incidence of measles had decreased to 2200 cases. Recent outbreaks have primarily affected two populations: nonvaccinated preschool-age children and previously vaccinated school-age children. Outbreaks affecting the latter are due to vaccine failure, waning immunity with age, and erroneous documentation of previous vaccination. Death, usually caused by pneumonia or encephalitis, occurs in 1 to 2 per 1000 reported cases.

The United States has also experienced a trend of increased incidence of mumps infection. Since 1990, 4000 to 5000 cases have been reported annually. Since vaccine licensure in 1967, there has been a shift in the peak incidence rate from the 5- to 9-year-old age group to the over 15-year-old age group. Orchitis occurs in up to 38% of cases in postpubertal males. Five in every 1000 reported cases are complicated by encephalitis.

In 1990, there were approximately 1100 reported cases of rubella. Use of rubella vaccine has led to a significant decrease in the overall incidence of rubella. There has, however, been little impact on rubella immunity in postpubertal women, 6% to 11% of whom are seronegative. Congenital rubella syndrome (CRS) develops in an estimated 85% of infants born to women acquiring rubella during the first trimester. There were 11 reported cases of CRS in 1991. The most frequently occurring clinical manifestations of CRS are deafness, low birth weight, hepatomegaly, splenomegaly, ocular lesions, psychomotor retardation, congenital heart disease, and petechiae. Half of noncongenital rubella infections are subclinical, with occasional serious complications such as thrombocytopenia (1 per 3000 cases) and encephalitis (1 per 6000 cases).

See chapter 50 for information about rubella immunization of adults.

### Recommendations of Major Authorities

*Normal-Risk Children*

- All major authorities, including the **Advisory Committee on Immunization Practices (ACIP), American Academy of Family Physicians (AAFP), American Academy of Pediatrics (AAP), American Medical Association (AMA),** and **U.S. Preventive Services Task Force (USPSTF)**—A primary measles-mumps-rubella (MMR) immunization should be given at 12-15 months of age. A booster dose should also be given. ACIP, AAFP, and USPSTF recommend that this booster be given at 4-6 years of age, before school entry. AAP and AMA recommend that this booster preferably be given at 11-12 years of age, before entry to middle school or junior high school.

## High-Risk Children

- **ACIP** and **AAP**—In areas at risk for recurrent measles transmission, the first MMR should be given at 12 months of age. Both authorities use the following two criteria to define a high-risk area: a county with more than five cases among preschool-age children during each of the last 5 years; a county with a recent outbreak among nonimmunized preschool-age children. AAP uses a third criterion: cities with a large nonimmunized preschool population. ACIP uses a slightly different third criterion: counties with a large urban population. In order to control outbreaks of measles among preschool-age children, the first immunization (either as monovalent measles vaccine or MMR) may be given as early as 6 months of age. Children immunized before 12 months of age should be revaccinated at 12-15 months of age and upon school entry, according to local policy.

## Postexposure

- **ACIP** and **AAP**—Exposure to measles is not a contraindication to vaccination. If live measles vaccine is given within 72 hours of measles exposure, it may provide some protection. ACIP states that use of vaccine is preferable to the use of immunoglobulin (IG) for children more than 12 months of age. The use of IG within 6 days of exposure can prevent or modify measles in susceptible individuals. IG may be particularly indicated for susceptible household contacts of measles patients, particularly contacts younger than 1 year of age, pregnant women, or immunocompromised individuals.

## Basics of Measles, Mumps, and Rubella Immunization and Measles Prophylaxis

### Immunization

1. *Vaccine Types:* Measles, mumps, and rubella are live attenuated vaccines. They are available as single antigen preparations and as combination preparations: measles-rubella, mumps-rubella, and measles-mumps-rubella (MMR). Unless a specific antigen is contraindicated, MMR should be used for children and adults.

2. *Indications:* Children and adolescents are considered susceptible to measles unless there is documentation of clinician-diagnosed measles, serological evidence of measles immunity, or documentation of receipt of adequate immunization. Patient or parental reports of measles illness or measles immunization are not adequate documentation.

   Children and adolescents are considered susceptible to mumps unless there is documentation of clinician-diagnosed mumps or laboratory evidence of immunity, or documentation of immunization with live mumps vaccine after the first birthday. Children for whom the immunization status is uncertain should be vaccinated. Testing for susceptibility is not necessary before vaccination of adolescents.

   Children and adolescents are considered susceptible to rubella unless there is documentation of immunity by laboratory testing or immunization after the first birthday. Patient or parental reports or clinician diagnosis are not adequate evidence of immunity. See chapter 50 for more information about indications for rubella immunization in adults.

3. *Schedule:* See Recommendations of Major Authorities section above. The primary immunization should be given at 12-15 months of age. Some high-risk children may

benefit from receiving this immunization earlier. Children receiving MMR before their first birthday should be revaccinated at 12-15 months of age. Major authorities recommend that a booster immunization be given either at 4-6 years (before school entry) or 11-12 years (before middle school or junior high school entry). Doses of MMR or other measles-containing vaccines should be separated by at least one month.

MMR may be given simultaneously with other childhood immunizations.

Patients who have received high doses of a systemically administered corticosteroid (2 mg/kg or 20 mg per day of prednisone or equivalent) should not receive MMR immunization until at least 3 months after discontinuation of the corticosteroid.

Immune globulin-containing preparations, such as IG, HBIG, VZIG, HRIG and packed red blood cell, whole blood, or plasma may interfere with immune response to MMR vaccination. MMR should not be given from 2 weeks before to 3-11 months (depending on the immune globulin content of the preparation) after such preparations are given. Vaccination should be repeated after the window of immune globulin interference has expired, or antibody testing should be performed to determine immunity status. See Advisory Committee on Immunization Practices (*MMWR*, in press) for more detailed information regarding this issue.

4. *Dosage and Administration:* The recommended dosage of MMR and the single-antigen preparations for both children and adults is 0.5 mL. The injection should be given subcutaneously into the thigh in infants and the deltoid area in children and adults, using a $5/8$ to $3/4$ inch 23-25 gauge needle.

5. *Precautions:* See Table ii-4 for a listing of appropriate and inappropriate contraindications and precautions for giving childhood immunizations. See Table 15-1 for a listing of appropriate and inappropriate contraindications specific for MMR vaccination.

6. *Adverse Reactions:* The measles component may cause a transient rash in 5% of vaccinees. Fever greater than 39.4°C (103°F) develops in 5% to 15% of individuals susceptible to measles, beginning 5 to 12 days after immunization and usually lasting 1 to 2 days (up to 5 days). Because of the late onset of fever, acetaminophen prophylaxis may not be practical in preventing febrile seizures. The rubella component is associated with the development of a mild rash lasting 1 to 2 days and mild pain and stiffness in the joints 1 to 2 weeks after the immunization, usually lasting up to 3 days. The joint problem affects 1% of children, about 25% of adults, and up to 40% of women. Rarely, pain or stiffness can last for months or longer and can recur. Joint swelling (arthritis) lasting a few days to a week develops in 1% of children and 10% of adults. Rarely, this arthritis may last longer or recur. Damage to joints is very rare. Both the rubella and mumps components can cause swollen anterior cervical, posterior auricular, or mandibular lymph nodes 1 to 2 weeks after the immunization. This happens rarely with the mumps component but may affect 1 in 7 children receiving the rubella component. The development of encephalitis is temporally related to the receipt of MMR in about 1 per 1 million immunizations given.

By law, the following adverse events following MMR vaccination must be reported to the Vaccine Adverse Event Reporting System (VAERS): anaphylaxis or anaphylactic shock within 24 hours; encephalopathy or encephalitis within 15 days; residual seizure disorder (fever less than 102°F, first seizure within 3 days and two seizures within 1 year); any acute complication or sequela (including death) of the preceding (without time limit); and events described in the manufacturer's package insert as contraindications to additional doses of vaccine. Providers are encouraged to report adverse reactions of all kinds, particularly if serious or unusual, to VAERS. VAERS forms and instructions are available in the *FDA Drug Bulletin* (Food and Drug Administration) and the *Physicians' Drug Reference*, or by calling the 24-hour VAERS information recording at 1-800 822-7967.

7. *Patient Education:* Effective April 15, 1992, as mandated by the National Childhood Vaccine Injury Act, every patient who receives an MMR immunization must receive

Table 15-1. Contraindications and Precautions for MMR Vaccination

| **True Contraindications and Precautions** | **NOT Contraindications (vaccine may be given)** |
|---|---|
| Anaphylactic reactions to egg ingestion and to neomycin* | Tuberculosis or positive PPD |
|  | Simultaneous TB skin testing** |
| Pregnancy | |
|  | Breast feeding |
| Known altered immunodeficiency (hematologic and solid tumors, congenital immunodeficiency, and long term immunosuppressive therapy) | Pregnancy of mother of recipient |
|  | Immunodeficient family member or household contact |
| ***Recent IG administration (within 3-11 months) | |
|  | Infection with HIV |
|  | Nonanaphylactic reactions to eggs or neomycin |

*Persons with a history of anaphylactic reactions following egg ingestion should be vaccinated only with extreme caution. Protocols have been developed for vaccinating such persons and should be consulted (Herman et al., 1983; Greenberg and Birx, 1988; and Lavi et al., 1990)

**Measles vaccination may temporarily suppress tuberculin reactivity. If testing cannot be done the day of MMR vaccination, the test should be postponed for 4-6 weeks.

***Precautions, although not contraindications, should be carefully reviewed. The benefits and risks of administering a specific vaccine to an individual under the circumstances should be considered. If the risks are believed to outweigh the benefits, the immunization should be withheld; if the benefits are believed to outweigh the risks (for example, during an outbreak or foreign travel), it should be given. It is prudent on theoretical grounds to avoid vaccinating pregnant women. (See also Advisory Committee on Immunization Practices, in press.)

Adapted from: National Vaccine Advisory Committee. *Standards for Pediatric Immunization Practices*. Atlanta, GA: Centers for Disease Control and Prevention; 1993.

written information about the nature of the diseases immunized against; manifestations of adverse reactions; precautionary measures that should be taken to reduce the risk for major adverse reactions; contraindications to, and the basis for delay of, administration of the vaccine; and notice of the availability of the National Vaccine Injury Compensation Program. The U.S. Department of Health and Human Services has developed a pamphlet for this purpose (see Family Resources). Clinicians may choose to use other patient educational materials, as long as they provide the information required by the National Childhood Vaccine Injury Act. For additional information about this requirement, contact the Training Coordinator, National Immunization Program, Centers for Disease Control and Prevention; (404) 639-8226.

8. *Vaccine Storage and Handling:* Measles, mumps, rubella, and MMR vaccines must be shipped at less than 10°C (50°F) and stored at 2° to 8°C (35° to 46°F) or colder and be protected from light exposure before reconstitution. After reconstitution, vaccine must be refrigerated at 2° to 8°C (35° to 46°F), protected from the light, and discarded if not used within 8 hours. Reconstituted vaccine and the diluent should never be frozen. Handle all vaccine preparations according to manufacturers' instructions.

## Postexposure Prophylaxis (for Measles Only)

1. *Dosage and Administration:* The recommended dosage of IG for immunocompetent individuals is 0.25 mL/kg of body weight (maximum dose: 15 mL) given intramuscularly. The recommended dosage for immunocompromised patients is 0.5 mL/kg of body weight (maximum dose: 15 mL).

   Preferred sites for administration of IG are the anterolateral thigh and the deltoid muscle. If the gluteal region must be used, injection must be limited to the ventrogluteal site or the upper outer quadrant. Large volumes should be divided and given in different sites for patient comfort. Ordinarily no more than 5 mL should be administered in one site to an adult or large child; smaller amounts (1 to 3 mL) should be given to smaller children and infants.

2. *Precautions:* The use of IG is contraindicated in patients with selective IgA deficiency or severe thrombocytopenia or coagulation disorders that would preclude an intramuscular injection. It should be used with caution in patients with a history of past allergic reactions after injections of IG.

3. *Adverse Reactions:* Local pain and swelling (often mistaken for an allergic reaction) are the most common adverse effects of IG injection. Urticaria, angioedema, and (rarely) anaphylaxis may occur.

## Family Resources

*Childhood Vaccines: What They Are and Why Your Child Needs Them.* American Academy of Family Physicians, 8880 Ward Parkway, Kansas City, MO 64114-2797; 1-800 944-0000.

*Immunization Protects Children.* American Academy of Pediatrics, PO Box 927, Elk Grove Village, IL 60009-0927; 1-800 433-9016.

*Measles, Mumps, and Rubella: What You Need to Know.* U.S. Department of Health and Human Services. Available from: state and local health departments; American Academy of Family Physicians, 8880 Ward Parkway, Kansas City, MO 64114-2797; 1-800 944-0000, or American Academy of Pediatrics, Division of Publications, PO Box 927, Elk Grove Village, IL 60009-0927; 1-800 433-9016.

*Parents Guide to Childhood Immunization.* U.S. Department of Health and Human Services. Available from state and local health departments.

## Selected References

Advisory Committee on Immunization Practices (ACIP). General recommendations on immunization. *MMWR.* In press.
Advisory Committee on Immunization Practices (ACIP). General recommendations on immunization. *MMWR.* 1989;38(13):205.
Advisory Committee on Immunization Practices (ACIP). Measles prevention. *MMWR.* 1989;38:1-13.
Advisory Committee on Immunization Practices (ACIP). Mumps prevention. *MMWR.* 1989;38:1-6.
Advisory Committee on Immunization Practices (ACIP). Rubella prevention. *MMWR.* 1990;39(RR-15):1-13.
American Academy of Family Physicians, Commission on Public Health and Scientific Affairs. *Age Charts for Periodic Health Examination.* Kansas City, Mo: American Academy of Family Physicians; 1993.
American Academy of Pediatrics, Committee on Infectious Diseases. *1991 Report.* Elk Grove Village, Ill: American Academy of Pediatrics; 1991.
Canadian Task Force on the Periodic Health Examination. The periodic health examination. *Can Med Assoc J.* 1979;121:119 3-1254.
Centers for Disease Control. Vaccine Adverse Event Reporting System—United States. *MMWR.* 1990;39:730-733.
Greenberg MA, Birx DL. Safe administration of mumps-measles-rubella vaccine in egg-allergic children. *J Pediatr.* 1988;113:504-506.
Herman JJ, Radin R, Schneiderman R. Allergic reactions to measles (rubeola) vaccine in patients hypersensitive to egg protein. *J Pediatr.* 1983;102:196-199.
Lavi S, Zimmerman B, Koren G, Gold R. Administration of measles, mumps, and rubella vaccine (live) to egg-allergic children. *JAMA* 1990;263:269-271.
National Vaccine Advisory Committee. *Standards for Pediatric Immunization Practices.* Atlanta, Ga: Centers for Disease Control and Prevention; 1993.
US Preventive Services Task Force. Childhood immunizations. In: *Guide to Clinical Preventive Services.* Baltimore, Md: Williams & Wilkins; 1989:chap 56.

Children/Adolescents — IMMUNIZATION/PROPHYLAXIS

# 16. Poliomyelitis

Polio vaccine has decreased dramatically the annual number of reported cases of paralytic poliomyelitis in the United States, from 21,269 in 1954 to 6 in 1991. A case of wild (not vaccine-related), indigenous polio has not occurred in the United States in over a decade. Poliomyelitis continues to be a problem in developing countries, with more than 100,000 cases of paralytic poliomyelitis estimated worldwide. The World Health Organization has established a goal of global eradication of poliomyelitis by the year 2000.

### Recommendations of Major Authorities

- **Advisory Committee on Immunization Practices, American Academy of Family Physicians, American Academy of Pediatrics**, and **U.S. Preventive Services Task Force**—All children should receive immunization with oral polio vaccine beginning at 2 months of age. See below for schedule.

### Basics of Poliomyelitis Immunization

1. *Vaccine Types:* Two types of trivalent vaccine are available for use in the United States: live oral poliovirus vaccine (OPV) and enhanced-potency inactivated poliovirus vaccine (IPV). Both vaccines contain antigens to poliovirus types I, II, and III. Both vaccines are highly effective, but the oral form has been preferred in this country because of ease of administration, induction of intestinal immunity, and secondary immunization of some contacts of vaccinated persons. OPV is the vaccine of choice for children in the United States. The principle roles for IPV are immunizing adults and immunizing children and adults for whom OPV vaccine is contraindicated, such as immunocompromised patients (including those with HIV infection) and their household contacts.

2. *Schedule:* According to ACIP, the OPV primary series should be given at 2, 4, and 6 months of age. The first dose may be given as early as 6 weeks of age, and the minimum interval between doses should be 6 weeks. AAP has recommended that the third dose of the primary series be received at 6-18 months of age. A booster dose should be received at 4-6 years of age, preferably at or before school entry.

    Children for whom the primary series is initiated late, but during the first year of life, should receive the second and third OPV doses 2 months and 4 months, respectively, after the first dose. The minimum interval between doses should be 6 weeks. A booster should be received at 4-6 years of age, preferably at or before school entry.

    Children who were not immunized during the first year of life should receive three doses of OPV 6 to 8 weeks apart. If the third dose is given before the age of 4 years, a booster dose should be given before school entry (4 to 6 years of age). If a child is partially immunized, the schedule of immunization should continue without repetition in order to complete the primary series of three doses.

The standard primary series of IPV consists of three injections, with a minimum of 4 weeks (but preferably 8 weeks) between the first two doses, and a minimum of 6 months (but preferably 12 months) between the second and third doses. The primary series may be started as early as 6 weeks of age, but preferably at 2 months of age. A booster injection should be given before school entry (4 to 6 years of age), unless the third injection was given after 4 years of age, in which case a booster is not needed.

OPV and IPV may be given simultaneously with other routine childhood immunizations at different sites.

3. *Dosage and Administration:* OPV is supplied in a disposable pipette containing a single dose of 0.5 mL. It is administered orally, either directly or mixed with distilled water, chlorine-free tap water, milk, or syrup NF. It may also be absorbed on foods, such as bread, cake, or sugar cubes. If a substantial amount of OPV is regurgitated or spit out within 5-10 minutes of administration, it may be regiven. If the repeat dose is also lost, readministration should be attempted at the next visit.

The recommended dosage of IPV is 0.5 mL, given subcutaneously in the skin of the thigh in infants and the deltoid area in older children and adults, with a $5/8$ to $3/4$ inch, 23-25 gauge needle.

4. *Precautions:* Because of the risk of inducing paralytic poliomyelitis (see Adverse Reactions), use of OPV vaccine is contraindicated in immunocompromised patients (including those with HIV infection) and their household contacts. For these patients and their household contacts, IPV should be used rather than OPV. Patients who have received high doses of a systemically administered corticosteroid (2 mg/kg or 20 mg per day of prednisone or equivalent) should not receive OPV immunization until at least 3 months after discontinuation of the corticosteroid. Hospitalized infants should not receive OPV until discharge, because of the theoretical risk of poliovirus transmission in the hospital. See Table ii-4 for a listing of appropriate and inappropriate contraindications and precautions for giving childhood immunizations. See Table 16-1 for a listing of appropriate and inappropriate contraindications specific to polio immunization.

5. *Adverse Reactions:* There is an extremely small risk of paralysis in recipients and their close contacts after OPV use. In immunologically normal recipients, the risk is 1 case per 6.8 million doses. The risk of paralysis to the close contacts of OPV recipients is approximately 1 case per 6.4 million doses. The greatest risk to both recipient and contacts occurs after the first dose. All adults who are not immunized or inadequately immunized against polio should be informed of the very small risk of developing paralytic poliomyelitis after a child with whom they have close contact has been immunized with the OPV vaccine. They should be advised to wash their hands well after diaper changes and avoid contact with feces. Nonimmunized and partially immunized adults may be

offered immunization with IPV. A child's immunization should not be significantly delayed due to an adult's inadequate immunization status.

IPV does not induce paralysis and its side effects are minor—such as local pain and swelling at the injection site.

By law, the following adverse events following polio immunization must be reported to the Vaccine Adverse Event Reporting System (VAERS): for OPV, paralytic poliomyelitis (within 30 days in a nonimmunodeficient recipient, 6 months in an immunodeficient recipient, or any time in a vaccine-associated community case); for IPV, anaphylaxis or anaphylactic shock within 24 hours of the immunization; and for OPV or IPV, any acute complication or sequela (including death) of the preceding (without time limit), or any events described in the manufacturer's package insert as contraindications to additional doses of vaccine. Providers are encouraged to report adverse reactions of all kinds, particularly if serious or unusual, to VAERS. VAERS forms and instructions are

**Table 16-1. Contraindications and Precautions for OPV/IPV Vaccination**

| Vaccine | True Contraindications and Precautions | NOT Contraindications (vaccines may be given) |
|---|---|---|
| OPV | Infection with HIV or a household contact with HIV<br><br>Known altered immunodeficiency (hematologic and solid tumors; congenital immunodeficiency, and long-term immunosuppressive therapy)<br><br>Immunodeficient household contact<br><br>*Pregnancy | Breast feeding<br><br>Current antimicrobial therapy<br><br>Diarrhea |
| IPV | Anaphylactic reaction to neomycin or streptomycin<br><br>*Pregnancy | Breast feeding<br><br>Current antimicrobial therapy<br><br>Diarrhea |

*Precautions, although not contraindications, should be carefully reviewed. The benefits and risks of administering a specific vaccine to an individual under the circumstances should be considered. If the risks are believed to outweigh the benefits, the immunization should be withheld; if the benefits are believed to outweigh the risks (for example, during an outbreak or foreign travel), the vaccination should be given. It is prudent on theoretical grounds to avoid vaccinating pregnant women. However, if immediate protection against poliomyelitis is needed, OPV is preferred, although IPV may be considered if full immunization can be completed before the anticipated imminent exposure. Pregnancy of a mother is not a contraindication to giving polio vaccine to her child.

Adapted from: National Vaccine Advisory Committee. *Standards for Pediatric Immunization Practices.* Atlanta, GA: Centers for Disease Control and Prevention; 1993.

available in the *FDA Drug Bulletin* (Food and Drug Administration) and the *Physicians' Drug Reference*, or by calling the 24-hour VAERS information recording at 1-800 822-7967.

6. *Patient Education:* Effective April 15, 1992, as mandated by the National Childhood Vaccine Injury Act, every patient who receives a polio immunization must receive written information about the nature of the disease immunized against; manifestations of adverse reactions; precautionary measures that should be taken to reduce the risk for major adverse reactions; contraindications to, and the basis for delay of, administration of the vaccine; and notice of the availability of the National Vaccine Injury Compensation Program. The U.S. Department of Health and Human Services has developed a pamphlet for this purpose (see Family Resources). Clinicians may choose to use other patient educational materials so long as they provide the information required by the National Childhood Vaccine Injury Act. For additional information about this requirement, contact the Training Coordinator, National Immunization Program, Centers for Disease Control and Prevention at (404) 639-8226.

7. *Vaccine Storage and Handling:* OPV should be stored at temperatures low enough to keep it solidly frozen. This may require temperatures below -14°C (+7°F). The vaccine must be completely thawed before use. A container of vaccine may be subjected to a maximum of ten cycles of thawing and refreezing as long as the temperature of the vaccine does not exceed 8°C (46°F) and the total cumulative time thawed is not greater than 24 hours. If it is thawed for more than 24 hours it should not be refrozen, but stored at 2° to 8°C (36° to 46°F) and used within 30 days. IPV should be stored at 2°to 8°C (36°to 46°F) and should not be frozen. IPV vaccine that has been frozen should not be used. Handle all vaccine preparations according to manufacturers' instructions.

**Family Resources**

*Childhood Vaccines: What They Are and Why Your Child Needs Them.* American Academy of Family Physicians, 8880 Ward Parkway, Kansas City, MO 64114-2797; 1-800 944-0000.

*Immunization Protects Children.* American Academy of Pediatrics, PO Box 927, Elk Grove Village, IL 60009-0927; 1-800 433-9016.

*Parents Guide to Childhood Immunization.* U.S. Department of Health and Human Services. Available from state and local health departments.

*Polio: What You Need to Know.* U.S. Department of Health and Human Services. Available from: state and local health departments; American Academy of Family Physicians, 8880 Ward Parkway, Kansas City, MO 64114-2797; 1-800 944-0000 or American Academy of Pediatrics, 141 Northwest Point Blvd., P.O. Box 927, Elk Grove Village, IL 60009-0927; 1-800 433-9016.

## Selected References

Advisory Committee on Immunization Practices (ACIP). General recommendations on immunization. *MMWR*. In press.

Advisory Committee on Immunization Practices (ACIP). Poliomyelitis prevention. *MMWR*. 1982;31:22-26,31-34.

Advisory Committee on Immunization Practices (ACIP). Poliomyelitis prevention: enhanced-potency inactivated poliomyelitis vaccine - supplementary statement. *MMWR*. 1987;36:795-798.

American Academy of Family Physicians, Commission on Public Health and Scientific Affairs. *Age Charts for Periodic Health Examination*. Kansas City, Mo: American Academy of Family Physicians; 1993.

American Academy of Pediatrics, Committee on Infectious Diseases. *1991 Report*. Elk Grove Village, Ill: American Academy of Pediatrics; 1991.

Canadian Task Force on the Periodic Health Examination. The periodic health examination. *Can Med Assoc J*. 1979;121:1193-1254.

Centers for Disease Control. Paralytic poliomyelitis—Senegal, 1986-1987: update on the N-IPV efficacy study. *MMWR*. 1988;37:257-259.

Centers for Disease Control. Vaccine Adverse Event Reporting System—United States. *MMWR* 1990;39:730-733.

Kimpen JLL, Ogra PL. Poliovirus vaccines: a continuing challenge. *Pediatr Clin North Am*. 1990;37(3):627-649.

LaForce FM. Poliomyelitis vaccines: success and controversy. *Infect Dis Clin North Am*. 1990;4:75-83.

National Vaccine Advisory Committee. *Standards for Pediatric Immunization Practices*. Atlanta, Ga: Centers for Disease Control and Prevention; 1993.

*Physician's Desk Reference*. Oradell, NJ: Medical Economics Co.; 1993: 1258-1259.

Strebel PM, Sutter RW, Coohi SL, et al. Epidemiology of poliomyelitis in the United States one decade after the last reported case of indigenous wild virus-associated disease. *Clin Infect Dis*. 1992;14:568-579.

US Preventive Services Task Force. Childhood immunizations. In: *Guide to Clinical Preventive Services*. Baltimore, Md: Williams & Wilkins; 1989:chap 56.

## Children/Adolescents — COUNSELING

# 17. Alcohol and Other Drug Abuse

Abuse of alcohol and other drugs is a major health problem for older children and adolescents. Unintentional injuries are the leading cause of death for adolescents, and approximately 40% of these are related to alcohol use. Alcohol use has also been implicated in a significant percentage of adolescent homicides and suicides—the second and third leading causes of death in this age group. Cocaine use leads to increased cardiovascular morbidity and mortality in adolescents and young adults, and indirectly contributes to a number of violent deaths of young people related to illegal drug activities. The use of illegal drugs by youth is related to a number of undesirable social characteristics, such as poor school performance, social withdrawal, and family dysfunction.

Drug abuse affects children in all cultural and socioeconomic groups, not just minorities, the poor, and the undereducated. A survey of high school seniors in 1990 found that the percentage of white youth reporting use of alcohol, marijuana, and cocaine in the month prior to the survey was equal to or higher than that of African American youth (alcohol: 62.2% versus 32.9%; marijuana: 15.6% versus 5.2%; cocaine: 1.8% versus 0.5%). In this same study, alcohol and marijuana use was found to be directly related to parental educational levels—that is, the higher the parental educational level, the more drug use by the child. In general, the prevalence of alcohol and other drug abuse among females is lower than among males.

See chapter 52 for information on counseling adults about abuse of alcohol and other drugs. See chapters 23 and 59 for information on counseling about tobacco and smoking cessation.

**Recommendations of Major Authorities**

- All major authorities, including the **American Academy of Family Physicians (AAFP), American Academy of Pediatrics (AAP), American Medical Association (AMA),** and **U.S. Preventive Services Task Force (USPSTF)**—Counseling regarding abuse of alcohol and other drugs should be included as a routine part of well-child care by primary care clinicians. **AAFP** and **AAP** recommend that counseling and education of parents and children begin in the prepubertal years. Parent counseling should include discussion of the parents' own alcohol and drug use. **USPSTF** recommends routine counseling beginning in adolescence. **AMA** recommends that adolescents receive annual screening and health guidance to promote avoidance of tobacco, alcohol, anabolic steroids, and other abusable substances.

- **Canadian Task Force on the Periodic Health Examination**—Active case-finding should be done through interviews, questionnaires, biomarkers, and the presence of physical signs to identify problem drinkers. A lower age limit for case-finding is not specified. Case-finding should be followed up by clarification of the problem, counseling to reduce alcohol consumption, and periodic monitoring of progress.

## Basics of Alcohol and Other Drug Abuse Counseling

1. Educational discussions with children and parents should begin during the preteen years. Sample questions for discussing drug use with children in this age group are listed in Table 17-1. Similar questions can be used to discuss alcohol use. All children and adolescents should be informed of the dangers of alcohol and other drug use. Emphasis should be given to the dangers of HIV exposure and of motor vehicle use while under the influence of alcohol and other drugs.

2. Parents should be asked about their own use of alcohol and other drugs and whether they discuss the use of alcohol and other drugs with their children. An assessment should be made of whether a family history of alcoholism or other drug use exists, and whether family stress places the child at increased risk. See chapter 52 for information on counseling adults about abuse of alcohol and other drugs.

3. The clinician should establish a caring and confidential relationship with adolescent patients. Both the parents and the adolescent must be clearly informed of the limits of this confidentiality.

4. Begin by asking children and adolescents about alcohol and drug use in their environment—at home, school (including use of drugs to enhance athletic ability), or work. This may be less threatening than first asking about their personal use. A set of questions developed using this indirect approach is listed in Table 17-2.

5. If a history of alcohol or other drug use is elicited, the adolescent should be asked in a nonjudgmental manner about the type of drugs used, the quantity and frequency of use, and the setting of use.

6. An evaluation should be made of the extent to which alcohol or other drug use is adversely affecting important aspects of the patient's life, such as school performance, peer relationships, family relationships, work performance, and sexual relationships. The CAGE Questionnaire (Table 52-1) and the Trauma Questionnaire (Table 52-3) are brief screening instruments developed for adults that may be adapted for this purpose. More extensive screening instruments have also been developed (Selzer 1971).

**Table 17-1. Sample Questions Concerning Drugs for School-aged Children**

| |
|---|
| Do you understand the word "drugs"? What does it mean? |
| Have your teachers ever talked about drugs at school? |
| What have you learned about drugs at school? |
| Have you and your friends ever talked about drugs? |
| Have you ever wondered why some people use drugs? |
| Why do you think grown-ups say that drugs are harmful? |
| Has anyone ever tried to sell you drugs or tried to force you to take drugs? |

Adapted from: Schonberg KS, ed. *Substance Abuse: A Guide for Health Professionals.* Elk Grove Village, Ill: American Academy of Pediatrics; 1988. Used with permission of the American Academy of Pediatrics; copyright © 1988.

**Table 17-2. Sample Questions Concerning Drug Use for Adolescents**

| |
|---|
| I know that many schools have drug problems. Does your school have a drug problem? |
| Do most of your friends drink alcohol or smoke marijuana at parties? |
| Do any of your friends use drugs other than alcohol or marijuana? |
| Where do most young people obtain drugs? |
| Do you smoke cigarettes? How many per day? |
| Have you ever tried alcohol? Marijuana? Other drugs? |
| Have you ever been ill as a result of using drugs or drinking? In what way? |
| Have you ever been in trouble with the law as a result of drugs or alcohol? |
| Do your parents know that you've used _____ ? What would (did) they say? |
| Have you ever worried about your _____ use? |
| Have you ever been drunk or stoned and driven a car (or motorcycle)? |

Adapted from: Schonberg KS, ed. *Substance Abuse: A Guide for Health Professionals.* Elk Grove Village, IL: American Academy of Pediatrics; 1988. Used with permission of the American Academy of Pediatrics; copyright © 1988.

7. The clinician should remain alert for signs and symptoms of physiological dependence or withdrawal, such as craving, compulsive alcohol- or drug-seeking behavior, tremulousness, agitation, weight loss, headaches, and changes in mental status.

8. The presence of significant psychosocial impairment or physiological dependence due to alcohol or other drug abuse should alert the clinician to the need for early referral of the patient for in-depth evaluation and treatment. The clinician should be familiar with the range of referral and treatment options in the community. Patients without serious impairment may be counseled by the primary care clinician.

9. Chapter 52 discusses basic principles of substance abuse counseling, including:

    - Establishing a therapeutic relationship.

    - Making the medical office or clinic off-limits for substance abuse.

    - Presenting information about negative health consequences.

    - Involving family and other support.

    - Setting goals.

    - Becoming familiar with community treatment services.

    - Providing follow-up.

## Family Resources

*Alcohol: Your Child and Drugs*; *Cocaine: Your Child and Drugs*; *Marijuana: Your Child and Drugs; Teens Who Drink and Drive: Reducing the Death Toll.* American Academy of Pediatrics, PO Box 927, Elk Grove Village, IL 60009-0927; 1-800 433-9016.

*Anabolic Steroids and Athletes.* American College of Sports Medicine, PO Box 1440, Indianapolis, IN 46202-1440; (317) 637-9200.

Other sources of materials include: National Clearinghouse for Alcohol and Drug Abuse Information, Dept. BSDS, Box 2345, Rockville, MD 20852; (800) 729-6686; and PRIDE, The Hurt Building, Suite 210, 50 Hurt Plaza, Atlanta, GA 30303; (404) 577-4500.

## Selected References

American Academy of Family Physicians, Commission on Public Health and Scientific Affairs. *Age Charts for Periodic Health Examination*. Kansas City, Mo: American Academy of Family Physicians; 1993.

American Academy of Pediatrics, Committee on Adolescence. Alcohol use and abuse: a pediatric concern. *Pediatrics*. 1987;79:450-453.

American Academy of Pediatrics, Committee on Adolescence, Committee on Substance Abuse. Marijuana: a continuing concern for pediatricians. *Pediatrics*. 1991;88:1070-1072.

American Academy of Pediatrics, Committee on Adolescence. The role of the pediatrician in substance abuse counseling. *Pediatrics*. 1983;72:251-252.

American Academy of Pediatrics, Committee on Adolescence, Committee on Bioethics, Provisional Committee on Substance Abuse. Screening for drugs of abuse in children and adolescents. *Pediatrics*. 1989;84:396-398.

American Academy of Pediatrics, American Academy of Family Physicians, American College of Obstetricians and Gynecologists, NAACOG—The Organization for Obstetric, Gynecologic, and Neonatal Nurses, National Medical Association (joint policy statement). Confidentiality in adolescent health care. In: *Policy Reference Guide: A Comprehensive Guide to AAP Policy Statements Published through December 1991*. Elk Grove Village, Ill: American Academy of Pediatrics; 1992: 97.

American Medical Association. *Guidelines for Adolescent Preventive Services (GAPS)*. Chicago, Ill: American Medical Association; 1992.

Canadian Task Force on the Periodic Health Examination. The periodic health examination: 2. 1989 update. *Can Med Assoc J*. 1989;141:4-11.

National Center for Health Statistics. *Health, United States, 1991 Prevention Profile*. Hyattsville, Md: Public Health Service; 1992. US Department of Health and Human Services Publication number (PHS) 92-1232.

Schonberg KS, ed. *Substance Abuse: A Guide for Health Professionals*. Elk Grove Village, Ill: American Academy of Pediatrics; 1988.

Selzer M. The Michigan Alcoholism Screening Test: the quest for a new diagnostic instrument. *Am J Psychiatry*. 1971;127:1653-1658.

US Preventive Services Task Force. Screening for alcohol and other drug abuse. In: *Guide to Clinical Preventive Services*. Baltimore, Md: Williams & Wilkins; 1989:chap 47.

Children/Adolescents — COUNSELING

# 18. Dental and Oral Health

Dental and oral health problems are common in children. Caries and periodontal disease occur most frequently, but other significant problems include malocclusion, trauma, congenital anomalies, and oral malignancies. Widespread use of fluoride and other preventive dental health practices have led to a significant decrease in the prevalence of dental caries. Nonetheless, by age 17, 84% of American children have decay in their permanent teeth and up to one third of all children have gingivitis. In most cases, these problems are preventable, and the dental and oral health status of adults is largely determined by the quality of preventive and treatment services received during childhood.

See chapter 53 for information on dental and oral health counseling for adults. See chapters 23 and 59 for information on counseling on tobacco and smoking cessation.

### Recommendations of Major Authorities

*Primary Care*

- **All major dental and medical authorities**—Dental and oral health counseling for children and parents should be provided routinely by primary care clinicians.

*Dental and Oral Care*

- **American Academy of Family Physicians** and **American Academy of Pediatrics**—Referral for the first dental visit should occur at 3 years of age, with frequency of subsequent visits determined by the dentist.

- **American Academy of Pediatric Dentistry**, **American Society of Dentistry for Children**, and **American Dental Association**—A child's first dental visit should occur at 6 months of age or when the first tooth erupts, whichever comes later, but no later than 1 year of age. Frequency of subsequent visits should be determined by the dentist.

- **Canadian Task Force on the Periodic Health Examination**—Dental visits should occur annually beginning at 2 years of age. This recommendation is currently under review.

- **U.S. Preventive Services Task Force**—All patients should be encouraged to visit a dental-care provider on a regular basis, with the optimal frequency determined by the patient's dentist.

### Basics of Dental and Oral Health Counseling

1. Oral health education and care should begin at an infant's first visit to a clinician and continue throughout childhood, adolescence, and adulthood.

2. During an infant's first visit to a clinician, the need for fluoride supplementation should be assessed. Approximately one-sixth of Americans live in areas without fluoridated

community water supplies. Infants who are exclusively breast-fed should receive fluoride supplementation. For children who live in an area without an optimally fluoridated community water supply, the child's water supply should be tested and other sources of fluoride determined prior to recommending supplementation. Information about fluoride content of community water supplies can be obtained from the local water department.

See Table 18-1 for the recommended dosage of fluoride supplementation. Fluoride supplementation should begin at 2 weeks of age and continue to approximately 13 years of age, if necessary. Fluoride supplements are available as drops (for infants and young children) and chewable tablets. These should be given in the recommended dosage once daily. When chewable tablets are used, children should be encouraged to chew and swish the resultant fluid in the mouth for 30 seconds before swallowing to increase its effectiveness.

3. Parents should be instructed to wipe their infant's gums and teeth after each feeding, using a moist washcloth or gauze pad. As multiple teeth appear, parents should begin daily brushing with a small toothbrush and a very small (pea-sized) amount of a toothpaste containing fluoride. This limitation is important because swallowing large amounts of toothpaste by infants and children may lead to enamel discoloration due to fluorosis. To avoid gum tissue injury, a brush with soft end-rounded or polished bristles should be used; it should be replaced when bristles are bent or worn. Although children should actively participate in their dental care, they should continue to receive assistance from parents or other caregivers until they are 7 or 8 years old.

4. During teething, an infant's irritability may be soothed by chewing on a cold teething ring, gently massaging the gums with a finger, or using acetaminophen. Fever is not a symptom of teething; if a fever is present, parents should be advised to contact their child's primary care provider.

5. Strategies to prevent tooth decay from breast- or bottle-feeding should be addressed. Infants should not be permitted to nurse throughout the night or fall asleep with a bottle containing anything other than water. If a bottle is required to quiet or comfort the infant before sleep, only water should be used. Infants should be encouraged to begin using a cup instead of a bottle at 1 year of age.

Table 18-1. Daily Fluoride Dosage (mg) According to Age and Water Supply Content

| Age, y | Fluoride Concentration in Local Water Supply (ppm) | | |
| --- | --- | --- | --- |
|  | <0.3 | 0.3-0.7 | >0.7 |
| 0-2 | 0.25 | 0 | 0 |
| 2-3 | 0.50 | 0.25 | 0 |
| 3-16 | 1.00 | 0.50 | 0 |

From: American Academy of Pediatrics, Committee on Nutrition. Fluoride supplementation. *Pediatrics.* 1986;77:758-761. Reproduced by permission of *Pediatrics*; copyright © 1986.

## Ch. 18. Dental and Oral Health — Children/Adolescents — COUNSELING

6. Parents should be advised to talk with their dentist or hygienist about when their child should begin using dental floss.

7. Thumb-sucking or use of a pacifier generally does not cause permanent dental problems for children under 4 years of age. Children who thumb-suck beyond age 5 years, however, may develop alignment problems of their permanent teeth. These children may need to be referred to a dentist for assessment.

8. Parents should receive counseling about the impact of dietary habits on oral health: Foods that are high in simple sugars or starches or are particularly sticky should be avoided. If snacks are eaten, they should be carefully chosen; raw fruits and vegetables, nuts, and low-sugar drinks should be encouraged. Sweets should be limited to once or twice a day, preferably with a meal.

9. If a child has a permanent tooth knocked out and it is intact and whole, it should be rinsed gently without removing any attached tissue and immediately reinserted into the socket. If this is not possible, it should be placed in cool water or milk. The child should see a dentist **as soon as possible** for emergency treatment. Replacement of the tooth within the first hour is critical for long-term retention. Primary teeth should not be reinserted.

10. Clinicians should recommend to parents that children between the ages of 5 and 13 years be evaluated by their dentist regarding the need for dental sealants on newly erupted molars. First molars usually erupt at about 6 years of age and second molars at about 12 years of age. The sealant is most effective if applied soon after eruption, before the decay process has had time to begin.

11. Children and adolescents should be given special counseling about dental and oral health problems, such as dental injuries and tobacco-related illnesses for which they are at increased risk. Those involved in contact sports should be advised to use appropriate mouth protectors and helmets. Adolescents should be advised of the cosmetic (yellowed teeth, bad breath) and health (lung cancer, heart disease, leukoplakia, and oral and pharyngeal cancers) problems caused by tobacco use. Smokeless tobacco (snuff and chewing tobacco) is a particular problem among adolescents, and its use should be seriously discouraged (see chapter 23).

12. When examining the oral cavity, primary care clinicians should remain alert for signs of oral disease, such as caries and inflamed or cyanotic gingiva, malalignment or crowding of teeth, and mismatching upper and lower dental arches.

13. Transient bacteremia is common during dental procedures, including cleaning. Antibiotic prophylaxis should be given to children prior to a dental cleaning or procedure if they have underlying great vessel or heart disease (see Tables 53-2 and 53-3).

# Ch. 18. Dental and Oral Health — Children/Adolescents — COUNSELING

## Family Resources

*A Guide to Children's Dental Health.* American Academy of Pediatrics, PO Box 927, Elk Grove Village, IL 60009-0927; 1-800 433-9016.

*A Healthy Mouth for Your and Your Baby*; *Prevent Baby Bottle Tooth Decay*; *Rx for Sound Teeth*; and other pamphlets and posters. National Institute of Dental Research, Public Information and Reports Section, PO Box 54793, Washington, DC 20032; (301) 496-4261.

*Baby's Bright Smile.* And other materials. American Society of Dentistry for Children, 211 E Chicago Ave., Suite 1430, Chicago, IL 60611; (312) 943-1244.

*Dental Emergency Procedures; Seal Out Decay; Your Child's Teeth.* American Dental Association, Dept. of Salable Materials, 211 E Chicago Ave., Chicago, IL 60611; 1-800 947-4746.

## Selected References

American Academy of Family Physicians, Commission on Public Health and Scientific Affairs. *Age Charts for Periodic Health Examination.* Kansas City, Mo: American Academy of Family Physicians; 1993.

American Academy of Pediatrics, Committee on Nutrition. Fluoride supplementation. *Pediatrics.* 1986;77:758-761.

American Academy of Pediatrics. Juice in ready-to-use bottles and nursing bottle caries. In: *Policy Reference Guide: A Comprehensive Guide to AAP Policy Statements Published through December 1991.* Elk Grove Village, Ill: American Academy of Pediatrics; 1992: 362.

American Academy of Pediatric Dentistry. *Reference Manual 1991-1992.* Chicago, Ill: American Academy of Pediatric Dentistry; 1991.

American Dental Association. *Baby Bottle Tooth Decay.* Chicago, Ill: American Dental Association; 1989.

American Dental Association. Fluoride compounds. In: *Accepted Dental Therapeutics.* 40th ed. Chicago, Ill: American Dental Association; 1984.

Canadian Task Force on the Periodic Health Examination. *Periodic Health Examination Monograph.* Hull, Quebec: Minister of Supply and Services Canada; 1980.

Canadian Task Force on the Periodic Health Examination. The periodic health examination: 2. 1984 update. *Can Med Assoc J.* 1984;130:1278-1285.

Greene JC, Louie R, Wycoff SJ. US Preventive Services Task Force: Preventive dentistry: I. Dental caries. *JAMA.* 1989;262:3459-3563.

Greene JC, Louie R, Wycoff SJ. US Preventive Services Task Force: Preventive dentistry: II. Periodontal diseases, malocclusion, trauma, and oral cancer. *JAMA.* 1990;263:421-423.

Helfetz SB. Amounts of fluoride in self-administered dental products: safety considerations for children. *Pediatrics.* 1986;77:876-882.

US Department of Health and Human Services. Oral Health of the United States Children. *The National Survey of Dental Caries in US School Children: 1986-1987. National and Regional Findings.* Bethesda, Md: National Institutes of Health; 1989. US Department of Health and Human Services publication NIH 89-2247.

US Preventive Services Task Force. Counseling to prevent dental disease. In: *Guide to Clinical Preventive Services.* Baltimore. Md: Williams & Wilkins; 1989:chap 55.

# Children/Adolescents — COUNSELING

## 19. Nutrition

Proper nutrition during childhood is essential for normal growth and development. Inadequate intake of nutrients is reflected in slow growth rates, inadequate mineralization of bones, and low body reserves of micronutrients. The mineral most commonly deficient in children is iron. Inadequate caloric intake is less of a problem for children in the United States than is excessive caloric intake. Many children are substantially overweight, physically inactive, and have high dietary intakes of total fat and saturated fat. These factors may lead to obesity and poor nutritional habits as adults, resulting in heart disease, Type II diabetes, high blood pressure, certain types of cancer, and other chronic diseases. The challenge primary care clinicians face is to help children develop dietary habits that promote growth and development and reduce the risk of chronic diseases later in life.

### Recommendations of Major Authorities

- All major authorities, including the **American Academy of Family Physicians, American Academy of Pediatrics, American Dietetic Association, American Medical Association,** and **U.S. Preventive Services Task Force**—Primary care providers should counsel children and adolescents and their parents about proper nutrition.

- All major authorities, including the **American Academy of Family Physicians, American Academy of Pediatrics, American Medical Association, Canadian Task Force on the Periodic Health Examination,** and **U.S. Preventive Services Task Force**—Parents should be counseled about the benefits and techniques of breast-feeding for infants.

### Basics of Nutrition Counseling

*Less than 2 Years of Age*

1. Breast milk is the best choice for feeding almost all infants. Mothers should be encouraged to breast-feed for 6 to 12 months if possible, but even a few weeks is desirable. Breast-feeding should be encouraged except in those few situations (ie. maternal use of certain drugs or medications, certain maternal infections) when it is contraindicated. Parents should be provided with education on the benefits of breast-feeding and techniques for successfully initiating and maintaining breast-feeding.

2. Parents should be counseled to begin the introduction of single-ingredient foods when infants are developmentally ready, usually at 4 to 6 months of age. A child should be able to sit up with some help, maintain good head and neck control, and accept soft food from a spoon. Infant cereal mixed with breast milk or formula is often a good first choice. Foods should be introduced one at a time, at 3 to 5 day intervals, to permit detection of food intolerances.

3. The use of iron-rich foods, such as iron-fortified infant formula and iron-fortified cereal, should be encouraged. Infants who are exclusively breast-fed may need iron supplementation beginning at 6 months of age. Many authorities recommend hemoglobin/hematocrit testing to detect iron-deficiency anemia prior to 1 year of age (see chapter 1).

4. Parents should be advised not to feed their children cow's milk until 1 year of age. Reduced-fat milk should not be used before 2 years of age.

5. Parents should be advised not to limit fat in children's diets during the first 2 years of life.

6. Parents should be counseled not to feed honey to infants during the first year of life because of the risk of infant botulism.

7. Parents should be counseled that vitamin supplements have not been proven to be necessary in healthy children who have balanced diets that include a variety of foods. Infants who are exclusively breast-fed, particularly if they are dark-skinned or are not regularly exposed to sunlight, may need vitamin D supplementation.

8. Infants and young children who are exclusively breast-fed or who live in areas with low fluoride content in the drinking water may need fluoride supplementation for prevention of dental caries (see chapter 18).

*Over 2 Years of Age*

1. Parents should be counseled that children, like adults, need a balanced diet that includes a wide variety of foods. The U.S. Departments of Agriculture and Health and Human Services have recently formulated the *Food Guide Pyramid* (see Fig 55-1) to assist the public in planning a balanced diet.

2. Parents and children should be instructed in choosing a diet low in total fat (30% or less of total calories), saturated fat (less than 10% of total calories), and cholesterol. Poultry (without skin), fish, lean meat, low-fat and skim milk products, cooked dry peas and beans, whole-grain breads and cereals, and fruits and vegetables should be encouraged.

3. Parents and children should be encouraged to use sugar, salt, and sodium only in moderation.

4. Children, particularly adolescent girls, and their families should be advised to eat foods rich in calcium (such as milk and milk products) and iron (such as lean meats, dry legumes, and whole-grain products).

5. Parents and children should be counseled on the importance of maintaining a healthy weight. Weight assessment in children needs to take into consideration many factors, including height, age, and body build. The limits of "healthy" weight are not well defined for children. As a rule of thumb, however, weight-for-height values from the 25th through

75th percentiles (see chapter 3) can be considered "healthy," provided there is neither a family history of obesity-related diseases nor the presence of conditions (such as high blood pressure or abnormal lipid patterns) that would make weight lower than the 75th percentile desirable.

6. Weight reduction through dieting or other means is not advisable for children who are still growing. Overweight children and their parents should be counseled on maintaining a constant weight as the child continues to grow, while increasing physical activity to improve fitness and avoid gaining weight. Parents and adolescents should also be asked about diets being followed for athletic teams, especially those including stringent weight standards.

7. Parents and children should be advised that vitamin supplements have not been proven to be necessary in normal children with balanced diets. Children up to approximately 13 years of age who live in areas with low fluoride content in the drinking water may need fluoride supplements to prevent dental caries (see chapter 18).

8. The U.S. Public Health Services recommends that all women of childbearing age in the United States consume 0.4 mg of folic acid per day to reduce their risk of having a pregnancy affected with spina bifida or other neural tube defects (NTDs). Adolescent females should be advised of the following options for complying with this recommendation:

- Consumption of a diet consistent with the *Food Guide Pyramid* (Fig 55-1) is likely to provide the proper amount of folic acid.

- Fortified foods, such as breakfast cereals, may help patients consume enough folic acid.

- Folic acid supplement pills and multivitamin preparations containing 0.4 mg folic acid are also available.

Patients should be cautioned against consuming more than 1 mg of folic acid daily because the effects of excess folic acid are not well known; they may include complicating the detection of vitamin $B_{12}$ deficiency. However, women who have had a previous NTD-affected pregnancy should talk with their doctor several months before planning to become pregnant about using a higher dose of folic acid. Public health measures to supplement the U.S. food supply with folic acid currently are being studied.

**Family Resources**

*The Gift of Love* (booklet on breast-feeding). American Academy of Pediatrics, PO Box 927, Elk Grove Village, IL 60009-0927; 1-800 433-9016.

*Nutrition and Sports Performance: A Guide for High School Athletes.* American College of Sports Medicine, PO Box 1440, Indianapolis, IN 46202-1440; (317) 634-7817.

*Feeding Kids Right Isn't Always Easy: Tips for Preventing Food Hassles*; *Growing Up Healthy: Fat, Cholesterol and More*; *Right from the Start: ABC's of Good Nutrition for Young Children*; *What's to Eat? Healthy Foods for Hungry Children.* American Dietetic Association, 216 West Jackson Blvd., Chicago, IL 60606-6995; (312) 899-0040.

*Nutrition and Your Health: Dietary Guidelines for Americans; The Food Guide Pyramid; Dietary Guidelines and Your Diet* [HG-232-1 through 7]; and *Dietary Guidelines and Your Diet* [HG-232-8 through 11]. U.S. Department of Agriculture and U.S. Department of Health and Human Services, 1990. Available through the Cooperative Extension System or contact Superintendent of Documents, U.S. Government Printing Office, Washington, DC 20402; (202) 783-3238.

*The Food Guide Pyramid: Beyond the Basic 4.* Food Marketing Institute, 800 Connecticut Ave. NW., Washington, DC 20006.

## Selected References

American Academy of Family Physicians, Commission on Public Health and Scientific Affairs. *Age Charts for Periodic Health Examination.* Kansas City, Mo: American Academy of Family Physicians; 1993.
American Academy of Pediatrics, Committee on Nutrition. Iron supplementation for infants. *Pediatrics.* 1976;58:765-768.
American Academy of Pediatrics, Committee on Nutrition. Nutrition and lactation. *Pediatrics.* 1981;68:470-478.
American Academy of Pediatrics, Committee on Nutrition. *Pediatric Nutrition Handbook.* 3rd ed. Elk Grove Village, Ill: American Academy of Pediatrics; 1993.
American Academy of Pediatrics, Committee on Nutrition. The promotion of breast-feeding. *Pediatrics.* 1982;69:654-661.
American Academy of Pediatrics, Committee on Nutrition. Prudent life-style for children: dietary fat and cholesterol. *Pediatrics.* 1986;78:521-525.
American Academy of Pediatrics, Committee on Nutrition. The use of whole cow's milk in infancy. *Pediatrics.* 1992;89:1105-1109.
American Medical Association. *Guidelines for Adolescent Preventive Services (GAPS).* Chicago, Ill: American Medical Association; 1992.
Canadian Task Force on the Periodic Health Examination. The periodic health examination: 2. 1984 update. *Can Med Assoc J.* 1984;130:1278-1285.
Cunningham AS. Morbidity in breast-fed and artificially fed infants. *J Pediatr.* 1977;90:726.
Freed GL, Landers S, Schanler RJ. A practical guide to successful breastfeeding management. *Am J Dis Child.* 1991;145:917-921.
Mallick MJ. Health hazards of obesity and weight control in children: a review of the literature. *Am J Public Health.* 1983;73:78-82.
National Cholesterol Education Program. Report of the Expert Panel on Blood Cholesterol Levels for Children and Adolescents. *Pediatrics.* 1992;89(suppl. 3):525-584.
US Public Health Service. *The Surgeon General's Report on Nutrition and Health.* Washington DC: US Department of Health and Human Services; 1988. DHHS (PHS) publication 88-50210.
US Preventive Services Task Force. Nutritional counseling. In: *Guide to Clinical Preventive Services.* Baltimore, Md: Williams & Wilkins; 1989:chap 50.
US Public Health Service. Recommendations for the use of folic acid to reduce the number of cases of spina bifida and other neural tube defects. *MMWR.* 1992;41:1-7.

## Children/Adolescents — COUNSELING

# 20. Physical Activity

Physical activity is vital to maintaining a healthy weight and cardiovascular and musculoskeletal fitness. Measurements of skin thickness taken over the last 30 years indicate that children in the United States are becoming increasingly obese (54% increase in prevalence of obesity in those 6 to 11 years old and 39% increase in obesity in those 12 to 17 years old). Many authorities believe that this is due to decreases in physical activity and increases in sedentary activities—such as watching television. In 1984, a national survey of children in grades 5 through 12 found that approximately half were not participating in adequate physical activity, which the survey defined as exercise involving large muscle groups in dynamic movement for 20 minutes or longer, three or more times weekly, at an intensity requiring 60% or more of cardiopulmonary capacity.

The health consequences of physical inactivity usually become increasingly apparent in adulthood—with the onset of heart disease, diabetes mellitus, and other chronic diseases—but these diseases may begin in childhood and adolescence. Fatty plaques have been found in the arterial walls of adolescents at autopsy. A recently published 55-year follow-up study that controlled for adult weight found that the relative risks of mortality from all causes and mortality from coronary heart disease were significantly increased for men who had been obese as adolescents. In fact, being overweight in adolescence was a more powerful predictor of these risks than was being overweight as an adult. It is believed that physical activity patterns developed in childhood and adolescence influence adulthood lifestyle habits. The primary care clinician has an opportunity to counsel children and their parents about the importance of adequate, appropriate physical activity.

See chapter 56 for information about physical activity counseling for adults. See chapters 19 and 55 for information on nutrition counseling for children and adolescents and adults, respectively.

**Recommendations of Major Authorities**

- **American Academy of Family Physicians** and **U.S. Preventive Services Task Force**—All patients (and parents) should receive counseling on the role of physical activity in disease prevention and assistance in selecting an appropriate exercise program.

- **American Academy of Pediatrics**—At each health supervision visit, the clinician should ask parents about their children's motor development and motor activities. Parents and other family members should be encouraged to serve as role models for their children by participating in regular physical activity programs themselves. In the preschool years, the clinician should advise parents to provide space and encouragement for physical activity appropriate for the developmental level and physical health status of the child. Beginning at school age, the clinician should advise the child to engage in regular physical activity and limit passive activity, such as viewing television and playing video games. In adolescence, assessment of sports fitness should become a routine part of health supervision visits.

- **American College of Sports Medicine**—The health-care professions need to become more actively involved in promoting physical fitness for children and youth. Health-care professionals can make a major impact by promoting and supporting physical fitness programs for children and youth.

- **American Medical Association**—Adolescents should receive annual counseling about the benefits of exercise and should be encouraged to engage in safe exercise on a regular basis.

## Basics of Physical Activity Counseling

1. Every visit should be used as an opportunity to inquire about the physical activity habits of both children and parents. The physical activity levels of parents and parental encouragement of physical activity can strongly influence children.

2. Preschool children generally do not need structured activities to achieve physical fitness; they need only a safe environment in which to express their innate curiosity and natural propensity for active exploration. School-age children should be encouraged to participate in a minimum of 20 to 30 minutes of vigorous activity at least three times weekly. As a rule of thumb, activity that elevates the heart rate to at least 60% of maximum for age (with maximum heart rate calculated as 220 minus age) can be considered vigorous. See chapter 56 for information on physiologic monitoring of activity. The American Academy of Pediatrics has published a classification of sports according to degree of strenuousness and contact (see Table 20-1). Depending on effort expended, activity levels during these sports can be considered vigorous, except those classified noncontact-moderately strenuous and noncontact-nonstrenuous.

3. Involvement in physical activities for enjoyment—not just competition—should be encouraged. Unpleasant experiences with competition in sports can discourage children from involvement in physical activity.

4. Involvement in physical activities that can be enjoyed into adulthood, such as swimming, hiking, running, tennis, or bicycle riding, should be encouraged.

5. Activities that can be easily incorporated into a child's daily routine and enjoyed all year should be encouraged. Activity levels tend to decrease significantly in the winter months.

6. Children and parents should be counseled on the importance of engaging in a variety of activities that help develop a range of abilities.

7. The appropriate use of safety equipment, such as helmets and pads, and the avoidance of alcohol or other drug use during sports participation, should be stressed.

8. Children with disabilities or disorders should be encouraged to participate fully in appropriate physical activities. The American Academy of Pediatrics has issued sports guidelines for children with certain medical conditions (see Table 20-2).

9. In order to reduce the risk of musculoskeletal injuries, it is prudent to advise children and adolescents to avoid weight lifting, power lifting, and body building until their development has attained Tanner growth stage 5.

10. Adolescents engaged in "power" sports, such as weight lifting or football, should be advised of the dangers of anabolic steroids and strongly counseled to avoid their use.

11. An office or clinic environment that conveys the message that physical activity is valued should be established through posters, pamphlets, and other means. Clinicians should be good role models by getting appropriate physical activity themselves.

Table 20-1. Classification of Sports According to Strenuousness and Contact

| Contact/ Collision | Limited Contact/Impact | Noncontact Strenuous | Noncontact Moderately Strenuous | Noncontact Non-strenuous |
|---|---|---|---|---|
| Boxing | Baseball | Aerobic dancing | Badminton | Archery |
| Field hockey | Basketball | Crew | Curling | Golf |
| Football | Bicycling | Fencing | Table tennis | Riflery |
| Ice hockey | Diving | Field | | |
| Lacrosse | Field |   Discus | | |
| Martial arts |   High Jump |   Javelin | | |
| Rodeo |   Pole vault |   Shot put | | |
| Soccer | Gymnastics | Running | | |
| Wrestling | Handball | Swimming | | |
| | Horseback riding | Tennis | | |
| | Skating | Track | | |
| |   Ice | Weight lifting | | |
| |   Roller | | | |
| | Skiing | | | |
| |   Cross-country | | | |
| |   Downhill | | | |
| |   Water | | | |
| | Softball | | | |
| | Squash | | | |
| | Volleyball | | | |

From: American Academy of Pediatrics, Committee on Sports Medicine and Fitness. Recommendations for participation in competitive sports. *Pediatrics*. 1988;81:737-739. Reproduced by permission of *Pediatrics*; copyright © 1988.

## Table 20-2. Recommendations for Participation in Competitive Sports

| Disorder/Condition | Contact/ Collision | Limited Contact/ Impact | Noncontact Strenuous | Noncontact Moderately Strenuous | Noncontact Non-Strenuous |
|---|---|---|---|---|---|
| **Atlantoaxial instability** [1]Swimming: no butterfly, breast stroke, or diving starts | No | No | Yes[1] | Yes | Yes |
| **Acute illnesses** [2]Needs individual assessment, e.g., contagiousness to others, risk of worsening illness | 2 | 2 | 2 | 2 | 2 |
| **Cardiovascular** | | | | | |
| Carditis | No | No | No | No | No |
| Hypertension | | | | | |
| Mild | Yes | Yes | Yes | Yes | Yes |
| Moderate | 3 | 3 | 3 | 3 | 3 |
| Severe | 3 | 3 | 3 | 3 | 3 |
| Congenital heart disease | 4 | 4 | 4 | 4 | 4 |

[3]Needs individual assessment
[4]Patients with mild forms can be allowed a full range of physical activities; patients with moderate to severe forms, or who are postoperative, should be evaluated by a cardiologist before athletic participation.

| | | | | | |
|---|---|---|---|---|---|
| **Eyes** | | | | | |
| Absence or loss of function of one eye | 5 | 5 | 5 | 5 | 5 |
| Detached retina | 6 | 6 | 6 | 6 | 6 |

[5]Availability of American Society for Testing and Materials (ASTM)-approved eye guards may allow competitor to participate in most sports, but this must be judged on an individual basis.
[6]Consult ophthalmologist

| | | | | | |
|---|---|---|---|---|---|
| **Inguinal hernia** | Yes | Yes | Yes | Yes | Yes |
| **Kidney: absence of one** | No | Yes | Yes | Yes | Yes |

## Table 20-2. Recommendations for Participation in Competitive Sports—Continued

| Disorder/Condition | Contact/ Collision | Limited Contact/ Impact | Noncontact Strenuous | Noncontact Moderately Strenuous | Noncontact Non- Strenuous |
|---|---|---|---|---|---|
| **Liver: enlarged** | No | No | Yes | Yes | Yes |
| **Musculoskeletal disorders** [7]Needs individual assessment | 7 | 7 | 7 | 7 | 7 |
| **Neurologic** | | | | | |
| History of serious head or spine trauma, repeated concussions, or craniotomy | 8 | 8 | Yes | Yes | Yes |
| Convulsive disorder | | | | | |
| Well controlled | Yes | Yes | Yes | Yes | Yes |
| Poorly controlled | No | No | Yes[9] | Yes | Yes[10] |
| [8]Needs individual assessment [9]No swimming or weight lifting [10]No archery or riflery | | | | | |
| **Ovary: absence of one** | Yes | Yes | Yes | Yes | Yes |
| **Respiratory** | | | | | |
| Pulmonary insufficiency | 11 | 11 | 11 | 11 | 11 |
| Asthma | Yes | Yes | Yes | Yes | Yes |
| [11]May be allowed to compete if oxygenation remains satisfactory during a graded stress test | | | | | |
| **Sickle cell trait** | Yes | Yes | Yes | Yes | Yes |
| **Skin: boils, herpes, impetigo, scabies** | 12 | 12 | Yes | Yes | Yes |
| [12]No gymnastics with mats, martial arts, wrestling or contact sports until not contagious | | | | | |
| **Spleen: enlarged** | No | No | No | Yes | Yes |
| **Testicle: absence or undescended** | Yes[13] | Yes[13] | Yes | Yes | Yes |
| [13]Certain sports may require a protective cup | | | | | |

From: American Academy of Pediatrics, Committee on Sports Medicine and Fitness. Recommendations for participation in competitive sports. *Pediatrics*. 1988;81:737-739. Reproduced by permission of *Pediatrics*; copyright © 1988.

## Family Resources

*Better Health Through Fitness.* American Academy of Pediatrics, PO Box 927, Elk Grove Village, IL 60009-0927; 1-800 433-9016.

*Anabolic Steroids and the Athlete*; *Weight Loss and Wrestlers*; *Youth Fitness.* American College of Sports Medicine, Public Information Department, PO Box 1440, Indianapolis, IN 46206-1440; (317) 637-9200.

*Get Fit: A Handbook for Youth Ages 6-17*; *Kids in Action: Fitness for Children Ages 2-17*; *Presidential Sports Awards: 4-Month Qualifications for Anyone Ages 6 and Up.* The President's Council on Physical Fitness and Sports, 701 Pennsylvania Ave. SW., Suite 250, Washington, DC 20004; (202) 272-3430.

## Selected References

American Academy of Family Physicians, Commission on Public Health and Scientific Affairs. *Age Charts for Periodic Health Examination.* Kansas City, Mo: American Academy of Family Physicians; 1993.

American Academy of Pediatrics, Committee on Sports Medicine and Fitness. Fitness, activity and sports participation in the pre-school child. *Pediatrics.* 1992;89:1002-1004.

American Academy of Pediatrics, Committee on Sports Medicine and Fitness. Recommendations for participation in competitive sports. *Pediatrics.* 1988;81:737-739.

American Academy of Pediatrics, Committee on Sports Medicine and Fitness. Strength training, weight and power lifting, and body building by children and adolescents. *Pediatrics.* 1990;86:801-803.

American Academy of Pediatrics, Committee on Sports Medicine. Counseling families. In: *Sports Medicine: Health Care for Young Athletes.* Elk Grove Village, Ill: American Academy of Pediatrics; 1983:chap 2.

American Academy of Pediatrics, Committee on Psychosocial Aspects of Child and Family Health. *Guidelines for Health Supervision.* 2nd ed. Elk Grove Village, Ill: American Academy of Pediatrics, 1988.

American College of Sports Medicine. Physical fitness in children and youth. *Med Sci Sports Exerc.* 1988;20:422-423.

American Medical Association. *Guidelines for Adolescent Preventive Services (GAPS).* Chicago, Ill: American Medical Association; 1992.

Baranowski T, Bouchard C, Bar-Or O, et al. Assessment, prevalence, and cardiovascular benefits of physical activity and fitness in youth. *Med Sci Sports Exerc.* 1992;24(suppl):S237-S247.

Must A, Jacques PF, Dallai GE, Bajema CJ, Dietz WH. Long-term morbidity and mortality of overweight adolescents: a follow-up of the Harvard Growth Study of 1922 to 1935. *N Engl J Med.* 1992;327:1350-1355.

Ross JG, Gilbert GG. The national children and youth fitness study: a summary of findings. *Journal of Physical Education, Recreation, and Dance.* 1985;56:45-50.

Ross JG, Pate RR. The national children and youth fitness study II: a summary of findings. *Journal of Physical Education, Recreation, and Dance.* 1987;58:51-56.

Sallis JF, Simons-Morton BG, Stone E, et al. Determinants of physical activity and interventions in youth. *Med Sci Sports Exerc.* 1992;24(suppl):S248-S257.

US Preventive Services Task Force. Exercise counseling. In: *Guide to Clinical Preventive Services.* Baltimore, Md: Williams & Wilkins; 1989:chap 49.

## Children/Adolescents — COUNSELING

# 21. Safety

Each year in the United States, childhood injuries cause 16 million emergency room visits, 600,000 hospitalizations, and 20,000 deaths. These injury deaths exceed childhood deaths from all other causes combined. Almost half of injury deaths are due to motor vehicle crashes, including occupant, bicycle, and pedestrian injuries. Other leading causes of unintentional childhood injury are drowning, burns and scalds, choking, firearms, falls, poisoning, and sports. Many of these injuries are preventable. Certain children are at higher risk of injury and should be targeted by clinicians: males; children with previous serious injuries; and children in families with low income, young mothers, and significant stressors. Among adolescents, alcohol use is an important risk factor for injuries of many types.

For additional information on safety, refer to chapter 25, which deals with counseling children and adolescents on violent behavior and firearms, and to chapter 54, on counseling on injury prevention for adults.

### Recommendations of Major Authorities

- All major authorities, including **American Academy of Family Physicians, American Academy of Pediatrics, Canadian Task Force on the Periodic Health Examination,** and **U.S. Preventive Services Task Force**—Age-specific safety counseling should be provided as a part of routine well-child care.

- **American Academy of Pediatrics**—Sleeping infants should be positioned on the side or back, instead of prone, to decrease the risk of sudden infant death syndrome (SIDS).

### Basics of Safety Counseling

*All Ages*

1. Parents should be encouraged to teach their children self-esteem and how to handle peer pressure that might interfere with making good safety decisions.

2. Parents should be encouraged to be good role models for safe behavior. In particular, parents should be counseled to avoid drinking before or while driving and to always wear seat belts.

3. Parents should be counseled about the importance of smoke alarms to prevent residential fire injuries, emphasizing proper installation, yearly battery changes, and monthly checks to make sure they work. The use of a family fire drill and escape plan should be discussed.

4. Parents should be encouraged to learn basic life-saving skills (CPR).

5. Parents should be encouraged not to keep a firearm in the home. If a gun is kept in the home, parents should be urged to keep it unloaded and locked up separately from the ammunition.

6. Parents should be counseled to teach their children to dial 911 or other local emergency numbers.

*Infants and Young Children*

1. Parents should be counseled about the legal requirements of child safety seat use. (They are required in all 50 states.) Only models made after January 1981 meet strict safety standards. All parents should be urged to install child safety seats on the rear seat of the car (preferably in the middle) and to use them every time children ride. Safety seats should be used until children weigh at least 40 lb (18 kg). Safety seats should face backward until children weigh 18 to 20 lb (8 to 9 kg) and are able to sit up well. Because it is not unusual for parents to fail to properly secure children in seats or the seats in the car, or both, parents should be urged to take particular care when securing both.

2. Parents should be advised to protect their children from drowning by installing fences at least 4 ft (1.2 m) high with self-latching gates completely around swimming pools. Parents should be made aware that children can drown in small amounts of water, such as may be contained in buckets, toilets, bathtubs, and wading pools.

3. To prevent falls, parents should be urged to use safety gates (preferably not the accordion type) across stairways (both top and bottom) and to install window guards above the first floor.

4. Parents should be counseled about the dangers of baby walkers, which are associated with more injuries each year than any other baby product (including strollers, high chairs, playpens, and cribs). National groups concerned about child safety have petitioned to prohibit the manufacture and sale of walkers in the United States.

5. Parents should be advised to keep objects that can cause suffocation (such as plastic bags) and choking (such as coins, small toy parts, and certain foods, including whole grapes, peanuts, raw carrots, and hot dogs) away from small children.

6. Parents should be counseled to protect their children from scald burns by reducing the temperature of their hot water heater to 49°C (120°F), if possible, or installing antiscald devices on bathroom and kitchen faucets, or both.

7. Parents should be reminded to keep medicines and other dangerous substances locked up and in child-resistant containers, to have the local poison center telephone number posted in a prominent place near the telephone, and to keep a 1-oz bottle of syrup of ipecac at home (and to replace it when it reaches its expiration date). Ipecac should not be used without first consulting with a poison control center or health professional.

8. Parents should be advised that **all** children should wear safety helmets when riding on bicycles, even as passengers.

9. Parents should be advised to keep unused electrical outlets covered with plastic guards or to install breaker outlets.

10. Parents should be advised that some authorities believe that positioning sleeping infants on their side or back, rather than prone, may decrease the risk of sudden infant death syndrome (SIDS).

*Older Children*

1. Parents should be advised to have their children sit in the rear seat of cars, if possible, and to use safety belts every time they ride. Children under 70 lb (32 kg) should use a properly secured booster seat. When a booster seat is not available, the lap belt should be worn low on the hips and adjusted snugly. If the shoulder belt crosses the child's face or neck when buckled, it should not be worn, but instead should be tucked **behind** the shoulders. Parents should be reminded that children should not ride in the cargo areas of pickup trucks, vans, or station wagons.

2. Parents should be encouraged to teach and demonstrate street safety to their children. They should be reminded that children under age 9 need supervision when crossing streets—particularly busy streets.

3. Parents should be advised that children should wear safety helmets **every** time they ride bicycles or use roller skates or in-line skates to prevent serious head injuries.

*Adolescents*

1. Adolescents and parents should be advised to use safety belts every time they operate or ride in a motor vehicle, even for short trips. Shoulder belts should be worn over the shoulder and across the chest; lap belts must ride low on the hips and fit snugly.

2. Adolescents should be advised to avoid alcohol and other drugs. They should be counseled to avoid drinking before or while driving and to avoid riding in a vehicle driven by anyone who has been or is drinking. Treatment or referral should be provided for adolescents with drug or alcohol abuse problems.

3. Adolescents should be advised of the importance of using safety helmets when on a bicycle or motorcycle, as operator or passenger, or when roller skating or in-line skating, in order to reduce the risk of serious head injuries.

**Family Resources**

*Child Safety: How to Keep Your Home Safe for Your Baby*. American Academy of Family Physicians, 8880 Ward Parkway, Kansas City, MO 64114-2797; 1-800 944-0000.

Injury prevention counseling materials, including *The Injury Prevention Program (TIPP)* and *Make Every Ride a Safe Ride.* American Academy of Pediatrics, PO Box 927, Elk Grove Village, IL 60009-0927; 1-800 433-9016.

Injury prevention magazines, brochures, posters, videos, and other material. National SAFE KIDS Campaign, 111 Michigan Ave. NE., Washington, DC 20010; (202) 939-4993.

Pamphlets on preventing injuries from toys, household goods, and other common items. U.S. Consumer Product Safety Commission, Publication Requests, Washington, DC 20207; 1-800 638-2772.

Brochures and information on prevention of motor vehicle trauma and alcohol-related traffic injuries. U.S. Department of Transportation National Highway Traffic Safety Administration; (202) 366-2705.

*Staying Healthy and Whole: A Consumer Guide to Product Safety Recalls.* U.S. Office of Consumer Affairs. Superintendent of Documents, Consumer Information Center—3C, PO Box 100, Pueblo, CO 81002.

**Provider Resources**

*HELP: Motor Vehicle Trauma*; *HELP Newsletter*, vol 2, no 1; *Prevention of Motor Vehicle Trauma Course: Is 40 Years Worth 3 Seconds of Your Time?* (kit with manual and videotape). American Academy of Family Physicians, 8880 Ward Parkway, Kansas City, MO 64114-2797; 1-800 944-0000.

*A Guide to Safety Counseling in Office Practice*; *Physician's Resource Guide for Bicycle Safety Education.* American Academy of Pediatrics, PO Box 927, Elk Grove Village, IL 60009-0927; 1-800 433-9016.

**Selected References**

Alpert JJ, Guyer B, eds. Symposium on injuries and injury prevention. *Pediatr Clin North Am.* 1985;32:1-270.
American Academy of Family Physicians, Commission on Public Health and Scientific Affairs. *Age Charts for Periodic Health Examination.* Kansas City, Mo: American Academy of Family Physicians; 1993.
American Academy of Pediatrics, Committee on Accident and Poison Prevention. *Injury Control for Children and Youth.* Elk Grove Village, Ill: American Academy of Pediatrics; 1987.
American Academy of Pediatrics, Committee on Accident and Poison Prevention. Injury Prevention. In: *Policy Reference Guide: A Comprehensive Guide to AAP Policy Statements Published through December 1990.* Elk Grove Village, Ill: American Academy of Pediatrics; 1991:315.
American Academy of Pediatrics. *The Injury Prevention Program (TIPP).* Elk Grove Village, Ill: American Academy of Pediatrics; 1989.
American College of Obstetricians and Gynecologists. *Automobile Passenger Restraints for Children and Pregnant Women.* Washington, DC: American College of Obstetricians and Gynecologists; 1991. ACOG Technical Bulletin 151.

American Medical Association. *Guidelines for Adolescent Preventive Services (GAPS)*. Chicago, Ill: American Medical Association; 1992.

Baker SP, O'Neill B, Karpf RS. *The Injury Fact Book*. Lexington, Mass: DC Heath & Co; 1984.

Centers for Disease Control. Childhood injuries in the United States. *AJDC*. 1990;144:627–646.

*Final Regulatory Impact Assessment on Amendments to Federal Motor Vehicle Safety Standard 208, Front Seat Occupant Protection*. Washington, DC: US Dept of Transportation, 1984. US DOT publication HS 806–572.

National Committee for Injury Prevention and Control. Injury Prevention: Meeting the Challenge. *Am J Prev Med*. 1989;5(3)(suppl).

National Highway Traffic Safety Administration and National Institute on Alcohol Abuse and Alcoholism. *Shifting into Action: Youth and Highway Safety*. Washington, DC: 1985. US DOT publication HS 806–798.

Rivara FP. Traumatic deaths of children in the United States: currently available prevention strategies. *Pediatrics*. 1985;75:456–462.

US Preventive Services Task Force. Counseling to prevent household and environmental injuries. In: *Guide to Clinical Preventive Services*. Baltimore, Md: Williams & Wilkins; 1989:chap 52.

## Children/Adolescents — COUNSELING

# 22. Sexually Transmitted Diseases and HIV Infection

Sexually transmitted diseases (STDs), including human immunodeficiency virus (HIV) infection, constitute a major health problem for adolescents. For the past three decades, the percentage of adolescents reporting sexual activity has steadily increased, with over 54% of all students in grades 9 to 12 now reporting being sexually active. This pattern of increased adolescent sexual behavior is paralleled by increased prevalence in adolescents of sexually transmitted diseases, including gonorrhea, chlamydia, syphilis, herpes simplex virus (HSV), human papilloma virus (HPV), and HIV. Among AIDS patients, 20% are in their midtwenties and probably became infected during their adolescence—predominantly by a sexual route. The consequences of non-HIV STDs can also be very serious for teenagers. Gonorrhea and chlamydia lead to pelvic inflammatory disease and potential sterility ten times more frequently in adolescent than in adult females. Syphilis, although relatively asymptomatic in the primary phase, may cause great damage to multiple organ systems in later stages. HPV, which may be the most prevalent sexually transmitted disease in adolescents, can lead to cervical neoplasia. HIV transmission may be facilitated by the presence of other STDs. STDs in pregnancy can lead to a number of serious consequences for the fetus or newborn child, including congenital infections and malformations, prematurity, low birth weight, and increased mortality.

Adolescents at high risk for HIV and other STDs include those: 1) with multiple sexual partners; 2) who reside in areas with a high prevalence of STD/HIV infection; 3) who are homosexual or bisexual males; 4) who have been sexually abused by or have had sexual contact with individuals with documented STD/HIV infection or injection drug use; 5) who have a past history of STDs; 6) who trade sex for money or drugs; 7) who use drugs (particularly if injected) or alcohol; 8) who are or have been pregnant and continue to be sexually active.

Refer to chapter 39 for information on screening for STDs and HIV infection. Material on counseling adults on STDs and HIV infection can be found in chapter 58. Related information on counseling adolescents and adults to prevent unintended pregnancy can be found in chapters 24 and 60.

**Recommendations of Major Authorities**

- **American Academy of Family Physicians (AAFP)** and **U.S. Preventive Services Task Force**—Clinicians should take a complete sexual and drug use history on all adolescent patients. Sexually active patients should be advised that abstaining from sex and maintaining a mutually faithful monogamous sexual relationship with a partner known to be uninfected are the most effective strategies to prevent infection with HIV and other STDs. Patients should also receive counseling about the indications and proper methods for using condoms and spermicides in sexual intercourse and about the health risks associated with anal intercourse. Injecting drug users should be encouraged to enroll in a drug treatment program and should be warned against sharing drug equipment and using unsterilized needles and syringes.

- **American Academy of Pediatrics**—As a routine part of health supervision, adolescents should be asked about sexual behavior and provided with counseling about responsible sexual behavior, including contraception and prevention of STDs and HIV. Condom use should be recommended to both males and females.

- **American College of Obstetricians and Gynecologists**—Adolescents should be routinely counseled about sexual practices and sexually transmitted diseases, including partner selection and use of barrier protection.

- **American Medical Association**—All adolescents should be asked annually about involvement in sexual behaviors that may result in unintended pregnancy and STDs, including HIV infection. This should include their use of and motivation to use condoms. All sexually active adolescents should be screened for gonorrhea and chlamydia; high-risk adolescents should be screened for syphilis; and HIV testing should be offered to high-risk adolescents.

- **American Nurses Association**—Education about the risks of HIV infection, basic sex information, including the option of abstinence, and the essential features of safer sex practices should be a major priority within community health practice with a special emphasis in school health settings and school-based clinics.

## Basics of STD and HIV Counseling

1. A trusting, caring relationship should be established with both patients and parents. Sensitivity to the cultural and personal needs of patients and families is essential.

2. Parents should be counselled about the role of emerging sexuality in teenagers' lives and the importance of methods to prevent STDs and HIV. It is very important to foster effective communication between adolescents and parents regarding responsible, safer sexual behavior.

3. An atmosphere in which adolescents feel comfortable disclosing their sexual behaviors should be provided. Interviews should be conducted without parents present. The importance and limits of confidentiality in the clinician's relationship with patients should be made explicit to both patients and parents.

4. It may be helpful to begin discussing sexual behavior and drug use indirectly, by asking patients about the behavior of their friends and peers, before moving to an explicit discussion of the patient's own knowledge, attitudes, behaviors, and beliefs. See Table 58-1 for examples of questions for taking clinical histories about sexual behavior, contraceptive use, and drug use.

5. All adolescents should be counseled that STD and HIV infections are most effectively prevented by abstinence. Adolescents who desire to abstain from sexual activity should be supported.

6. Adolescents should be educated explicitly about sexual practices and drug use behavior that will put them and their partners at high risk for STDs and HIV infections, and about those measures that will minimize risk (e.g., use of condoms). They should also be educated explicitly about the long- and short-term consequences of STD and HIV infections. As appropriate, this education should be provided to preadolescents as well.

7. It is essential that adolescents understand that their partners' sexual and drug behaviors can put them at risk. A thorough drug use history is important not only because HIV can be transmitted through injection drug use, but also because of the "disinhibiting" effects of alcohol and other drug use, which can lead to unsafe behaviors responsible for transmission of STDs and HIV.

8. The state or local health agency responsible for communicable disease reporting should be contacted to determine local prevalence of STD and HIV infections. This agency also can provide information regarding state and local laws regulating patient testing, confidentiality, and reporting cases of infection.

9. All adolescents should be counseled about the importance of properly using condoms (see Table 22-1) during sexual activity to help prevent STDs and HIV. Many adolescents, particularly at younger ages, are hesitant to purchase condoms on their own. Adolescents should be counseled about how to purchase condoms and about access to other sources of condoms. Some authorities advocate providing condoms at office visits.

10. Educational materials about prevention of STDs and HIV should be provided to patients and parents. (See Family Resources.)

### Table 22-1. Guidelines for Proper Condom Use

| |
|---|
| Condoms made of latex, rather than natural membrane, should be used. |
| Torn condoms, those in damaged packages, or those with signs of age (brittle, sticky, discolored, past expiration date) should not be used. |
| The condom should be put on an erect penis, unrolled completely to the base, before the penis comes in contact with a body opening. |
| A space should be left at the tip of the condom to collect semen; air pockets in the space should be removed by pressing the air out towards the base. |
| Only water-based lubricants should be used. Those made with petroleum jelly, mineral oil, cold cream, vegetable oil, and other oils should not be applied because they may damage the condom. |
| Nonoxynol 9 inside the condom or inside the vagina may increase protection against STDs and HIV. However, if spermicides cause local irritation, they may increase risk of HIV. Nonoxynol 9 does not give added protection in anal intercourse. |
| If a condom breaks, it should be replaced immediately. |
| After ejaculation and while the penis is still erect, the penis should be withdrawn while the condom is carefully held against the base of the penis so that the condom remains in place. |
| Condoms should not be reused. |

Adapted from: U.S. Preventive Services Task Force. Counseling to prevent human immunodeficiency virus infection and other sexually transmitted diseases. In: *Guide to Clinical Preventive Services*. Baltimore, MD: Williams & Wilkins; 1989:chap. 53.

## Family Resources

*AIDS: How To Reduce Your Risk of Catching It*; *AIDS: A Guide for Survival*. American Academy of Family Physicians, 8880 Ward Parkway, Kansas City, MO 64114-2797; 1-800 944-0000.

*Being a Teenager: You and Your Sexuality*; *Sexually Transmitted Diseases*. American College of Obstetricians and Gynecologists, 409 12th Street SW., Washington, DC 20024-2188; 1-800 762-2264.

*Caring for Your Adolescent: Age 12 to 21*; *Sex Education for Adolescents: A Bibliography of Low Cost Materials*. American Academy of Pediatrics, PO Box 927, Elk Grove Village, IL 60009-0927; 1-800 433-9016.

*Condoms and Sexually Transmitted Diseases...Especially AIDS*. Food and Drug Administration, Center for Devices and Radiological Health. HHS publication FDA 90-4239; available from National AIDS Clearinghouse: 1-800 458-5231.

*Jimmy and the Eggs Virus*, parent information booklets, and other materials on pediatric AIDS. National Pediatric HIV Resource Center, 15 South Ninth Street, Newark, NJ 07107; (201) 268-8251.

*9 Common Sexually Transmitted Diseases*. American Council for Healthful Living, 39 Main St., Orange, NJ 07050; (201) 674-7476.

*Teenagers and AIDS; AIDS Prevention Program for Youth: Information for Students*. American Red Cross, contact local chapter or National Office of HIV-AIDS Education; (202) 973-6000.

*National AIDS Information Hot Line*. 1-800 342-AIDS (English speaking); 1-800 344-SIDA (Spanish speaking); 1-800 AIDS-TTY (hearing impaired). All phone calls are confidential.

*National AIDS Information Clearinghouse*, P.O. Box 6003, Rockville, MD 20850; 1-800 458-5231 (English and Spanish).

*National STD Hot Line*: 1-800 227-8922.

## Provider Resources

*AIDS: A slide show for early adolescents*—A 45-minute scripted slide show for presentations to adolescents; *HIV Infection and AIDS* (monograph); *HIV Infection in the Family Physician's Office* (brochure); and *Clinical and Psychosocial Aspects of Caring for HIV Patients* (audiotape). American Academy of Family Physicians, 8880 Ward Parkway, Kansas City, MO 64114-2797; 1-800 944-0000.

*Caring for Families with HIV*; *HIV and AIDS in Children: Questions and Answers*; and others. National Pediatric HIV Resource Center, 15 South Ninth Street, Newark, NJ 07107; (201) 268-8251.

Information on hemophilia and HIV. Hemophilia and AIDS Network for the Dissemination of Information, 110 Green Street, New York, NY 10012; 1-800 424-2634.

**Selected References**

AIDS & Adolescents Network of New York. *HIV Antibody Counseling and Testing for Adolescents: Policy Recommendations and Practical Guidelines*. New York, NY: AIDS & Adolescents Network of New York; 1992.

American Academy of Family Physicians, Commission on Public Health and Scientific Affairs. *Age Charts for Periodic Health Examination*. Kansas City, Mo: American Academy of Family Physicians; 1993.

American Academy of Pediatrics, Committee on School Health. Acquired immunodeficiency syndrome education in schools. *Pediatrics*. 1988;82:278-280.

American Academy of Pediatrics, Committee on Adolescence. Contraception and adolescents. *Pediatrics*. 1990;86:134-138.

American Academy of Pediatrics, Committee on Psychosocial Aspects of Child and Family Health. *Guidelines for Health Supervision*. 2nd ed. Elk Grove Village, Ill: American Academy of Pediatrics; 1988.

American Academy of Pediatrics, Committee on Adolescence. Homosexuality and adolescence. *Pediatrics* 1983;72:249-250.

American Academy of Pediatrics, Committee on Adolescence. Role of the pediatrician in the management of sexually transmitted disease in children and adolescents. *Pediatrics*. 1987;79:454-456.

American Academy of Pediatrics, Committee on Adolescence. Sexuality, contraception, and the media. *Pediatrics*. 1986;78:535-536.

American College of Obstetricians and Gynecologists. *The Obstetrician-Gynecologist and Primary-Preventive Health Care*. Washington, DC: American College of Obstetricians and Gynecologist; 1993.

American College of Obstetricians and Gynecologists. *The Adolescent Obstetric-Gynecologic Patient*. Washington, DC: American College of Obstetricians and Gynecologists; 1990. ACOG Technical Bulletin 145.

American Medical Association. *Guidelines for Adolescent Preventive Services (GAPS)*. Chicago, Ill: American Medical Association; 1992.

Brookman RR. Adolescent Sexual Behavior. In: Holmes KK, Mardh P, Sparling PF, Wiesner PJ, eds. *Sexually Transmitted Diseases*. New York, NY: McGraw-Hill Book Co.; 1990:chap. 8.

Cates W. The epidemiology and control of sexually transmitted diseases in adolescents. *Adolescent Medicine: State of the Art Reviews*. 1990;1:409-427.

Centers for Disease Control. Sexual behavior among high school students—United States, 1990. *MMWR*. 1992;40:885-888.

Hatcher, RA, Stewart F, Trussell J, et al. *Contraceptive Technology 1990-1992*. New York, NY: Irvington Publishers; 1990.

US Department of Health and Human Services. Sexually transmitted diseases. In: *Healthy People 2000: National Health Promotion and Disease Prevention Objectives*. Washington, DC: US Dept of Health and Human Services, Public Health Service; 1991:chap 19. DHHS publication PHS 91-50212.

US Preventive Services Task Force. Counseling to prevent human immunodeficiency virus infection and other sexually transmitted diseases. In: *Guide to Clinical Preventive Services*. Baltimore, Md: Williams & Wilkins; 1989:chap 53.

## Children/Adolescents — COUNSELING

# 23. Tobacco

Tobacco use continues to be the single largest cause of preventable illness and death in the United States. Cigarette smoking, smokeless tobacco use, and exposure to environmental tobacco smoke create significant health hazards for all children and adolescents.

The morbidity and mortality of smoking and the benefits of smoking cessation are well known (see Fig 59-1). Approximately 19% of high school students report daily smoking of cigarettes—a figure that has remained unchanged in recent years. Use among female adolescents remains higher than among male adolescents. Cigarette smoking is increasingly common in younger children; in 1990, the average age of initial cigarette use was 11.6 years. Approximately 95% of regular adult cigarette smokers initiate smoking before 20 years of age. Children from families in which one or both parents smoke are twice as likely to smoke as those whose parents do not smoke.

Smokeless tobacco use in children and adolescents is increasing. Users have an increased risk of oral cancer and leukoplakia. Some case studies also have reported gingival recession at the site of tobacco placement and increased periodontal disease. Use of smokeless tobacco is estimated at 10% among high school students and is significantly higher among males in some regions of the country. More than half of all smokeless tobacco users begin by 13 years of age, and some begin as early as 4 or 5 years of age.

Exposure to environmental tobacco smoke is a potential health hazard to infants and young children. An estimated 39% of households with one or more children aged 6 or younger contain at least one smoker. Passive smoking can exacerbate the symptoms of asthma and allergies and decrease pulmonary function and the rate of lung growth. Children who are exposed to passive smoking also have higher rates of lower respiratory tract infections, middle ear infections, and lung cancer.

See chapter 59 for additional information about smoking cessation.

### Recommendations of Major Authorities

- **All major authorities**—Primary care clinicians should counsel both parents and children about the importance of avoiding initiating tobacco use and of stopping tobacco use after initiation.

- **American Academy of Pediatrics**—Clinicians should obtain a history of environmental tobacco smoke exposure when encountering a child with a respiratory illness, and should inform both patients and parents about the hazards of tobacco use.

- **American Medical Association**—Adolescents should receive annual screening and health guidance to promote avoidance of tobacco use. A cessation plan should be provided for adolescents who use tobacco products.

- **National Cancer Institute**—Clinicians treating children should follow five principles that start with the letter *A* in counseling about smoking prevention/cessation:

  1. Anticipate the risk for tobacco use at each developmental stage.
  2. Ask about exposure to tobacco smoke and tobacco use at each visit.
  3. Advise all smoking parents to stop and all children not to use tobacco products.
  4. Assist children in resisting tobacco use; assist tobacco users in quitting.
  5. Arrange follow-up visits as required.

**Basics of Tobacco Counseling**

1. A smoke-free environment should be maintained in the medical office or clinic. Smoking by staff, patients, or their parents should not be allowed in the office or waiting room. No-smoking signs should be posted and literature about the importance of avoiding tobacco use and stopping smoking should be made readily available.

2. Clinicians should obtain a history for all patients regarding tobacco use in the child's household and day-care or school settings. If parents or other family members smoke, the importance of stopping should be stressed. Emphasizing the negative health consequences for the child can be an effective strategy in dealing with parents. Parents who desire to quit smoking should receive proper counseling and support, either by the clinician or by referral (see chapter 59). Use of ineffective measures, such as blowing smoke away from a child, attempting to increase ventilation in a room, or smoking in another but contiguous room, should be discouraged.

3. All children should be asked about tobacco use. It is probably never too early to start talking about tobacco use, only too late—if a child has already started using tobacco. Information should be elicited in a nonthreatening manner. The absence of parents from the room is often helpful. Discussion during a physical examination is often well-received by children and adolescents. Adolescents may be able to complete a previsit questionnaire. They often find this to be a nonthreatening way to reveal information about tobacco use and other sensitive issues.

4. Discussion of tobacco use avoidance or cessation with children or adolescents should emphasize the unattractive cosmetic (stained teeth and fingernails, oral sores, and foul-smelling breath and clothes) and athletic (decreased endurance, shortness of breath) consequences of tobacco use. The negative social consequences, such as disapproval by peers, should also be emphasized. These strategies are generally more effective with children and adolescents than discussing long-term health consequences.

5. Children and adolescents should be advised that, contrary to popular belief, use of smokeless tobacco is not safer and can be more addicting than cigarette use. Smokeless tobacco causes many health problems, some of which may be life-threatening, such as oral cancer.

6. Clinicians should work with children and adolescents who use tobacco to set a quit date. A written "contract" may be helpful. Pamphlets and other informational materials of an appropriate reading level may also be of use.

7. Smokers who have quit should be supported with positive feedback and suggestions of ways to avoid negative peer pressure and deal with withdrawal symptoms. Exercise and other healthful activities should be encouraged. Scheduling follow-up visits and phone calls may help encourage continued abstinence from tobacco.

8. The use of nicotine gum and dermal patches has not been tested adequately in children and adolescents. Their use with children and adolescents should, in general, be avoided.

**Family Resources**

*Chew or Snuff Is Real Bad Stuff; Why Do You Smoke?* National Cancer Institute. Superintendent of Documents, Consumer Information Center—3C, PO Box 100, Pueblo, CO 81002.

*Through with Chew.* American Academy of Otolaryngology, 1 Prince St., Alexandria, VA 22314; (703) 836-4444.

*Smoking: Guidelines for Teens*; *Tobacco Abuse—A Message to Parents and Teens.* American Academy of Pediatrics, PO Box 927, Elk Grove Village, IL 60009-0927; 1-800 433-9016.

*Smokeless Tobacco: Think Before You Chew.* American Dental Association, Dept. of Salable Materials, 211 E. Chicago Ave., Chicago, Il 60611; 1-800 947-4746.

**Provider Resources**

*Clinical Interventions To Prevent Tobacco Use by Children and Adolescents*; *How To Help Your Patients Stop Smoking: A National Cancer Institute Manual for Physicians.* National Cancer Institute; 1-800 4-CANCER.

**Selected References**

American Academy of Family Physicians, Commission on Public Health and Scientific Affairs. *Age Charts for Periodic Health Examination.* Kansas City, Mo: American Academy of Family Physicians; 1993.
American Academy of Pediatrics, Committee on Environmental Hazards. Involuntary smoking—a hazard to children. *Pediatrics.* 1986;77:755-757.
American Academy of Pediatrics, Committee on Environmental Hazards. Smokeless tobacco—a carcinogenic hazard to children. *Pediatrics.* 1985;75:1009-1011.
American Academy of Pediatrics, Committee on Adolescence. Tobacco use by children and adolescents. *Pediatrics.* 1987;79:479-481.
American Medical Association. *Guidelines for Adolescent Preventive Services (GAPS).* Chicago, Ill: American Medical Association; 1992.
Epps RP, Manley MW. Clinical Interventions to Prevent Tobacco Use by Children and Adolescents. Bethesda, Md: National Cancer Institute, US Dept of Health and Human Services; 1991.

Epps RP, Manley MW. A physician's guide to preventing tobacco use during childhood and adolescence. *Pediatrics*. 1991;88:140-144.

McGinnis JM, Shopland D, Brown C. Tobacco and health: trends in smoking and smokeless tobacco consumption in the United States. *Annu Rev Public Health*. 1987;8:441-67.

Schonberg KS, ed. *Substance Abuse: A Guide for Health Professionals*. Elk Grove Village, Ill: American Academy of Pediatrics; 1988.

US Preventive Services Task Force. Counseling to prevent tobacco use. In: *Guide to Clinical Preventive Services*. Baltimore, Md: Williams & Wilkins; 1989:chap 48.

## Children/Adolescents — COUNSELING

# 24. Unintended Pregnancy

The teenage pregnancy rate in the United States is the highest of any country in the Western world. Every year, more than 1 million U.S. teenagers become pregnant. By 18 years of age, 24% of U.S. female teenagers have become pregnant at least once. The majority of teenage pregnancies are unplanned, and less than half (47%) of these pregnancies result in a live birth. Forty percent are terminated by elective abortion; 13% end in miscarriage. Unintended pregnancy affects nonwhite teenagers at a rate approaching twice that of white teenagers.

Teenagers are becoming sexually active at increasingly younger ages. In 1982, 19% of unmarried females 15 years of age reported sexual activity. By 1988, this had increased to 27%. In 1990, 48% of female and 61% of male high school students reported having experienced sexual intercourse. Teenagers are less likely than adults to use contraception, particularly at younger ages and during initial sexual encounters. About half of teenagers use a contraceptive method (almost exclusively condoms) during first intercourse. Seventy-eight percent of teenagers report using some form of contraception during their most recent intercourse. Teenagers who use contraceptives do so less effectively than adults. Teenagers who use birth control pills are almost twice as likely to become pregnant as adults who use birth control pills.

Teenage pregnancy is more likely to result in adverse health outcomes for mother and baby than adult pregnancy, largely as a result of later prenatal care, poor nutrition, and other life-style factors. Teenage mothers are at an increased risk of being socioeconomically disadvantaged compared with those who delay childbearing until their twenties. The Center for Population Options estimated societal costs of adolescent parenthood in 1989 at $21.55 billion (50% for Aid-to-Dependent Children payments, 35% for food stamp payments, and 15% for Medicaid payments).

For information on counseling to prevent unintended pregnancy in adults, see chapter 60. Also, refer to related information on counseling to prevent sexually transmitted diseases (STDs) and HIV infection among adolescents (chapter 22) and adults (chapter 58).

**Recommendations of Major Authorities**

- All major authorities, including **American Academy of Family Physicians (AAFP), American Academy of Pediatrics (AAP), American College of Obstetricians and Gynecologists (ACOG), American Medical Association (AMA)**, and **U.S. Preventive Services Task Force (USPSTF)**—Primary care providers should routinely counsel adolescents in the prevention of unintended pregnancies. **AAP** recommends that all pediatricians who choose to see teenagers should be able to provide counseling about sexual behavior, education on contraceptive methods and prevention of STDs, and assistance with access to contraception, preferably in the office or, if necessary, by referral. **ACOG** recommends that special attention be given to ensure that sexually active adolescents have access to suitable methods of contraception. **AMA** recommends that all adolescents should be asked annually about involvement in sexual behaviors that may result in unintended pregnancy and STDs, including HIV infection. **AAFP** and **USPSTF** recommend that clinicians should obtain a complete sexual history from adolescents and that detailed counseling on methods to prevent unintended pregnancy be given to those who do not want to have a child. Counseling on sexual development and behavior should also be routinely provided. This is often best performed early in adolescence and with the involvement of parents. **AAFP** recommends that sex education be included in the periodic health examination for children beginning at 7 years of age.

## Basics of Counseling To Prevent Unintended Pregnancy

1. All adolescents should be asked about their sexual experiences and use of contraceptive methods. An attempt should be made by the clinician to maintain a nonjudgmental, empathetic manner. It may be helpful to begin this discussion with questions about the patient's peer group before moving on to more explicit questions about the patient's own sexual behavior. The clinician's willingness to answer any questions and to provide contraceptive advice and prescriptions should be stated. Explicit information should be provided to adolescents about the consequences of pregnancy and STDs, and about effective methods to prevent them.

2. Adolescents should be spoken to without parents in the room, assuring confidentiality to the maximum extent possible. State laws vary regarding the minimum age for consenting to treatment or receiving prescription contraceptives, or both. Clinicians should familiarize themselves with the laws in their state regarding these issues. Adolescents should be informed about their legal rights to confidentiality regarding pregnancy prevention and STD testing and treatment.

3. Parents should be counselled about the role of emerging sexuality in teenagers' lives and the options for contraception. It is very important to foster effective communication between adolescents and their families regarding responsible sexual behavior.

4. Adolescents who are sexually abstinent should be supported in remaining abstinent, if they so desire. All patients should be supported in resisting unwelcome or coercive sexual relationships.

5. Sexually active adolescents should be assisted in choosing an effective, appropriate primary method of contraception. This should take into consideration their personal preferences and motivation, religious beliefs, cultural norms, and relationship with their partner(s).

The pregnancy ("failure") rates for women in the first year of use of contraceptives are given in Table 60-1. The failure rates for adolescent use may be considerably higher than those given. The two most popular methods among adolescents are birth control pills and condoms. Implants or injectable contraceptives may also be appropriate choices for teens.

In general, diaphragms, cervical caps, withdrawal, and periodic abstinence are technically more difficult for teenagers to use effectively. Intrauterine devices (IUDs) are not recommended for adolescents because of increased risk of pelvic inflammatory disease, which may lead to sterility. Permanent sterilization procedures are not appropriate for adolescents. In situations of unprotected intercourse, it may be appropriate to suggest emergency contraceptive pills ("morning after pills") if treatment can be initiated within 72 hours after sexual contact. See the discussion on emergency contraception in chapter 60.

6. All sexually active adolescents, except perhaps those in a mutually monogamous relationship, should be encouraged to use condoms as a means of preventing STDs and HIV—even if they are using another form of contraception. Many teenagers, particularly at younger ages, are hesitant to purchase condoms. Educating teenagers about their rights to purchase condoms and about access to other sources of condoms can be helpful. Some authorities recommend making condoms available to teenagers during office visits.

7. Adolescents of both genders should be encouraged to talk frankly with their partners about STDs, HIV, and the use of contraceptives. Assertiveness with their partners about the use of contraception and protective measures against STDs should be supported. It should also be stressed that saying "no," without coercion or fear, is every person's right each and every time.

8. Males should be provided with as much counseling as females about contraception and STD prevention. The young adolescent male should be taught responsible sexual behavior at an early age—particularly regarding the importance of condom use.

9. Close follow-up should be provided to adolescents after beginning contraceptive use. Contraceptives are often unnecessarily discontinued by adolescents because of concerns about side effects and misconceptions about proper technique. Many of these concerns and misconceptions can be easily dealt with in follow-up counseling. Table 24-1 provides sample responses to some common concerns of adolescents about oral contraceptives.

**Family Resources**

*Being a Teenager: You and Your Sexuality; Teaching Your Children About Sexuality, Growing Up.* American College of Obstetricians and Gynecologists, 409 12th St. SW, Washington, DC 20024; 1-800 762-2264.

*Birth Control: Choosing the Method That's Right for You.* American Academy of Family Physicians, 8880 Ward Parkway, Kansas City, MO 64114-2797; 1-800 944-0000.

*How to Talk With Your Child About Sexuality, Decisions About Sex; How to Talk to Your Teenagers About the Facts of Life.* Planned Parenthood, 810 Seventh Ave., New York, NY 10019; (212) 541-7800.

*Making the Right Choice: Facts Young People Need to Know About Avoiding Pregnancy.* American Academy of Pediatrics, 141 Northwest Point Blvd., P.O. Box 927, Elk Grove Village, IL 60009-0927; 1-800 433-9016.

### Table 24-1. Addressing Adolescents' Common Concerns About Oral Contraceptives

| Concern | Response |
| --- | --- |
| Weight gain | Women are as likely to lose weight as gain weight while using oral contraceptives. |
| Irregular bleeding | This is a common side effect that tends to resolve after a few cycles of use. |
| Nausea, acne, vaginal discharge | These are uncommon side effects. They can usually be eliminated by changing to a different type of pill. |
| Cancer risk | Oral contraceptive use decreases risk of endometrial and ovarian cancer. An increased risk of breast cancer is unproven. |
| Sexually transmitted diseases | Oral contraceptive use does not prevent STDs but does decrease the risk of developing pelvic inflammatory disease. Latex condoms are the only form of birth control that can help prevent STDs and HIV. |
| Ovarian cysts, benign breast disease | The incidence and severity of these are decreased by oral contraceptive use. |
| Blood clots | The risk of death is very small for adolescents using low-dose oral contraceptives—less than from an abortion or continuing a pregnancy. |

Adapted from: American College of Obstetricians and Gynecologists. *Safety of Oral Contraceptives for Teenagers*. Washington, DC: American College of Obstetricians and Gynecologists; 1991. ACOG Committee Opinion No. 90. Reproduced by permission of the publisher; copyright © 1991.

## Provider Resources

*The Adolescent and Young Adult Fact Book*; *Evaluating Your Adolescent Pregnancy Program: How to Get Started*; *Teenage Pregnancy Prevention Strategies*; *What About the Boys?*; posters and other materials on adolescents and pregnancy. Children's Defense Fund, 25 E Street NW., Washington, DC 20001; (202) 628-8787.

## Selected References

American Academy of Family Physicians, Commission on Public Health and Scientific Affairs. *Age Charts for Periodic Health Examination*. Kansas City, Mo: American Academy of Family Physicians; 1993.

American Academy of Pediatrics. Committee on Adolescence: Contraception and Adolescents. *Pediatrics*. 1990;86:134-138.

American College of Obstetricians and Gynecologists. *Safety of Oral Contraceptives for Teenagers*. Washington, DC: American College of Obstetricians and Gynecologists; 1991. ACOG Committee Opinion No. 90.

American College of Obstetricians and Gynecologists. *The Adolescent Obstetric-Gynecologic Patient.* Washington, DC: American College of Obstetricians and Gynecologists; 1990. ACOG Technical Bulletin No. 145.

American Medical Association. *Guidelines for Adolescent Preventive Services (GAPS).* Chicago, Ill: American Medical Association; 1992.

Canadian Task Force on the Periodic Health Examination. The periodic health examination: 2. 1987 update. *Can Med Assoc J.* 1988;138:618-626.

Center for Population Options. *Teenage Pregnancy and Too-Early Childbearing: Public Costs, Personal Consequences.* 5th ed. Washington, DC: Center for Population Options; 1990.

Centers for Disease Control. Sexual behavior among high school students: United States, 1990. *MMWR.* 1991;40:85-88.

Hatcher RA, Stewart F, Trussell J, et al. *Contraceptive Technology 1990-1992.* New York, NY: Irvington Publishers; 1990.

Hatcher RA, Trussell J, Stewart F, et al. *Contraceptive Technology.* 16th Rev. Ed. New York, NY: Irvington Publishers; 1994.

US Preventive Services Task Force. Counseling to prevent unintended pregnancy. In: *Guide to Clinical Preventive Services.* Baltimore, Md: Williams & Wilkins; 1989:chap 54.

Ventura SJ, Taffel SM, Mosher WD, Henshaw S. Trends in pregnancies and pregnancy rates, United States, 1980-88. *Monthly Vital Statistics Report.* 41;6(suppl). Hyattsville, Md: National Center for Health Statistics; 1993. US Dept of Health and Human Services publication PHS 93-1120.

# Children/Adolescents — COUNSELING

## 25. Violent Behavior and Firearms

Violence is a major health and social problem affecting children and adolescents in the United States. Homicide is the third leading cause of death for 15- to 24-year-olds and the leading cause of death for African-American males in that age group. Firearms are involved in at least two-thirds of homicides involving children and adolescents. A large proportion (41%) of school-age boys report easy access to a gun, and in the past decade more than 7000 people have died as a result of homicides committed by teenagers using firearms. There are handguns in one out of four homes in the United States. For every instance in which a gun is used in self-defense, there are 40 shooting deaths of family members or acquaintances in suicides, nonjustifiable homicides, and accidents.

For adolescent males, the risk of dying from homicide is twice that of adolescent females, and the risk of victimization from other violent crimes is three times greater. Urban males of low socioeconomic status and low educational achievement are at the highest risk of being affected by violence. Other risk factors include a history of juvenile detention or incarceration, alcohol or other drug use, access to firearms, homelessness, mental illness, social isolation, and violence in the home. The risk factors for victims and perpetrators of violence are similar.

For information about depression and suicide, see chapter 5 (for children and adolescents) and chapter 32 (for adults). For information about alcohol and other drug abuse, see chapter 17 (for children and adolescents) and chapter 52 (for adults). For information about safety and injury prevention, see chapter 21 (for children and adolescents) and chapter 54 (for adults).

**Recommendations of Major Authorities**

- **American Academy of Family Physicians** and **U.S. Preventive Services Task Force**—Teenagers (especially boys) should be routinely counseled about violent behavior and firearms. Clinicians should ask adolescent males to discuss previous violent behavior, current alcohol and drug use, and the availability of firearms. Patients with evidence of violent behavior should be counseled regarding nonviolent alternatives for conflict resolution and about the risks of violent injury associated with easy access to firearms and intoxication with alcohol or other drugs.

- **American Academy of Pediatrics**—Adolescents and their parents should be questioned about impulsiveness, antisocial behavior, and methods of dealing with anger. The clinician should be concerned about adolescents who display aggressive or acting-out behaviors, such as lying, stealing, temper outbursts, vandalism, excessive fighting, and destructiveness. All adolescent-health-care providers should promote the responsibility of every family to create a gun-safe home environment, with particular emphasis placed on high-risk homes—those with alcohol or drug-prone or drug-addicted individuals—and those with adolescent boys. This should include asking about the presence of guns in the home; counseling patients, parents, and relatives (particularly male relatives) on the dangers of having a gun, especially a handgun, in the home; advising the removal or reduction of guns in the household; providing office literature on the risks of guns; and emphasizing gun safety rules when patients visit friends' homes. Asking about the presence of a gun in the home and, if one is present, counseling on its removal or secured storage may be the most effective action the primary care clinician can take.

- **American Medical Association**—Parents or other adult care-givers of adolescents should be given health guidance during their children's early, middle, and late adolescence (more often if necessary) to avoid having weapons in the home and, if weapons are kept in the home, to make them inaccessible to adolescents. Weapons should be removed from homes of adolescents with suicidal intent.

## Basics of Violent Behavior and Firearms Counseling

1. Prevention of violence-related injuries should be made a priority. Every child and family should be assessed for the potential for injury from violence. Some factors to consider include:

    - Is there a history of violent injury to the child or other family members?
    - Is there a history of alcohol or other drug abuse by the child or other family members?
    - Are there guns or other weapons in the home?
    - Is violent injury a prevalent problem in the community?

2. All parents should be advised about the dangers of keeping a gun in the home. This advice may be better accepted if given as part of general counseling on safety-related issues. The following model intervention has been suggested by the American Academy of Pediatrics and the Center To Prevent Handgun Violence (1992):

    > You are doing all you can to make sure your children are not hurt—by using a car seat, buckling up safety belts in the car, locking away poisonous chemicals, and putting safety latches on kitchen cabinets. Along with these safety measures, I urge you to take another. Easy-to-reach, loaded guns at home are risky. The safest thing for your family is not to have a gun at home. If your keep a gun at home, be sure to empty it out and lock it up at all times. Lock the bullets in a separate location.

    From: American Academy of Pediatrics, Center To Prevent Handgun Violence. *Rx for Safety: Preventing Firearms Injuries among Children and Adolescents.* Washington DC: Center To Prevent Handgun Violence; 1992. Reproduced by permission of the publisher; copyright © 1992.

3. If parents keep a gun in the home, they should be urged to follow basic rules of safety :

    - Never keep a loaded gun in the house or car.
    - Keep guns and ammunition locked in separate places.
    - Always treat a gun as if it were loaded and ready to fire.

Ch. 25. Violent Behavior and Firearms    Children/Adolescents — COUNSELING

- Never allow children access to guns.

- Have a gunsmith check antique and souvenir guns to be sure they are not loaded; these guns should be fixed so they cannot be fired.

From: American Academy of Pediatrics, Committee on Injury Control for Children and Youth. Firearms. In: *Injury Control for Children and Youth*. Elk Grove Village, Ill: American Academy of Pediatrics; 1987. Reproduced by permission of the American Academy of Pediatrics; copyright © 1987.

4. Parents should be advised to inquire about the availability of guns in places their children spend time, such as at friends' houses, schools, and recreation facilities. It may be wise for parents to limit their children's access to these places until guns are no longer available. Parents should be encouraged to take an active role in limiting the availability of guns in their children's environment.

5. It may be less threatening to adolescents to first ask about violence in their environment (school, friends, etc.) before asking specifically about their personal experiences.

6. When treating patients with injuries that may have been caused by violence, it is important to ask specific questions about the cause of the injury. If the injury has been caused by violence, an attempt should be made to determine if the conflict has been settled or has the potential to lead to further violence. The following sample questions have been suggested for use in this situation:

    - Have you settled it?

    - Is there anyone who can settle this—someone who can talk for you and explain your side?

    - Do you know where to go if this is not settled?

    - Are you safe?

From: Violence Prevention Project. *Identification and Prevention of Youth Violence: A Protocol for Health Care Providers*. Boston, MA: Violence Prevention Project, Department of Health & Hospitals; 1992. Reproduced by permission of the publisher; copyright © 1992.

7. Despite the desirability of maintaining confidentiality, it may be necessary to consult with parents, police, and other authorities in order to protect the safety of children and adolescents involved in potentially violent situations.

8. Patients should be asked about how they deal with anger. It may be helpful to:

    - Emphasize that anger is a normal emotion

    - Encourage young people to consider alternative ways for dealing with anger

- Offer positive ways to deal with anger and arguments, the leading precipitators of homicide

From: Violence Prevention Project. *Identification and Prevention of Youth Violence: A Protocol for Health Care Providers*. Boston, MA: Violence Prevention Project, Department of Health & Hospitals; 1992. Reproduced by permission of the publisher; copyright © 1992.

9. Parents and children should be given the facts about violence through a variety of media in the office or clinic, such as posters, videotapes, and brochures.

## Provider Resources

*Identification and Prevention of Youth Violence: A Protocol for Health Care Providers*. Also available are audiotapes, slides, and a script on the process of interviewing youth on violence-related issues, and office posters on violence prevention. Violence Prevention Project, Department of Health & Hospitals, 1010 Massachusetts Ave., 2nd Floor, Boston, MA 02118; (617) 534-5196.

*Rx for Safety: Preventing Firearm Injuries among Children and Adolescents*. American Academy of Pediatrics and the Center To Prevent Handgun Violence. Available from: Center To Prevent Handgun Violence, 1225 I St. NW., Suite 1150, Washington, DC 20005; (202) 289-7319.

## Selected References

American Academy of Family Physicians, Commission on Public Health and Scientific Affairs. *Age Charts for Periodic Health Examination*. Kansas City, Mo: American Academy of Family Physicians; 1993.

American Academy of Pediatrics, Committee on Adolescence. Firearms and adolescents. *Pediatrics*. 1992;89:784-787.

American Academy of Pediatrics, Committee on Injury and Poison Prevention. Firearm injuries affecting the pediatric population. *Pediatrics*. 1992;89:788-790.

American Academy of Pediatrics, Committee on Psychosocial Aspects of Child and Family Health. *Guidelines for Health Supervision*. 2nd ed. Elk Grove Village, Ill: American Academy of Pediatrics; 1988.

American Academy of Pediatrics, Committee on Injury Control for Children and Youth. Firearms. In: *Injury Control for Children and Youth*. Elk Grove Village, Ill: American Academy of Pediatrics; 1987.

American Academy of Pediatrics, Center To Prevent Handgun Violence. *Rx for Safety: Preventing Firearms Injuries among Children and Adolescents*. Washington DC: Center To Prevent Handgun Violence; 1992.

American Medical Association. *Guidelines for Adolescent Preventive Services (GAPS)*. Chicago, Ill: American Medical Association; 1992.

American Psychiatric Association Task Force. *Clinical Aspects of the Violent Individual*. Washington, DC: American Psychiatric Association; 1974.

Centers for Disease Control. Weapon-carrying among high school students. *MMWR*. 1991;40:681.

Children's Safety Network. *A Data Book of Child and Adolescent Injury*. Washington, DC: National Center for Education in Maternal and Child Health; 1991.

Christoffel KK. Violent death and injury in US children and adolescents. *AJDC*. 1990;144:697-706.

Cohall AT, Mayer R, Cohall K, et al. Teen violence: the reasons why. *Contemporary Pediatrics.* October 1991:54-77.

Cohall AT, Mayer R, Cohall K, et al. Teen violence: the new mortality. *Contemporary Pediatrics.* September 1991:76-86.

Rosenberg ML, Gelles RJ, Holinger PC, et al. Violence: homicide, assault, and suicide. In: Amber RW, Dull HB, eds. *Closing the Gap: The Burden of Unnecessary Illness.* New York, NY: Oxford University Press; 1987.

US Dept of Health and Human Services, US Dept of Justice. *Report of the Surgeon General's Workshop on Violence and Public Health.* Leesburg, Va: Health Resources and Services Administration, US Dept of Health and Human Services; 1986.

US Preventive Services Task Force. Screening for violent injuries. In: *Guide to Clinical Preventive Services.* Baltimore, Md: Williams & Wilkins; 1989:chap 46.

# Adults/Older Adults

## Adults/Older Adults — SCREENING

# 26. Anemia and Hemoglobinopathies

Anemia in adults, defined as a hemoglobin level below the 95% reference range for age and gender, is most prevalent in young women (4.5%) and elderly men (4.8%). It is also more common in individuals of low socioeconomic status and in African Americans. Common causes include iron and vitamin deficiencies, occult blood loss, chronic illness, and hemoglobinopathies. Although most forms of anemia are treatable, it is not clear that treatment of asymptomatic individuals is beneficial. For this reason, most authorities either recommend against routinely screening adults for anemia or recommend screening high-risk adults only.

The hemoglobinopathies are genetic disorders that affect the production and function of hemoglobin molecules. They include sickle cell disease and trait, the thalassemias, and other rarer conditions. Hemoglobinopathies tend to occur in defined ethnic and racial groups. Approximately 50,000 African Americans are affected by sickle cell disease and another 2 million carry the trait. Fewer than 1000 Americans have beta-thalassemia major, but sizable numbers of Italian-Americans, Greek-Americans, and immigrants from Southeast Asia carry the genetic trait. Screening in adult populations is primarily useful in the provision of preconception and prenatal genetic counseling to carriers.

See chapters 1 and 8 for discussions of screening for anemia and hemoglobinopathies in children and adolescents.

### Recommendations of Major Authorities

*Screening for Anemia*

- **American Academy of Family Physicians**, **American College of Physicians**, **Centers for Disease Control and Prevention**, and **U.S. Preventive Services Task Force**—Routine screening for anemia is not recommended in adults without clinical indications.

- **American College of Obstetricians and Gynecologists**—Hemoglobin levels should be measured as part of routine preventive care for women with a history of excessive menstrual flow, and for women 65 years of age or older.

- **Canadian Task Force on the Periodic Health Examination**—Individuals of low socioeconomic status may be tested for anemia as part of the periodic health examination at the discretion of the clinician.

*Screening for Hemoglobinopathies*

- **American Academy of Family Physicians** and **U.S. Preventive Services Task Force**—Hemoglobin testing should be discussed with adolescents and young adults at risk for sickle cell trait, thalassemia, and other hemoglobinopathies. Counseling should include a description of the significance of the disease in question, how it is inherited, the availability of a screening test, and the implications to the individual and offspring of having a positive test.

- **American College of Obstetricians and Gynecologists**—Screening should be provided to women of reproductive age who are of Caribbean, Latin American, Asian, Mediterranean, or African descent.

- **Canadian Task Force on the Periodic Health Examination**—Because of the serious complications of homozygous thalassemia and because screening and case-finding are harmless (except for the possibility of labeling), it is recommended that people of Asian, African, and Mediterranean ancestry who are of parenting age be encouraged to submit to detection maneuvers.

## Basics of Screening for Anemia and Hemoglobinopathies

### Anemia

1. The primary screening tests for anemia are measurements of hemoglobin concentration (Hb) and hematocrit (Hct). If possible, a venous blood specimen should be obtained and analyzed by an automated cell counter. This will yield more accurate and reliable results than analysis of a capillary sample by centrifuge.

2. In men, anemia is defined as a Hb level of less than 13 g/dL or a Hct level of less than 41%. In nonpregnant women, the cut points are 12 g/dL for Hb and 36% for Hct. Cigarette smokers and individuals living at altitudes greater than 3000 feet (1000 meters) tend to have higher levels of Hb and Hct. Cut points for anemia in smokers and those living at high altitudes should be adjusted by the correction factors given in Tables 26-1 and 26-2.

### Hemoglobinopathies

1. Hemoglobin electrophoresis is the test of choice in screening for hemoglobinopathies. This test is very accurate in identifying the types of hemoglobin in a blood sample. It can distinguish among affected homozygotes, heterozygous carriers, and those unaffected by sickle cell disease, beta-thalassemia, and other hemoglobin disorders. (Alpha-thalassemia trait may not be detectable.) Sickle cell disease and trait can also be detected by demonstrating red blood cell sickling under reduced oxygen concentration. This is accomplished through the widely used sickle preparation (or Sickledex). Hemoglobin electrophoresis

Table 26-1. Smoking Adjustments for Hemoglobin and Hematocrit Cut Points for Anemia

| Smoking Status | Hb (g/dL) | Hct (%) |
| --- | --- | --- |
| Nonsmoker | 0.0 | 0.0 |
| Smoker (all) | +0.3 | +1.0 |
| 0.5-<1.0 packs per day | +0.3 | +1.0 |
| 1.0-2.0 packs per day | +0.5 | +1.5 |
| >2.0 packs per day | +0.7 | +2.0 |

From: Centers for Disease Control. Reference criteria for anemia screening. *MMWR*. 1989;38:400-404.

## Table 26-2. Altitude Adjustments for Hemoglobin and Hematocrit Cut Points for Anemia

| Altitude (Ft) | Hb (g/dL) | Hct (%) |
|---|---|---|
| <3000 | 0.0 | 0.0 |
| 3000-3999 | +0.2 | +0.5 |
| 4000-4999 | +0.3 | +1.0 |
| 5000-5999 | +0.5 | +1.5 |
| 6000-6999 | +0.7 | +2.0 |
| 7000-7999 | +1.0 | +3.0 |
| 8000-8999 | +1.3 | +4.0 |
| 9000-9999 | +1.6 | +5.0 |
| ≥10,000 | +2.0 | +6.0 |

From: Centers for Disease Control. Reference criteria for anemia screening. *MMWR*. 1989;38:400-404.

is still necessary, however, to distinguish between the carrier and affected state, and to determine the presence of other hemoglobins. Measurement of mean corpuscular volume (MCV) can also be used to screen for thalassemia, but it is much less sensitive than hemoglobin electrophoresis.

2. Adults who are screened for hemoglobinopathies should receive appropriate genetic counseling—before and after laboratory testing. At a minimum, this counseling should address: 1) a description of the disease process and its pattern of inheritance; 2) the availability and accuracy of screening and prenatal detection techniques; 3) the implications of possible results for the individual, partner, and potential offspring.

## Selected References

American Academy of Family Physicians, Commission on Public Health and Scientific Affairs. *Age Charts for Periodic Health Examination*. Kansas City, Mo: American Academy of Family Physicians; 1993.

American College of Obstetricians and Gynecologists. *The Obstetrician-Gynecologist and Primary-Preventive Health Care*. Washington, DC: American College of Obstetricians and Gynecologists. 1993.

Canadian Task Force on the Periodic Health Examination. The periodic health examination. *Can Med Assoc J*. 1979; 121:1194-532.

Centers for Disease Control. Reference criteria for anemia screening. *MMWR*. 1989;38:400-404.

Dallman, P, Ray, Y, Johnson, C. Prevalence and causes of anemia in the United States, 1976 to 1980, *Am J Cl Nutr*. 1984;39:437-445.

Lipkin M, Fisher L, Rowley PT, Loader S, Iker HP. Genetic counseling of asymptomatic carriers in a primary care setting. *Ann Intern Med*. 1985;105:115-123.

Shapiro MF, Greenfield S. The complete blood count and leukocyte differential count: an approach to their rational application. *Ann Intern Med*. 1987;106:65-74.

US Preventive Services Task Force. Screening for anemia. In: *Guide to Clinical Preventive Services*. Baltimore, Md: Williams & Wilkins; 1989:chap 28.

US Preventive Services Task Force. Screening for hemoglobinopathies. In: *Guide to Clinical Preventive Services*. Baltimore, Md: Williams & Wilkins; 1989:chap 29.

## Adults/Older Adults — SCREENING

# 27. Blood Pressure

Approximately 50 million Americans have elevated blood pressure warranting monitoring or drug therapy. These persons are at increased risk for coronary artery disease, peripheral vascular disease, stroke, renal disease, and retinopathy. Treatment for hypertension is very effective. Antihypertensive therapy has contributed to a 57% reduction in stroke mortality and a 50% reduction in mortality from coronary artery disease since 1972. The benefits of antihypertensive therapy are greatest in those with the most marked elevations in blood pressure; however, even patients with Stage 1, or mild, hypertension benefit from treatment. Recent research has demonstrated the importance of treating "isolated" systolic hypertension, especially in older adult patients.

**Recommendations of Major Authorities**

- **American Academy of Family Physicians**–Blood pressure should be measured at every visit, with a minimum frequency of every 2 years.

- **American College of Obstetricians and Gynecologists**–Blood pressure should be measured as part of periodic evaluation visits, which should occur yearly or as appropriate.

- **American College of Physicians**–Blood pressure should be measured in adults every 1 to 2 years. Normotensive patients should have blood pressure measurements at least yearly if any of the following pertains: 1) diastolic blood pressure between 85 and 89 mm Hg; 2) African-American heritage; 3) moderate or extreme obesity; 4) a first-degree relative with hypertension; 5) a personal history of hypertension.

- **National High Blood Pressure Education Program (NHBPEP) of the National Heart, Lung, and Blood Institute**–Blood pressure measurements should be performed on adults at least every 2 years, and at each patient visit if possible. Patients with diastolic blood pressures of 85 to 89 mm Hg should have their blood pressure rechecked within 1 year. See Tables 27-1 and 27-2 for classification of blood pressure and recommendations for follow-up.

- **U.S. Preventive Services Task Force**–Adults should have blood pressure measured regularly, with the optimal interval left to clinical discretion. For those whose diastolic blood pressure is 85 to 89 mm Hg, measurement should be performed at least yearly.

**Basics of Blood Pressure Screening**

1. The patient should be advised to avoid using tobacco and caffeine for 30 minutes prior to the measurement.

2. The patient should be seated in a quiet environment free from temperature extremes for at least 5 minutes before the measurement is performed.

3. The measurement should be performed with a mercury sphygmomanometer, if available. An aneroid manometer may be used if it is periodically calibrated according to manufacturer's recommendations. A validated electronic device meeting the requirements of the American National Standard for Electronic or Automated Sphygmomanometers set forth by the Association for the Advancement of Medical Instruments may also be used.

4. The manometer should be positioned at the clinician's eye level, if possible, to assure accuracy in reading.

5. An appropriate sized cuff should be used. The bladder of the cuff should encircle 80% to 100% of the arm. The cuff width should be 40% of the circumference of the upper arm. Narrow cuffs lead to falsely elevated readings; wide cuffs may falsely lower the reading.

6. The patient's arm should be bare. Constriction of the upper arm by a rolled shirt sleeve should be avoided. The arm should be supported horizontally so the cuff is positioned at heart level (the fourth intercostal space). If the arm cannot be positioned appropriately, a correction factor should be utilized: For each 1 cm above or below heart level, 0.8 mm Hg should be added or subtracted, respectively.

7. The stethoscope must be lightly applied to the antecubital fossa. Excess pressure results in falsely low diastolic blood pressure readings.

8. The cuff pressure should be rapidly increased to about 30 mm Hg beyond the point at which the radial pulse is no longer palpable. The pressure indicator's rate of descent should be no greater than 2 to 3 mm Hg per second.

9. In adults, the systolic (SBP) and diastolic (DBP) pressure readings should be identified by the pressures corresponding to the first of two consecutive sounds and the disappearance of sound (not muffling), respectively. Disappearance should be confirmed by listening for 10 to 20 mm Hg below the last sound heard.

10. The average of at least two readings should be used unless the first two differ by more than 5 mm Hg, in which case additional readings should be obtained. To allow blood to be released from arm veins, there should be an interval of 1 to 2 minutes before pressure measurements are repeated in the same arm.

11. Blood pressure should be measured in both arms initially and remeasured at subsequent visits using the arm with the highest initial pressures.

12. Diagnosis of hypertension requires confirmation during at least two subsequent visits (unless SBP is 210 mm Hg or greater, or DBP is 120 mm Hg or greater, or both). See Table 27-2 for recommendations for follow-up from the Joint National Committee on Detection, Evaluation, and Treatment of High Blood Pressure.

## Ch. 27. Blood Pressure — Adults/Older Adults — SCREENING

**Table 27-1. Classification of Blood Pressure for Adults Aged 18 Years and Older***

| Category | Systolic (mm Hg) | Diastolic (mm Hg) |
|---|---|---|
| Normal** | <130 | <85 |
| High normal | 130-139 | 85-89 |
| Hypertension*** | | |
| Stage 1 (Mild) | 140-159 | 90-99 |
| Stage 2 (Moderate) | 160-179 | 100-109 |
| Stage 3 (Severe) | 180-209 | 110-119 |
| Stage 4 (Very Severe) | ≥210 | ≥120 |

*Not taking antihypertensive drugs and not acutely ill. When systolic and diastolic pressures fall into different categories, the higher category should be selected to classify the individual's blood pressure status. For instance, 160/92 mm Hg should be classified as Stage 2, and 180/120 mm Hg should be classified as Stage 4. Isolated systolic hypertension (ISH) is defined as SBP ≥140 mm Hg and DBP <90 mm Hg and staged appropriately (e.g., 170/85 mm Hg is defined as Stage 2 ISH)

**Optimal blood pressure with respect to cardiovascular risk is SBP <120 mm Hg and DBP <80 mm Hg. However, unusually low readings should be evaluated for clinical significance.

***Based on the average of two or more readings taken at each of two or more visits following an initial screening.

Note: In addition to classifying stages of hypertension based on average blood pressure levels, the clinician should specify presence or absence of target-organ disease and additional risk factors. For example, a patient with diabetes and a blood pressure of 142/94 mm Hg plus left ventricular hypertrophy should be classified as "Stage 1 hypertension with target-organ disease (left ventricular hypertrophy) and with another major risk factor (diabetes)." This specificity is important for risk classification and management.

From: Joint National Committee on Detection, Evaluation, and Treatment of High Blood Pressure. The Fifth Report of the Joint National Committee on Detection, Evaluation, and Treatment of High Blood Pressure. *Arch Int Med*. 1993;153:154-188.

13. Because blood pressure readings obtained in a medical setting may not be typical of a patient's usual blood pressure, monitoring at home or work by the patient, family, or friends may be valuable. If this is done, measurement devices must be calibrated initially and rechecked at least yearly. The person taking the blood pressure should be instructed in proper technique and the technique rechecked periodically. In certain clinical situations, continuous ambulatory blood pressure monitoring may provide a useful adjunct to episodic blood pressure monitoring performed by the provider or patient. Clinical situations in which ambulatory blood pressure monitoring may be useful are given in Table 27-3. Its use in these situations is controversial (Appel and Stason 1993).

14. Life-style modifications can help prevent the development of hypertension and should be the initial treatment modality for the first 3-4 months for patients with Stage 1 (mild) or Stage 2 (moderate) hypertension. See Table 27-4 for a list of the basic life-style modifications for controlling blood pressure.

**Table 27-2. Recommendations for Follow-Up Based on Initial Set of Blood Pressure Measurements for Adults Age 18 and Over**

| Initial Screening Blood Pressure (mm Hg)* | | Follow-up Recommended** |
|---|---|---|
| Systolic | Diastolic | |
| <130 | <85 | Recheck in 2 years |
| 130-139 | 85-89 | Recheck in 1 year*** |
| 140-159 | 90-99 | Confirm within 2 months |
| 160-179 | 100-109 | Evaluate or refer to source of care within 1 month |
| 180-209 | 110-119 | Evaluate or refer to source of care within 1 week |
| ≥210 | ≥120 | Evaluate or refer to source of care immediately |

*If the systolic and diastolic categories are different, follow recommendations for the shorter time follow-up (e.g., 160/85 mm Hg should be evaluated or referred to source of care within 1 month).

**The scheduling of follow-ups should be modified by reliable information about past blood pressure measurements, other cardiovascular risk factors, or target-organ disease.

***Consider providing advice about lifestyle modifications.

From: Joint National Committee on Detection, Evaluation, and Treatment of High Blood Pressure. The Fifth Report of the Joint National Committee on Detection, Evaluation, and Treatment of High Blood Pressure. *Arch Int Med.* 1993;153:154-188.

**Table 27-3. Situations In Which Automated Noninvasive Ambulatory Blood Pressure Monitoring Devices May Be Useful**

| |
|---|
| "Office" or "white-coat" hypertension: blood pressure repeatedly elevated in office setting but repeatedly normal out of office |
| Evaluation of drug resistance |
| Evaluation of nocturnal blood pressure changes |
| Episodic hypertension |
| Hypotensive symptoms associated with antihypertensive medications or autonomic dysfunction |
| Carotid sinus syncope and pacemaker syndromes (along with electrocardiographic monitoring) |

From: Joint National Committee on Detection, Evaluation, and Treatment of High Blood Pressure. The Fifth Report of the Joint National Committee on Detection, Evaluation, and Treatment of High Blood Pressure. *Arch Int Med.* 1993;153:154-188.

**Table 27-4. Life-style Modifications for Hypertension Control**

| |
|---|
| Lose weight if overweight |
| Limit alcohol intake to no more than 2 drinks daily for men and 1 drink daily for women |
| Exercise (aerobic) regularly (3-5 times a week) |
| Reduce sodium intake to less than 100 mmol per day (<2.3 grams of sodium or <6 grams of sodium chloride, 1 teaspoon of salt = 2 grams of sodium) |
| Maintain adequate dietary potassium, calcium, and magnesium intake |

Adapted from: Joint National Committee on Detection, Evaluation, and Treatment of High Blood Pressure. The Fifth Report of the Joint National Committee on Detection, Evaluation, and Treatment of High Blood Pressure. *Arch Int Med.* 1993;153:154-188.

## Patient Resources

*Blacks and High Blood Pressure*; *Eating Right to Lower Your Blood Pressure*; *High Blood Pressure and What You Can Do About It*; *Six Good Reasons to Control Your High Blood Pressure*. National Heart, Lung, and Blood Institute Information Center, P.O. Box 30105, Bethesda, MD 20824-0105; (301) 251-1222.

## Provider Resources

*The Fifth Report of the Joint National Committee on Detection, Evaluation, and Treatment of High Blood Pressure.* (NIH Publication 93-1088). National Heart, Lung, and Blood Institute Information Center, P.O. Box 30105, Bethesda, MD 20824-0105; (301) 251-1222.

## Selected References

American Academy of Family Physicians, Commission on Public Health and Scientific Affairs. *Age Charts for Periodic Health Examination*. Kansas City, Mo: American Academy of Family Physicians; 1993.

American College of Obstetricians and Gynecologists. *The Obstetrician-Gynecologist and Primary-Preventive Health Care*. Washington, DC: American College of Obstetricians and Gynecologists, 1993.

American College of Physicians. Guidelines. In: Eddy DM, ed. *Common Screening Tests*. Philadelphia, Pa: American College of Physicians; 1991:396-397.

American College of Physicians. Automated ambulatory blood pressure and self-measured blood pressure monitoring devices: their role in the diagnosis and management of hypertension (position paper). *Ann Intern Med.* 1993;118:889-892.

Appel LJ, Stason WB. Ambulatory blood pressure monitoring and blood pressure self-measurement in the diagnosis and management of hypertension. *Ann Intern Med.* 1993;118:867-882.

Frohlich ED, Grim C, Lavarthe DR, et al. Recommendations for human blood pressure determination by sphygmomanometers: report of a special task force appointed by the Steering Committee, American Heart Association. *Hypertension.* 1988;11:209A-222A.

Joint National Committee on Detection, Evaluation, and Treatment of High Blood Pressure. The Fifth Report of the Joint National Committee on Detection, Evaluation, and Treatment of High Blood Pressure. *Arch Int Med.* 1993;153:154-188.

National High Blood Pressure Education Program (NHBPEP) Working Group. Report on ambulatory blood pressure monitoring. *Arch Int Med.* 1990;150:2270-2280.

SHEP Cooperative Research Group. Prevention of stroke by antihypertensive drug treatment in older persons with isolated systolic hypertension. *JAMA*. 1991; 265:3255-3264.

US Preventive Services Task Force. Screening for hypertension. In: *Guide to Clinical Preventive Services*. Baltimore, Md: Williams & Wilkins; 1989;chap 3.

Webster J, Newnham D, Petrie JC, Lovell HG. Influence of arm position on measurement of blood pressure. *Br Med J*. 1984;288:1574-157.

# Adults/Older Adults — SCREENING

## 28. Body Measurement

Approximately 32 million American adults (24% of men and 27% of women) are overweight. Mortality rates are increased for individuals with weights only 10% above desirable weight. Most authorities recognize weights 20% or more above desirable weight to constitute obesity and to be associated with multiple attendant health risks. Hypertension and noninsulin dependent diabetes mellitus (Type II) are three times more prevalent in the obese. The risks of hypercholesterolemia and coronary artery disease are also increased, as are the risks of several types of cancer including colon, rectal, prostate, gallbladder, biliary tract, breast, cervical, endometrial, and ovarian cancers. Abdominal adiposity, measured by waist-to-hip circumference ratio (WHR), is associated with increased risk of diabetes, hypertension, coronary heart disease, stroke, and death from all causes. Recent research indicates that WHR may be a stronger predictor of mortality than measures of general body adiposity.

Weight loss, through changes in diet, increased physical activity, and other interventions, can decrease the risk of most forms of morbidity associated with obesity. In order for weight loss to be beneficial it must be sustained. Recent research indicates that fluctuations in weight may be an independent risk factor for increased total mortality and mortality from coronary artery disease.

See chapter 3 for information on body measurement of children and adolescents. See chapters 55 and 56 for information on counseling adults about nutrition and physical activity.

### Recommendations of Major Authorities

- **American Academy of Family Physicians** and **U.S. Preventive Services Task Force**—All adults should receive periodic measurement of height and weight. The optimal frequency for measuring height and weight in adults is a matter of clinical discretion. Those individuals who are 20% or more above desirable weight should receive appropriate nutritional and exercise counseling.

- **Canadian Task Force on the Periodic Health Examination**—Height and weight measurements should be made at the discretion of the clinician.

- **U.S. Department of Agriculture**, **U.S. Department of Health and Human Services**—Calculation of the ratio of waist circumference to hip circumference should be used, in addition to height and weight measurements, to determine if a person's weight is "healthy."

### Basics of Body Measurement Screening

1. Height is most accurately measured with the patient barefoot or in socks or stockings only. Care should be taken to make sure that the patient is standing as erect as possible with feet flat on the floor. If a height-measuring rod attached to a scale is used, its accuracy should be checked regularly, as such rods tend to become inaccurate with use.

## Ch. 28. Body Measurement — Adults/Older Adults — SCREENING

2. Weight is most accurately measured with the patient wearing minimal or no clothing. A balance beam or electronic scale (not a spring-type scale) should be used for measurements.

3. There is currently considerable debate about the definition of a "healthy" weight. Two basic methods are used for evaluating weight: 1) reference to standardized height-weight tables and 2) calculation of body mass index (BMI).

- Clinicians have been most accustomed to using height-weight tables. Tables 28-1 and 28-2 give height-weight tables for men and women adapted from those that were developed by the Metropolitan Life Insurance Company in 1959 from mortality data of its insured population. These have been the most widely used height-weight tables, but they have certain limitations. In practice, body frame cannot be easily measured and must be estimated visually. Also, these tables are based on an insured population, which may not be totally representative of the general population. A separate column

### Table 28-1. Height and Weight Tables for Men Aged 25 and Over

| Height* | Small Frame | Medium Frame | Large Frame | 20% Overweight*** |
|---|---|---|---|---|
| 5'1" | 105-113 | 111-122 | 119-134 | 140 |
| 5'2" | 108-116 | 114-126 | 122-137 | 144 |
| 5'3" | 111-119 | 117-129 | 125-141 | 148 |
| 5'4" | 114-122 | 120-132 | 128-145 | 151 |
| 5'5" | 117-126 | 123-136 | 131-149 | 155 |
| 5'6" | 121-130 | 127-140 | 135-154 | 160 |
| 5'7" | 125-134 | 131-145 | 140-159 | 166 |
| 5'8" | 129-138 | 135-149 | 144-163 | 170 |
| 5'9" | 133-143 | 139-153 | 148-167 | 175 |
| 5'10" | 137-147 | 143-158 | 152-172 | 181 |
| 5'11" | 141-151 | 147-163 | 157-177 | 186 |
| 6'0" | 145-155 | 151-168 | 161-182 | 191 |
| 6'1" | 149-160 | 155-173 | 168-187 | 197 |
| 6'2" | 153-164 | 160-178 | 171-192 | 203 |
| 6'3" | 157-168 | 165-183 | 175-197 | 209 |

Weight in Pounds**

*without shoes
**without clothing
***20% over midpoint of medium frame weight; not in original Metropolitan table

Adapted from: Metropolitan Life Insurance Company. New weight standards for men and women. *Stat Bull Metropol Life Insur Co.* 1959;40:1-4 and Metropolitan height and weight tables. *Stat Bull Metropol Life Insur Co.* 1983:64:2-9. Reproduced by permission of the publisher; copyright © 1959 and 1983.

has been added to both of these tables to give values for 20% above desirable weight (of the midpoint weight for a medium-frame person), because some authorities (National Institutes of Health Consensus Development Conference, 1985, and US Preventive Services Task Force, 1989) have designated this weight as the threshold of overweight at which negative health consequences occur.

- In recent years, some authorities have endorsed using BMI to evaluate healthy weight. BMI values are believed to correlate more accurately with total body fat content. The formula for calculation of BMI is:

$$\frac{\text{Weight (kg)}}{\text{Height}^2 \text{ (m)}}$$

Table 28-2. Height and Weight Tables for Women Aged 25 and Over

| Height* | Weight in Pounds** Small Frame | Medium Frame | Large Frame | 20% Overweight*** |
|---|---|---|---|---|
| 4'9" | 90-97 | 94-106 | 102-118 | 120 |
| 4'10" | 92-100 | 97-109 | 106-121 | 124 |
| 4'11" | 95-103 | 100-112 | 108-124 | 127 |
| 5'0" | 98-106 | 103-116 | 111-127 | 131 |
| 5'1" | 101-109 | 106-118 | 114-130 | 134 |
| 5'2" | 104-112 | 109-122 | 117-134 | 139 |
| 5'3" | 107-115 | 112-126 | 121-138 | 141 |
| 5'4" | 110-119 | 116-131 | 125-142 | 148 |
| 5'5" | 114-123 | 120-136 | 129-146 | 154 |
| 5'6" | 118-127 | 124-139 | 133-150 | 158 |
| 5'7" | 122-131 | 128-143 | 137-154 | 163 |
| 5'8" | 126-136 | 132-147 | 141-159 | 167 |
| 5'9" | 130-140 | 136-151 | 145-164 | 172 |
| 5'10" | 134-144 | 140-155 | 149-169 | 177 |

*without shoes
**without clothing
***20% over midpoint of medium frame weight; not in original Metropolitan table

Adapted from: Metropolitan Life Insurance Company. New weight standards for men and women. *Stat Bull Metropol Life Insur Co.* 1959;40:1-4 and Metropolitan height and weight tables. *Stat Bull Metropol Life Insur Co.* 1983:64:2-9. Reproduced by permission of the publisher; copyright © 1959 and 1983.

## Ch. 28. Body Measurement — Adults/Older Adults — SCREENING

Fig 28-1 is a nomogram that can be used quickly to calculate BMI. Its author's recommended cut points for overweight and obesity are on the nomogram. Values above 26.4 for men and 25.8 for women correspond to the 20% over desirable weight limits derived from the Metropolitan Life Insurance tables, and are commonly cited by some other experts as constituting overweight.

- Some authorities believe that the normal ranges of BMI and weight increase with age. The National Academy of Sciences (1989) published a table (see Table 28-3) of

**Figure 28-1. Body Mass Index (BMI) Nomogram**

*Instructions for use:* Place a straightedge across the scales for weight and height. BMI is found where the straightedge crosses the middle scale.

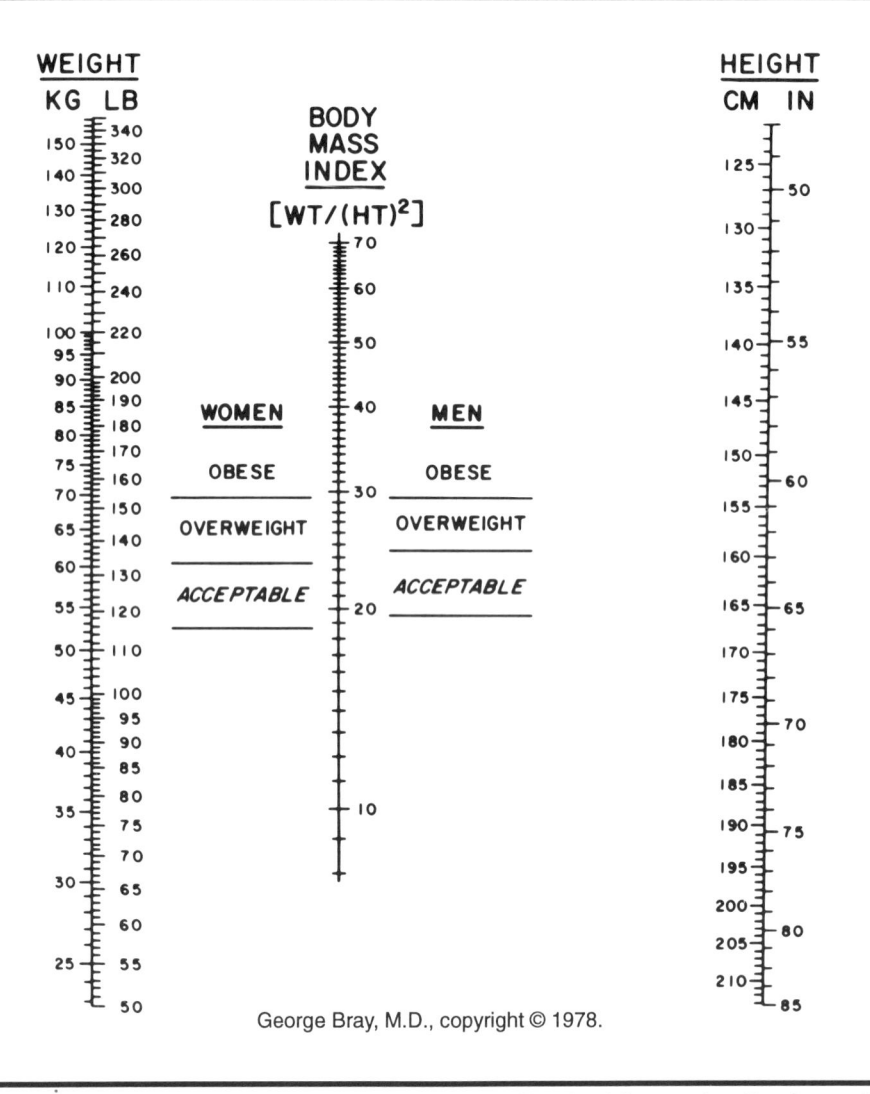

George Bray, M.D., copyright © 1978.

Ch. 28. Body Measurement                    Adults/Older Adults — SCREENING

**Table 28-3. Desirable Body Mass Index (BMI) in Relation to Age**

| Age Group, y | BMI (kg/m$^2$) |
|---|---|
| 19-24 | 19-24 |
| 25-34 | 20-25 |
| 35-44 | 21-26 |
| 45-54 | 22-27 |
| 55-65 | 23-28 |
| >65 | 24-29 |

From: National Academy of Sciences, Committee on Diet and Health, Food and Nutrition Board, Commission on Life Sciences, National Research Council. *Diet and Health: Implications for Reducing Chronic Disease Risk.* Washington, DC: National Academy Press; 1989:564-565. Reproduced by permission of the publisher; copyright © 1989.

desirable BMI values in relation to age. Other authorities have questioned the validity of age adjustments.

4. The determination of WHR is also useful for assessing patients, particularly those with borderline high weight who have personal or family medical histories placing them at increased health risk. WHR is determined by measuring the abdominal (waist) circumference and the hip circumference. The abdominal circumference is measured at the level of the umbilicus (or the level of greatest anterior extension of the abdomen) with the patient standing. The hip circumference is determined by measuring the greatest circumference at the level of the buttocks. Both measurements should be performed at the end of a normal expiration and without indenting the skin. The formula for calculating WHR is:

$$\frac{\text{Abdominal Circumference}}{\text{Hip Circumference}}$$

WHR values above 1.0 for men and above 0.8 for women are associated with increased risk of diabetes, hypertension, heart disease, and stroke.

**Patient Resources**

*Nutrition and Your Health: Dietary Guidelines for Americans* (3rd ed, 1990). US Dept of Agriculture and US Dept of Health and Human Services. Available from: Consumer Information Center—3C, Dept 514-X, Pueblo, CO 81009.

*Check Your Weight and Heart Disease I.Q.* National Heart, Lung, and Blood Institute Information Center, P.O Box 30105, Bethesda, MD 20824-0105; (301) 251-1222.

*Weight Control: Losing Weight and Keeping It Off.* American Academy of Family Physicians, 8880 Ward Parkway, Kansas City, MO 64114-2797; 1-800 944-0000.

**Selected References**

American Academy of Family Physicians, Commission on Public Health and Scientific Affairs. *Age Charts for Periodic Health Examination.* Kansas City, Mo: American Academy of Family Physicians; 1993.

American College of Obstetricians and Gynecologists. *The Obstetrician-Gynecologist and Primary-Preventive Health Care.* Washington, DC: American College of Obstetricians and Gynecologists, 1993.

Bjorntorp P. Regional patterns of fat distribution. *Ann Intern Med.* 1985;103:994-995.

Bray GA, Gray DS. Obesity: part 1—pathogenesis. *West J Med.* 1988;149:429-441.

Folsom AR, Kaye SA, Sellers TA, et al. Body fat distribution and 5-year risk of death in older women. *JAMA.* 1993;269:483-487.

Hubert HB, Feinlieb M, McNamara PM, Castelli WP. Obesity as an independent risk factor for cardiovascular disease: a 26-year follow-up of participants in the Framingham Heart Study. *Circulation.* 1983;67:968-977.

Lissner L, Odell PM, D'Agostino RB, et al. Variability of body weight and health outcomes in the Framingham population. *N Eng J Med.* 1991;324:1839-1844.

Lohman TG, Roche AF, Martorell R. *Anthropometric Standardization Reference Manual.* Champaign, Ill: Human Kinetics Books; 1988.

Manson JE, Stampler MJ, Hennekens CH, Willet WC. Body weight and longevity: a reassessment. *JAMA.* 1987;257:353-358.

Metropolitan Life Insurance Company. New weight standards for men and women. *Stat Bull Metropol Life Insur Co.* 1959;40:1-4.

Metropolitan Life Insurance Company. Metropolitan height and weight tables. *Stat Bull Metropol Life Insur Co.* 1983;64:2-9.

National Academy of Sciences, Committee on Diet and Health, Food and Nutrition Board, Commission on Life Sciences, National Research Council. *Diet and Health: Implications for Reducing Chronic Disease Risk.* Washington, DC: National Academy Press; 1989: 564-565.

National Institutes of Health. National Institutes of Health Consensus Development Conference Statement: health implications of obesity. *Ann Int Med.* 1985;103:1073-1077.

Rowland ML. A nomogram for computing body mass index. *Dietetic Currents.* 1989;16:5-12.

Simpoulos AP, Van Itallie TB. Body weight, health and longevity. *Ann Int Med.* 1984;100:285-295.

US Department of Agriculture, US Dept of Health and Human Services. *Nutrition and Your Health: Dietary Guidelines for Americans.* Washington DC: US Government Printing Office; 1990. Home and Garden Bulletin 232.

Van Itallie TB. Health implications of overweight and obesity in the United States. *Ann Int Med.* 1985; 103:983-988.

Willet WC, Stampfer M, Manson J, et al. New weight guidelines for Americans: justified or injudicious? *Am J Clin Nutr.* 1991;53:1102-3.

## Adults/Older Adults — SCREENING

# 29. Cancer Detection by Physical Examination

Approximately 30% of Americans will eventually develop cancer. Three of every four families in the United States will be affected. Early detection may be important because many cancers can be cured if detected and treated in the early stages. By one estimate, 42,500 cancer deaths could be prevented yearly through early detection and treatment. Table 29–1 provides data on the incidence of and numbers of deaths from the major types of cancer.

This chapter presents information on detection of cancers through physical examination. Topics covered include examinations of the breast, oral cavity, pelvic organs, rectum and prostate, skin, testes, and thyroid. Screening tests for early detection of cancer are addressed in separate chapters in this handbook. These include fecal occult blood testing (chapter 33), mammography (chapter 35), Papanicolaou smear (chapter 36), prostate-specific antigen (chapter 38), and sigmoidoscopy (chapter 40).

## ■ Breast Examination ■

Breast cancer is the most common type of cancer among women in the United States, accounting for an estimated 182,000 new cases in 1994. It is the second leading cause of cancer death in women (after lung cancer), and will cause an estimated 46,000 deaths in 1994. The average woman has one chance in nine of developing breast cancer during her lifetime. Major risk factors for breast cancer are age over 50 and personal or family (first-degree relative) history of breast cancer. Other factors associated with very modest increases in risk include first pregnancy after 30 years of age, nulliparity, menarche before 12 years of age, menopause after 50 years of age, postmenopausal obesity, some types of benign breast disease, high socioeconomic status, and a personal history of ovarian or endometrial cancer. Women with localized disease have a 5-year survival rate of approximately 93%. If distant metastasis has occurred, the 5-year survival rate is 18%. When performed by a clinician, breast examination has a sensitivity of approximately 45%.

**Recommendations of Major Authorities**

*Women Under 40 Years of Age*

- **American Academy of Family Physicians**—Clinical breast examination should be performed every 1 to 3 years on women aged 30 to 39.

- **American Cancer Society**—Women should have clinical breast examinations every 3 years from age 20 to 39 years.

- **American College of Obstetricians and Gynecologists**—Women over age 18 years should have clinical breast examination during the periodic evaluation, yearly, or as appropriate.

- **Canadian Task Force on the Periodic Health Examination** and **U.S. Preventive Services Task Force**—Physicians may elect to perform clinical breast examination on women under age 40 who are at high risk, especially those whose first-degree relatives have had breast cancer diagnosed before menopause.

## Women 40 Years of Age and Over

- **American Academy of Family Physicians, American Cancer Society, American College of Obstetricians and Gynecologists,** and **American College of Physicians**—Annual clinical breast examination should be performed on women 40 years of age and older.

Table 29-1. Leading Sites of Cancer Incidence and Death—1994 Estimates

| Rank | Cancer Incidence* Male | Cancer Incidence* Female | Cancer Deaths Male | Cancer Deaths Female |
|---|---|---|---|---|
| 1 | Prostate 200,000 | Breast 182,000 | Lung 94,000 | Lung 59,000 |
| 2 | Lung 100,000 | Colon/Rectum 74,000 | Prostate 38,000 | Breast 46,000 |
| 3 | Colon/Rectum 75,000 | Lung 72,000 | Colon/Rectum 27,800 | Colon/Rectum 28,200 |
| 4 | Bladder 38,000 | Uterus 46,000 | Pancreas 12,400 | Ovary 13,600 |
| 5 | Lymphoma 29,400 | Ovary 24,000 | Lymphoma 12,100 | Pancreas 13,500 |
| 6 | Oral 19,800 | Lymphoma 23,500 | Leukemia 10,500 | Lymphoma 10,650 |
| 7 | Melanoma 17,000 | Melanoma 15,000 | Stomach 8,400 | Uterus 10,500 |
| 8 | Kidney 17,000 | Pancreas 14,000 | Esophagus 7,800 | Leukemia 8,600 |
| 9 | Leukemia 16,200 | Bladder 13,200 | Liver 7,200 | Liver 6,000 |
| 10 | Stomach 15,000 | Leukemia 12,400 | Bladder 7,000 | Brain 5,800 |
| 11 | Pancreas 13,000 | Kidney 10,600 | Brain 6,800 | Stomach 5,600 |
| 12 | Larynx 9,800 | Oral 9,800 | Kidney 6,800 | Multiple Myeloma 4,800 |
| All Sites** | 632,000 | 576,000 | 283,000 | 255,000 |

*Excluding basal and squamous cell skin cancer and in situ carcinomas except bladder
**Including sites not listed in the table

Adapted from: Boring CC, Squires TS, Tong T, Montgomery S. Cancer Statistics, 1994. CA. 1994;4:7-26. Reproduced by permission of the authors and the American Cancer Society; copyright © 1994.

- **Canadian Task Force on the Periodic Health Examination** and **U.S. Preventive Services Task Force**—Clinical breast examination should be performed on women aged 50 and over every 1 to 2 years. Physicians may elect to perform clinical breast examination on women under age 50 who are at high risk, especially those whose first-degree relatives have had breast cancer diagnosed before menopause. These recommendations are under review.

## Basics of Breast Examination

1. *General Considerations*: Breast examination involves bilateral inspection and palpation of the breasts (and areolae) and the axillary and supraclavicular areas. Examination should be performed in both the upright and supine positions.

2. *Inspection*: The breasts should be visually examined under good lighting with the patient sitting or standing with her hands on her hips. Focus should be on symmetry and contour of the breasts; position of the nipples; skin changes such as puckering, dimpling, or scaling of the skin; scars; nipple discharge; nipple retraction; and appearance of a mass. Any bulging, discoloration, or edema of the lymphatic drainage areas (i.e., the supraclavicular and axillary regions) should be noted.

3. *Screening for Retraction*: The breast tissue should be observed for signs of retraction while the patient lifts her arms slowly over her head. Both breasts should move symmetrically. With the patient's arms lowered and palms pressed together at waist level, signs of retraction should again be observed for. The patient with large breasts should be asked to lean forward and the symmetric forward movement of the breasts should be noted. There should be no evidence of fixation to the chest wall.

4. *Breast Palpation*: It is very important that palpation be systematic. Two commonly used patterns of palpation are to start with the nipple and move out radially to the periphery—much like spokes on a wheel—or to move outward from the nipple and around the breast in a spiral, or corkscrew, pattern. Regardless of the pattern used, the clinician should be thorough and not miss any areas. One of the best predictors of examination accuracy is the length of time spent by the examiner. Care should be taken to palpate the tail of Spence, which extends from the upper outer quadrant to the axilla. The first three fingers should be used to press firmly in a small circular motion. The amount of pressure should vary from firm, to detect deep masses, to light, to detect superficial ones. All of the breast tissue should be palpated with the patient both upright and supine. First, with the woman in an upright position, the breast should be palpated using a bimanual technique. The inferior aspect of the breast should be supported with one hand while the other hand palpates the breast. Each breast should next be palpated with the patient in a supine position with the arm on the side to be examined raised over her head.

5. *Axillary and Supraclavicular Node Palpation*: The axillary and supraclavicular areas should be palpated for adenopathy while the patient is sitting. While lifting and supporting the woman's arm, the clinician's fingers should be placed high into the axilla and moved down firmly to palpate in four directions: along the chest wall, along the anterior border of the axilla, along the posterior border of the axilla, and along the inner aspect of the upper arm. It may be helpful to move the patient's arm through the full range of motion

to increase the surface area that can be reached. The supraclavicular nodes should be palpated while the patient is sitting and relaxed, with neck flexed slightly forward. It may help to have the patient's head turned slightly toward the side being examined. The supraclavicular nodes may be felt in the angle formed by the clavicle and sternocleidomastoid muscle.

6. *Areolae*: The examiner should check for nipple discharge by gently squeezing the nipple. Discharge is easier to elicit when the patient is in an upright position. Nipple inversion may be normal. However, changes in nipple inversion should not occur after puberty and inverted nipples should not be fixed (i.e., it should be possible to pull the nipple out).

7. *Breast Self-Examination:* The American Academy of Family Physicians, the American Cancer Society, the American College of Obstetricians and Gynecologists, and the National Cancer Institute recommend that clinicians encourage women to examine their breasts every month. Clinicians may wish to instruct their female patients in breast self-examination. Pamphlets on breast self-examination are listed in Patient Resources at the end of this chapter.

## ■ Oral Cavity Examination ■

An estimated 29,600 new cases of oral cavity and pharyngeal cancer will be diagnosed in 1994, with an estimated 7925 deaths during that period. Most deaths occur within 3 or 4 years of diagnosis. Incidence is twice as high in men as in women, with the highest incidence rates among African-American males. In high-risk populations, such as heavy smokers and drinkers over 40 years of age, the detection rate can be as high as 1 cancer in every 200 to 250 individuals examined.

### Recommendations of Major Authorities

- **American Academy of Family Physicians** and **U.S. Preventive Services Task Force**— A complete oral cavity examination should be a part of routine preventive care for adults at high risk due to exposure to tobacco or excessive amounts of alcohol.

- **American Cancer Society**—Individuals 20 to 39 years of age should have a cancer checkup, including examination of the oral region, every three years; those 40 years of age and older should have one yearly.

- **American College of Obstetricians and Gynecologists**—Examinations of the oral cavity in women 40 years of age and older should be part of periodic health examinations performed annually, as appropriate.

- **Canadian Task Force on the Periodic Health Examination**—Oral examination for adults should be part of an annual dental check-up.

- **National Cancer Institute** and **National Institute of Dental Research**—Starting at 50 years of age, individuals should have a complete oral examination as part of the periodic health examination, with special attention given to those at high risk due to tobacco and alcohol use or lower socioeconomic status.

## Basics of Oral Cavity Examination

1. *General Considerations*: Examination of the oral cavity is intended to identify the presence of lesions that are precancerous or may predispose to cancer. Lesions that have the potential for malignant transformation tend to be flat white (leukoplakia), white-red (erythroleukoplakia), and red (erythroplakia). The examination should include inspection and palpation of the lips, gingivae, buccal mucosa, palate, floor of the mouth, tongue, and pharynx. If the patient is wearing dentures, these should be removed prior to the examination. The examiner should work systematically from anterior to posterior so that no areas are omitted. A bright light should be used for optimal visualization.

2. *Lips*: The lips should be inspected closely, with note made of symmetry, color, moisture, and the presence of cracking and lesions.

3. *Gingivae*: The gums should be inspected for bleeding, sponginess, and discoloration. Normally, the gums appear pink or coral with a stippled surface.

4. *Buccal Mucosa*: The patient should be asked to hold his or her mouth open widely. Holding the cheek open with a wooden tongue blade, the examiner should inspect the buccal mucosa, noting color and the presence of nodules and lesions. The buccal surface normally appears pink, smooth, and moist. Leukoplakia appears as white plaque on the mucous membranes of the cheeks, gums, and tongue. Squamous cell carcinoma in its earliest stages may present as an erythematous, indurated lesion.

5. *Palate*: The palate should be inspected for plaques, ulceration, and masses. A normal variation is the *torus palatinus*, a nodular bony ridge down the middle of the hard palate.

6. *Floor of the Mouth*: The entire U-shaped area under the tongue should be examined closely, as this is the most common location for oral malignancies. The examiner should inspect for white patches, nodules, and ulcerations. The floor of the mouth should be palpated bimanually with one finger under the tongue and the other hand under the jaw to stabilize the tissue, feeling for induration, thickening, and masses.

7. *Tongue*: Color, surface characteristics, and moisture should be noted. The patient should be asked to touch the tongue to the roof of the mouth to permit examination of the undersurface of the tongue. With the tongue protruded, the examiner should gently grasp it with a piece of gauze, using the other hand to palpate the tongue. Over 85% of all lingual cancers arise in the lateral margins of the tongue. Neoplasms may limit a patient's ability to protrude the tongue. Induration and ulceration are suggestive of carcinoma.

8. *Pharynx*: The middle third of the tongue should be depressed with a tongue blade to increase visualization of the posterior pharynx. Any asymmetry, discharge, mass, or ulceration of the pharynx should be noted.

# ■ Pelvic Organ Examination ■

One of every 70 women will develop ovarian cancer. Approximately 24,000 new cases of ovarian cancer will occur in 1994 in the United States, with an estimated 13,600 deaths in that period. A woman's risk of ovarian cancer is increased by nulliparity; older age at the time of first pregnancy or live birth; fewer pregnancies; and a personal history of breast, endometrial, or colorectal cancer. Pelvic examination is used in the detection of cancers of the female genital tract—the ovaries, cervix, and endometrium. Ovarian cancer often shows no signs or symptoms until late in its development and is often of considerable size by the time it is detectable by pelvic examination.

Pelvic examination is usually performed in conjunction with Pap smear testing for cervical neoplasms and premalignant lesions (see chapter 36). Although much less sensitive than Pap smear testing, bimanual palpation may detect some neoplasms of the cervix as well as benign lesions. Bimanual examination may also detect some cases of endometrial cancer, although the efficacy and effectiveness of such detection has not been well studied.

## Recommendations of Major Authorities

- **American Academy of Family Physicians**—Pelvic examination should be performed as part of routine periodic preventive care for adult women.

- **American Cancer Society**—Pelvic examination should be performed every 1 to 3 years for women aged 18 to 39 and annually for women over age 40.

- **American College of Obstetricians and Gynecologists** and **National Cancer Institute**—Women who have become sexually active or are 18 years of age and older should have annual pelvic examinations as part of a periodic health examination.

- **U.S. Preventive Services Task Force**—Routine pelvic examination is not recommended for the detection of ovarian cancer.

## Basics of Pelvic Organ Examination

1. *General Considerations*: Good lighting and a proper examination table should be used. The patient should empty her bladder and rectum prior to the examination.

2. *Inspection*: A general inspection of the external genitalia should be performed with the patient in the lithotomy position. The skin of the vulva should be inspected for redness, excoriation, masses, leukoplakia, and pigmentation.

3. *Femoral Nodes*: The horizontal chain of nodes inferior to the inguinal ligament and the vertical chain along the upper inner thigh should be palpated. Nodes less than 1 cm in this area may be normal if soft, discrete, and movable.

4. *Vagina and Cervix*: A speculum should be used to inspect the vagina and cervix. Water, rather than a lubricating jelly, should be used to warm and lubricate the speculum because

the jelly may interfere with interpretation of cervical cytology. The labia should be separated with two fingers and pressure applied posteriorly in the introitus. The speculum should be introduced at an oblique angle, avoiding pain-sensitive anterior structures, then rotated to the transverse position. The blades are then opened slowly and the speculum locked open. Any discharge that obscures the vaginal walls or cervix should be removed with cotton-tipped applicators. The vagina and cervix should be inspected for erosion, ulceration, leukoplakia, and masses. A Pap smear may be taken at this point (see chapter 36). As the speculum is removed, the vaginal sidewalls should once again be examined for leukoplakia, masses, and other abnormalities.

5. *Bimanual Palpation*: The lubricated index and middle fingers of one hand should be placed into the vaginal vault with the other hand on top of the abdomen. The fingers within the vaginal vault are used to palpate the cervix and sidewalls of the vagina for induration, masses, and tenderness. The fingers within the vagina are next used to lift the reproductive organs out of the pelvis so that they can be palpated by the abdominal hand. The size, location, contour, and mobility of the uterus, ovaries, and adnexa should be noted.

6. *Rectovaginal Septum*: The hand is partially withdrawn so that the middle finger can be removed from the vagina and inserted into the rectum. This allows for palpation of the rectovaginal septum to detect tumors, inflammatory or granulomatous masses, and for better evaluation of the uterus in obese individuals or in those in whom the uterus is retroverted.

## ■ Rectum and Prostate Examination ■

Colorectal cancer is the second leading cause of death from cancer in the United States. An estimated 149,000 new cases will be diagnosed, and 56,000 deaths will occur in 1994. Invasive colorectal cancer is the most preventable visceral cancer. Most cases arise from adenomatous polyps that take approximately 10 years to progress to an invasive stage. Patients presenting with regional disease have a 5-year survival rate of approximately 50%, whereas those presenting with localized disease have a 5-year survival rate of 85% for rectal cancer and 91% for colon cancer. Increased incidence is noted with familial syndromes; ulcerative colitis; first-degree family history of adenomas or colorectal cancer; and a personal history of adenomas or of ovarian, endometrial, or breast cancer. It is estimated that fewer than 10% of colorectal cancers can be palpated by digital rectal examination.

Prostate cancer is the most common type of cancer in men, after skin cancer. It is estimated that 1 of every 10 men in the United States will develop prostate cancer. There will be approximately 200,000 new cases in 1994 in the United States, with approximately 38,000 deaths in that period. Risk factors include advanced age and African-American race. Dietary fat may also be associated with prostate cancer. Digital rectal examination has a sensitivity of 33% to 69% and a specificity of 49% to 97% for detecting prostate cancer. There is little evidence that screening by digital rectal examination decreases mortality from prostate cancer. Some authorities believe this may be due to either its inability to detect tumors at an early,

## Ch. 29. Cancer Detection/Physical Examination — Adults/Older Adults — SCREENING

treatable stage or to the fact that some tumors grow so rapidly that yearly screening cannot detect most of them at an early, treatable stage, or both.

### Recommendations of Major Authorities

- **American Academy of Family Physicians**—Digital rectal examination should be included in the periodic health examination of individuals 40 years of age and older.

- **American Cancer Society**—Annual digital rectal examination should be performed for all patients starting at 40 years of age.

- **American College of Obstetricians and Gynecologists**—Digital rectal examination should be included in the periodic health examination of women 40 years of age and older as part of the pelvic exam.

- **American Society of Colon and Rectal Surgeons**—Annual digital rectal examination should be performed for asymptomatic, low-risk individuals 40 years of age and older and for asymptomatic individuals over 35 years of age with either a family history of colorectal adenomatous polyps or cancer in one or more first-degree relatives.

- **American Urological Association**—Digital rectal examination should be performed annually for men 40 to 49 years of age who have a family history of prostate cancer, and for all men over 50.

- **Canadian Task Force on the Periodic Health Examination**—Digital rectal examination is feasible, relatively cost-effective, and acceptable for detecting prostate cancer and can be adapted to case-finding in the primary care setting. However, the use of digital rectal examination is not recommended for screening for colorectal cancer.

- **National Cancer Institute**—A rectal examination should be included as a part of the periodic health examination. The clinician should identify high-risk patients for special surveillance, including those with a strong family history of colon cancer or a personal history of adenomas or inflammatory bowel disease.

- **U.S. Preventive Services Task Force**—There is insufficient evidence to recommend for or against routine digital rectal examination as an effective screening test for prostate cancer in asymptomatic men. No recommendation has been made regarding the use of the examination for colorectal cancer screening.

### Basics of Rectum and Prostate Examination

1. *General Considerations*: Male and female patients may be examined in the left lateral decubitus position or standing, bent over the examination table. Female patients may also be examined in the lithotomy position during a pelvic examination. The postexamination testing of fecal matter on the gloved finger for occult blood is of unknown value because trauma caused by the examination potentially may produce false-positive results.

2. *Inspection*: The anal opening should be visually inspected, with note made of any skin breakdown, fissures, and protrusions from the anal opening.

3. *Palpation*: The exam is performed by inserting the lubricated, gloved index finger into the anal opening. The gloved finger should be inserted just past the rectal sphincter and not advanced until the sphincter relaxes. When this procedure is followed, rectal exams may be uncomfortable, but most are not painful. All sides of the rectum should be palpated for polyps, which may be sessile (attached by a base) or pedunculated (attached by a stalk). Intraperitoneal metastases may be felt anterior to the rectum as hard, shelf-like projections into the rectum. In men, the posterior and lateral lobes of the prostate gland should be thoroughly palpated. The normal prostate gland is approximately 2.5 cm x 4 cm and does not protrude into the rectum by more than 1 cm. It should feel smooth and rubbery throughout and have a palpable central groove. Asymmetry of the prostate gland or the presence of a hard, irregular nodule, or both, are typical presentations of prostate cancer.

## ■ Skin Examination ■

Skin cancer is the most common type of cancer in the United States. Approximately 700,000 new cases of basal and squamous cell carcinoma, as well as 32,000 cases of malignant melanoma, will be diagnosed in 1994. An estimated 6900 deaths from malignant melanoma and approximately 2300 deaths from other types of skin cancer will occur in 1994. The incidence of malignant melanoma is increasing at the rate of 4% per year. Virtually 100% of skin cancers are curable if diagnosed and excised early. Skin cancers occur more commonly in fair-skinned individuals who have been exposed to the sun, X-rays, or ultraviolet light for prolonged periods of time. Chronic overexposure to sunlight is the cause of 95% of all basal cell carcinomas. Other risk factors for basal cell and squamous cell carcinomas include exposure to radiation, as complications of burns or scars, and contact with arsenic. Basal cell cancer is more common in older adults and affects men more frequently than women. Both basal cell and squamous cell cancers can occur in anyone with a history of prolonged sun exposure, and both are most likely to occur in sun-exposed areas. Factors placing individuals at increased risk for malignant melanoma include the presence of pigmented nevi and a personal or family history of skin cancer or dysplastic nevi.

**Recommendations of Major Authorities**

- **American Academy of Dermatology** and **Skin Cancer Foundation**—Annual skin examinations are recommended for all patients.

- **American Academy of Family Physicians, American College of Obstetricians and Gynecologists,** and **U.S. Preventive Services Task Force**—Skin examination should be performed for individuals with a family or personal history of skin cancer, increased occupational or recreational exposure to sunlight, or clinical evidence of precursor lesions (e.g., dysplastic nevi and certain congenital nevi).

- **American Cancer Society**—Patients should undergo a cancer checkup that includes examination of the skin every 3 years for those 20 to 39 years of age, and yearly after age 40.

- **Canadian Task Force on the Periodic Health Examination**—There is fair evidence for exclusion of cancer of the skin from specific consideration in a periodic health examination for the general population, but fair justification for inclusion of inspection of the skin in the periodic health examination for those at high risk, such as outdoor workers and those in contact with polycyclic aromatic hydrocarbons. It may be prudent to monitor more closely the relatives of patients afflicted with dysplastic nevi.

- **National Cancer Institute**—Primary care physicians are encouraged to examine the skin as part of the periodic health examination and other patient encounters, with special attention given to individuals at high risk and those with pigmented nevi.

**Basics of Skin Examination**

1. *General Considerations*: The room should be comfortably warm. Lighting should be adjusted to produce optimal illumination. Basal cell or squamous cell carcinomas are likely to present in one of the following ways: as an open sore that bleeds, oozes, or crusts and is present for more than 3 weeks; as an irritated red patch that may itch or hurt; as a growth with a rolled border and central indentation; as a shiny bump or nodule; as a scarlike area. Characteristics that may make a lesion suspicious for malignant melanoma may be remembered by following the ABCDs: **A**—asymmetry; **B**—irregular borders; **C**—variation in color from one area to another within the same lesion; and **D**—a diameter greater than 6 mm, about the size of a pencil eraser. Additional warning signs for malignant melanoma include sudden or continuous enlargement; elevation of a previously macular pigmented lesion; surface changes, such as bleeding, crusting, erosion, oozing, scaliness, or ulceration; changes in the surrounding skin, such as redness, swelling, or satellite pigmentation; changes in sensation, such as itching, tenderness, or pain; changes in consistency, such as softening or friability; and the development of a new pigmented lesion, particularly in patients more than 40 years of age. All pigmented lesions should be evaluated carefully.

2. *With the Patient Seated*: The skin of the head, upper torso, and upper extremities is easily examined with the patient in this position. Parting the hair will aid a thorough and careful inspection of the scalp. When examining the skin of the face and neck, special note should be taken of the eyelids, forehead, ears, nose, and lips. The upper extremities should be examined completely, as should the shoulders and back.

3. *With the Patient Supine*: The skin of the chest and abdomen should be inspected, with particular attention to the inguinal and genital areas. The scrotum should be elevated to allow inspection of the perineal area. The feet, including the soles and the area between the toes, should be examined carefully.

4. *With the Patient Lying on the Left Side*: The remaining skin of the back, legs, gluteal, and perianal areas may be examined with the patient in this position.

■ **Testis Examination** ■

Testicular cancer causes 1% of all cancers in men. It is the most common cancer in white men aged 20 to 34 years and will account for an estimated 6800 new cases and 325 deaths in 1994. The prognosis for testicular cancer is very good, especially if treated early. Increased incidence is noted in males with a history of cryptorchidism, gonadal dysgenesis, Klinefelter's syndrome, or in utero exposure to diethylstilbestrol (DES). Testicular cancer is more common in white men than in African Americans, with intermediate incidence rates in Hispanics, American Indians, and Asians.

## Recommendations of Major Authorities

- **American Academy of Family Physicians**—Testicular examination should be a routine part of the periodic health examination for men 19 to 39 years of age. Adolescents 13 to 18 years of age with a history cryptorchidism, orchiopexy, or testicular atrophy should also be examined.

- **American Cancer Society**—Testicular examination should be a part of the cancer checkup received by men every 3 years from 20 to 39 years of age and annually beginning at age 40.

- **American Urological Association**—Yearly clinical examinations should begin at age 15.

- **Canadian Task Force on the Periodic Health Examination**—Testicular examination should be part of the periodic health examination for men with a history of cryptorchidism, infertile or atrophic testes, or ambiguous genitalia.

- **National Cancer Institute**—Routine palpation of the testicles should continue to be a part of the periodic physical examination, but high-risk individuals with a history of cryptorchidism, gonadal dysgenesis, and Klinefelter's syndrome should receive special attention.

- **U.S. Preventive Services Task Force**—Clinical testicular examination should be performed for males aged 13 to 39 with a history of cryptorchidism, orchiopexy, or testicular atrophy.

## Basics of Testicular Examination

1. *Inspection*: With the patient standing, the genital area should be inspected for swelling, edema, and other visible abnormalities. The scrotum should be elevated to permit inspection of the perineum.

2. *Femoral Nodes*: The horizontal chain of nodes inferior to the inguinal ligament and the vertical chain along the upper inner thigh should be palpated. Nodes less than 1 cm may be normal if soft, discrete, and movable.

3. *Palpation*: With the patient standing, both hands should be used to examine each testicle individually. One hand holds the superior and inferior poles of the testicle while the other hand palpates the anterior, posterior, medial, and lateral surfaces. If any masses are noted, an attempt should be made to place a finger between the mass and the testicle. This will help differentiate between masses that originate from the testicle and those that arise from other structures within the scrotum. Next, an attempt should be made to transilluminate the mass. A tumor should not transilluminate. When a neoplasm is present, the testicle is usually enlarged, firm, and heavier than normal. If any abnormalities are noted, the patient should then be examined in the supine position to try to distinguish between solid masses (which will remain) and varicoceles (which may resolve).

4. *Testicular Self-Examination*: There is disagreement among authorities about whether to encourage patients to examine their testes regularly. Clinicians wishing to do so may refer to pamphlets on self-examination listed in Patient Resources at the end of this chapter.

# ■ Thyroid Examination ■

Approximately 13,000 cases of thyroid cancer will be diagnosed in 1994 in the United States, with approximately 1025 deaths attributed to the disease. Increased risk occurs in those who have had radiation to the head and neck as children or a family history of multiple endocrine neoplasia, type II. Thyroid malignancy occurs twice as frequently in women as in men.

## Recommendations of Major Authorities

- **American Academy of Family Physicians** and **U.S. Preventive Services Task Force**—Palpation for thyroid nodules should be performed in adults with a history of upper body irradiation.

- **American Cancer Society**—A cancer checkup, including palpation of the thyroid, should be performed every 3 years on individuals 20 to 39 years of age and yearly for individuals aged 40 years and over.

- **American College of Obstetricians and Gynecologists**—Thyroid palpation should be part of the periodic health examination for all women over the age of 18 years.

## Basics of Thyroid Examination

1. *Inspection*: The patient should be seated with the neck flexed slightly in order to relax the sternocleidomastoid muscles. A standing lamp may be positioned to shine tangentially across the neck in order to highlight any swelling. The neck should be observed as the patient takes a sip of water. Thyroid masses will move up and down with swallowing because of the thyroid's location within the fascial sheath of the trachea. A midline mass may also be a thyroglossal duct cyst.

2. *Palpation*: The patient should be sitting straight with the neck flexed slightly forward and to the right. Standing behind the patient, the examiner should use the fingertips of the left hand to push the trachea slightly to the right and the fingers of the right hand to retract the sternocleidomastoid muscle. While the patient takes a sip of water, the medial and lateral margins of the thyroid should be palpated with the fingertips of the right hand. The procedure is reversed for the left side. A malignancy may be palpated as a discrete area of firmness or hardness. Thyroid gland tenderness may also be suggestive of malignancy.

3. *Lymph Nodes*: Examination of the thyroid should include a determination of the presence of lymphadenopathy. The uppermost pretracheal node that lies above or over the thyroid isthmus is called the Delphian node. An enlarged Delphian node may be the earliest sign of metastatic papillary cancer. The pre- and postauricular nodes should also be examined, as well as the anterior and posterior cervical nodes. The anterior cervical nodes are clustered in a 7-shaped configuration with the horizontal axis just below the body of the mandible and the vertical axis along the anterior border of the sternocleidomastoid muscle. The posterior cervical nodes are clustered in an L-shaped configuration with the horizontal axis along the clavicle and the vertical axis along the anterior margin of the trapezius. The lymph nodes may be palpated by using a gentle circular motion of the

fingerpads. It is usually most efficient to palpate with both hands so that a comparison of the two sides can be made. Normal nodes should feel movable, discrete, soft, and nontender.

**Patient Resources**

*Breast Cancer: Steps to Finding Breast Lumps Early*; *Skin Cancer: Saving Your Skin From Sun Damage.* American Academy of Family Physicians, 8880 Ward Parkway, Kansas City, MO 64114-2797; 1-800 944-0000.

*Detecting and Treating Breast Problems.* American College of Obstetricians and Gynecologists, 409 12th Street, SW, Washington, DC 20024-2188;(202) 638-5577.

*Head & Neck Cancer: Know What the Warning Signs Are. . .*; *Your Thyroid Gland: A Guide for the Patient.* American Academy of Otolaryngology-Head and Neck Surgery, Order Dept., 1 Prince St., Alexandria, VA 22314; (703) 836-4444.

*For Men Only: Testicular Cancer and How To Do TSE (A Self Exam)*; *How To Do Breast Self Examination.* American Cancer Society, 1559 Clifton Rd. NE, Atlanta, GA 30329-4251; 1-800 ACS-2345.

*Preventing Cancer*; *Cancer of the Ovary.* American College of Obstetricians and Gynecologists, 409 12th St. SW, Washington, DC 20024; 1-800 762-2264.

*Colorectal Cancer, Questions & Answers.* American Society of Colon and Rectal Surgeons, 800 E Northwest Highway, Suite 1080, Palatine, IL 60067; (708) 359-9184.

*Testicular Cancer & Testicular Self-Examination.* American Urological Association, Inc., 1120 N Charles St., Baltimore, MD 21201-5559.

*Breast Exams: What You Should Know*; *Questions and Answers about Breast Lumps*; *Smart Advice for Women 40 and Over*; *What You Need To Know About Breast Cancer*; *What You Need To Know About Cancer of the Colon and Rectum*; *What You Need To Know About Ovarian Cancer*; *Question and Answers About the Pap Smear.* Office of Cancer Communications, National Cancer Institute, Bldg 31, Rm 10A24, Bethesda, MD 20892; 1-800 4-CANCER.

*Prostate Cancer: What Every Man over 40 Should Know.* Prostate Health Council, c/o American Foundation for Urologic Disease, Inc., 1120 N Charles St., Suite 401, Baltimore, MD 21201; 1-800 242-2383.

*The ABCDs of Moles & Melanomas*; *Dysplastic Nevi and Malignant Melanoma: A Patient's Guide*; *Skin Cancer: If You Can Spot It, You Can Stop It.* The Skin Cancer Foundation, PO Box 561, New York, NY 10156; (212) 725-5176.

## Provider Resources

*Nonmalignant Conditions of the Breast* (ACOG Technical Bulletin 156; 1991). American College of Obstetricians and Gynecologists, 409 12th St. SW, Washington, DC 20024; 1-800 762-2264.

*PDQ: The Physician Data Query System for Cancer Information.* PDQ is the National Cancer Institute's computerized database providing the most up-to-date cancer information available. Access to the system can be gained 24 hours a day, 7 days a week, using a personal computer and standard telephone line, or through medical libraries. Ask a medical librarian or call 1-800 4-CANCER. In Hawaii, on Oahu, call 524-1234.

## Selected References

American Academy of Family Physicians, Commission on Public Health and Scientific Affairs. *Age Charts for Periodic Health Examination.* Kansas City, Mo: American Academy of Family Physicians; 1993.

American Cancer Society. *Summary of American Cancer Society Recommendations for the Early Detection of Cancer in Asymptomatic People.* Atlanta, Ga: American Cancer Society; 1992.

American College of Obstetricians and Gynecologists. *Report of Task Force on Routine Cancer Screening.* Washington, DC: American College of Obstetricians and Gynecologists; 1989. ACOG Committee Opinion 68.

American College of Obstetricians and Gynecologists. *The Obstetrician-Gynecologist and Primary-Preventive Health Care.* Washington, DC: American College of Obstetricians and Gynecologists, 1993.

American College of Physicians. Guidelines. In Eddy, DM ed., *Common Screening Tests.* Philadelphia, Pa: American College of Physicians;19191:411-416.

American Society of Colon and Rectal Surgeons. *Practice Parameters for the Detection of Colorectal Neoplasms.* Palatine, Ill: American Society of Colon and Rectal Surgeons; 1992.

American Urological Association. *Early Detection of Prostate Cancer and Use of Transrectal Ultrasound.* Baltimore, Md: American Urological Association; 1992.

Boring CC, Squires TS, Tong T, Montgomery S. Cancer Statistics, 1994. *CA.* 1994;4:7-26.

Canadian Task Force on the Periodic Health Examination. The periodic health examination, 1979. *Can Med Assoc J.* 1979;121:18.

Canadian Task Force on the Periodic Health Examination. The periodic health examination: 2. 1984 update: cancer of the skin (including melanoma). *Can Med Assoc J.* 1984;130:7.

Canadian Task Force on the Periodic Health Examination. The periodic health examination: 2. 1984 update: cancer of the testis. *Can Med Assoc J.* 1984;130:9–10.

Canadian Task Force on the Periodic Health Examination. The periodic health examination: 2. 1985 update: breast cancer. *Can Med Assoc J.* 1986;134:724–725.

Canadian Task Force on the Periodic Health Examination. The periodic health examination: 2. 1987 update: endometrial cancer. *Can Med Assoc J.* 1988;138:620–621.

Canadian Task Force on the Periodic Health Examination. The periodic health examination: 2. 1989 update: early detection of colorectal cancer. *Can Med Assoc J.* 1989;141:4–7.

Canadian Task Force on the Periodic Health Examination. The periodic health examination: 3. 1991 update: secondary prevention of prostate cancer. *Can Med Assoc J.* 1991;144:15–30.

DeGowin EL, DeGowin RL. *Bedside Diagnostic Examination.* 5th ed. New York, NY: Macmillan Publishing Co; 1987.

Fink DJ. Cancer detection: the cancer-related checkup guidelines. In: *American Cancer Society Textbook of Clinical Oncology.* Atlanta, Ga: American Cancer Society; 1991.

Friedman RJ, Rigel DS, Silverman MK, Kopf AW, Vossaert KA. Malignant melanoma in the 1990s: the continued importance of early detection and the role of physician examination and self-examination of the skin. *CA*. 1991;41:201–227.

Gerber GS, Thompson IM, Thisted R, Chodak GW. Disease-specific survival following routine prostate cancer screening by digital rectal examination. *JAMA*. 1993;269:61–64.

Jarvis C. *Physical Examination and Health Assessment*. Philadelphia, Pa: WB Saunders Co; 1992.

MacLeod J, Munro J, eds. *Clinical Examination*. 7th ed. New York, NY: Churchill Livingstone; 1986.

Moloy PJ. How to (and how not to) manage the patient with a lump in the neck. In: *Common Problems of the Head and Neck Region*. Philadelphia, Pa: WB Saunders Co;1992:129–150.

Rhodes AR, Weinstock MA, Fitzpatrick TB, Mihm MC, Sober AJ. Risk factors for cutaneous melanoma: a practical method of recognizing predisposed individuals. *JAMA*. 1987;258:3146–3153.

Smart CR, Chu K, Conley V, Henson DE, Pommerenke F, Srivastova S. Cancer Screening and Early Detection. In: Holland JF, Frei III EF, Bast Sr. RC, Kufe DW, Morton DL, Weichselbaum RR, eds. *Cancer Medicine*. 3rd ed. Vol.1. Philadelphia: Lea and Febiger, 1993; 408-431.

Swartz MH. *Textbook of Physical Diagnosis*. Philadelphia, Pa: WB Saunders Co; 1989.

US Preventive Services Task Force. Neoplastic diseases. In: *Guide to Clinical Preventive Services*. Baltimore, Md: Williams & Wilkins, 1989:chaps 6-9, 11-13, 15.

Wartofsky L. Examination of the thyroid. In: Becker KL, ed. *Principles and Practice of Endocrinology & Metabolism*. New York, NY: JB Lippincott; 1990

## Adults/Older Adults — SCREENING

# 30. Cholesterol

High blood cholesterol is a major modifiable risk factor for coronary heart disease (CHD)—the leading cause of death for both men and women in the United States. Approximately 1.25 million myocardial infarctions and 500,000 deaths from CHD occur each year. In large population-based studies, total cholesterol levels are directly related to CHD incidence. In the Multiple Risk Factor Intervention Trial (MRFIT), the 6-year risk of death from CHD in normotensive, nonsmoking, middle-aged men with blood cholesterol levels less than 182 mg/dL was one fourth that of men with blood cholesterol levels greater than or equal to 245 mg/dL. Epidemiologic studies have shown that cholesterol lipoprotein subfractions play an important role in CHD. LDL-cholesterol is directly and HDL-cholesterol is inversely associated with CHD incidence.

A meta-analysis of cholesterol-lowering trials performed mainly in middle-aged men has shown that lowering blood cholesterol through diet or drug therapy significantly reduces the risk of CHD death and nonfatal myocardial infarction. In secondary prevention trials among those who have had a myocardial infarction, the reduction in CHD mortality is associated with a reduction in total mortality. In primary prevention trials, however, reduced total mortality has not been shown, and there have been variable increases in different causes of noncardiac mortality offsetting the decline in CHD deaths. It is unclear whether this is a chance finding reflecting the limited statistical power of the primary prevention studies for observations on total mortality or whether it reflects effects of cholesterol lowering.

See chapter 4 for information on cholesterol screening in children and adolescents.

### Recommendations of Major Authorities

- **American Academy of Family Physicians**—Adults (19 years of age and older) should have measurement of nonfasting or fasting total blood cholesterol performed at least every 5 years.

- **American College of Obstetricians and Gynecologists**—Adults (19 years of age and older) should have cholesterol measured every 5 years until 64 years of age, and then every 3 to 5 years thereafter.

- **American College of Physicians**—Total cholesterol measurement is recommended at least once in early adulthood and at intervals of 5 or more years up to age 70. The LDL and HDL cholesterol and serum triglyceride levels should be measured in individuals with an elevated total serum cholesterol level. The decision to perform these additional tests should be individualized. Factors to be taken into account include age, gender, number of other cardiovascular risk factors, and the patients' willingness to comply with drug and dietary treatment of hypercholesterolemia.

- **Canadian Task Force on the Periodic Health Examination**—There is insufficient evidence for the inclusion or exclusion of universal screening for hypercholesterolemia in a periodic health examination. Nonetheless, case-finding through repeated measurements of the nonfasting total blood cholesterol level should be considered in men 30 to 59 years of age. Individual clinical judgment on whether testing is appropriate should be exercised in all other circumstances.

- **National Cholesterol Education Program (NCEP) of the National Heart, Lung, and Blood Institute**—Adults (20 years of age and older) should have a measurement of total blood cholesterol at least once every 5 years; HDL-cholesterol should be measured at the same time if accurate results are available. Lipoprotein analysis should be performed for all patients with CHD. In patients without CHD, lipoprotein analysis should be performed in any of the following circumstances: 1) if the total cholesterol is 240 mg/dL or above; 2) if the total cholesterol is 200 to 239 mg/dL and the patient also has two or more CHD risk factors; 3) if the patient has an HDL-cholesterol less than 35 mg/dL. See Table 30-1 and Figs 30-1, 30-2, and 30-3 for NCEP recommendations on CHD risk factors and patient classification and identification.

- **U.S. Preventive Services Task Force**—Periodic measurement of total serum cholesterol (nonfasting) is most important for middle-aged men, and it may also be clinically prudent in young men, women, and the elderly. The optimal frequency for cholesterol measurement in asymptomatic individuals has not been determined on the basis of scientific evidence and is left to clinical discretion. This recommendation is currently under review.

## Basics of Cholesterol Screening

1. Patients who are acutely ill, losing weight, pregnant, or nursing should not be screened, as their cholesterol levels may not be representative of usual levels. Because cholesterol levels in patients who have had myocardial infarction within the last 3 months are likely to be lower than usual, results obtained during this period should be rechecked.

2. Patients need not vary their usual eating habits before undergoing screening for total blood cholesterol or HDL-cholesterol. Patients undergoing lipoprotein analysis should fast (water and black coffee are acceptable) for 12 hours before testing.

3. If possible, cholesterol tests should be performed on venous blood samples, as cholesterol concentrations measured from finger-stick blood samples may be unreliable. The NCEP cut points for diagnostic and therapeutic actions refer to venous serum samples.

4. To prevent an effect of posture or stasis on the cholesterol value, venipuncture should be carried out only after the patient has been in the sitting position for at least 5 minutes, and the tourniquet should be applied for as brief a period as possible.

5. In interpreting results, clinicians should be familiar with the effects of medications on cholesterol levels. Anabolic steroids, progestins, bile salts, and chlorpromazine increase blood cholesterol. Clinicians should also be knowledgeable about conditions that may cause increased cholesterol levels, such as hypothyroidism, nephrotic syndrome, diabetes mellitus, and obstructive liver disease.

6. Cholesterol tests should be analyzed by an accredited laboratory that meets current standards for precision and accuracy. The Laboratory Standardization Panel of the National Cholesterol Education Program has set a goal that laboratories have systematic and precision errors of less than 3% in processing total cholesterol samples. Clinicians

## Table 30-1. NCEP Coronary Heart Disease Risk Factors Other Than LDL-Cholesterol*

**Postive Risk Factors**

Age
　Male ≥45 years
　Female ≥55 years or premature menopause without estrogen replacement therapy

Family history of premature CHD (definite myocardial infarction or sudden death)
　father/first degree male relative <55 years
　mother/first degree female relative <65 years

Cigarette smoking

Hypertension
　≥140/90 mmHg**, or on anti-hypertensive medication

Low HDL-cholesterol (<35 mg/dL)

Diabetes mellitus

**Negative Risk Factors***

HDL Cholesterol ≥60 mg/dL

*High risk, defined as two or more CHD risk factors (after positive and negative factors have been summed), leads to more vigorous intervention in Figs. 30-1 and 30-2. Age (defined differently for men and for women) is treated as a risk factor because rates of CHD are higher in the elderly than in the young, and in men than in women of the same age. Obesity is not listed as a risk factor because it operates through other risk factors that are included (hypertension, hyperlipidemia, decreased HDL-cholesterol, and diabetes mellitus), but it should be considered a target for intervention. Physical inactivity is similarly not listed as a risk factor, but it too should be considered a target for intervention, and physical activity is recommended as desirable for everyone. High risk due to coronary or peripheral atherosclerosis is addressed directly in Fig. 30-3.

**Confirmed by measurements on several occasions

***If the HDL-cholesterol level is ≥60 mg/dL subtract one risk factor (because high HDL-cholesterol levels decrease CHD risk)

Adapted from: National Cholesterol Education Program. *Second Report of the National Cholesterol Education Program Expert Panel on Detection, Evaluation, and Treatment of High Blood Cholesterol in Adults (Adult Treatment Panel II)*. Bethesda, MD: National Institutes of Health, National Heart, Lung, and Blood Institute. USDHHS Pub. No. NIH 93-3095, 1993.

should inquire about a laboratory's performance history and quality-control methods before using it for screening.

7. Cholesterol values in plasma samples tend to be lower than serum samples because of the effects of EDTA in plasma samples. NCEP has determined cholesterol level cut points based on serum samples and has designated that cholesterol levels obtained from plasma samples be multiplied by 1.03 to arrive at a serum equivalent.

8. Cholesterol values in mg/dL can be converted to mmol/L by multiplying by 0.02586. Triglyceride levels can be similarly converted by multiplying by 0.01129.

9. See Table 55-2 for information about NCEP's Step I and Step II Diet for treatment of patients with elevated cholesterol levels.

10. All patients who are obese, regardless of cholesterol level, should receive dietary and weight reduction counseling (see chapters 28 and 55). All patients who are physically inactive, regardless of cholesterol level, should receive counseling on increasing physical activity (see chapter 56).

**Patient Resources**

*Cholesterol: What You Can Do to Lower Your Level.* American Academy of Family Physicians, 8880 Ward Parkway, Kansas City, MO 64114-2797; 1-800 944-0000.

*Cholesterol and Your Health.* American College of Obstetricians and Gynecologists, 409 12th St. SW, Washington, DC 20024-2188; 1-800 762-2264.

*Cholesterol and Your Heart; Dietary Treatment of Hypercholesterolemia: A Manual for Patients; Eat Less Fat and High Cholesterol Foods*; and many other materials. American Heart Association, 7320 Greenville Ave., Dallas, TX 75231; 1-800 242-8721.

*Eating to Lower Your High Blood Cholesterol; So You Have High Blood Cholesterol.* National Heart, Lung, and Blood Institute Information Center, PO Box 30105, Bethesda, MD 20824-0105; (301) 251-1222.

**Provider Resources**

*Summary of the Second Report of the National Cholesterol Education Program Expert Panel on Detection, Evaluation, and Treatment of High Blood Cholesterol in Adults (Adult Treatment Panel II, or ATP II).* National Heart, Lung, and Blood Institute Information Center, P.O. Box 30105, Bethesda, MD 20824-0105; (301) 251-1222.

*Heart Rx.* American Heart Association, 7320 Greenville Ave., Dallas, TX 75231. A kit of materials for patients, providers, and office staff; 1-800 242-8721.

**Selected References**

American Academy of Family Physicians, Commission on Public Health and Scientific Affairs. *Age Charts for Periodic Health Examination.* Kansas City, Mo: American Academy of Family Physicians; 1993.
American College of Obstetricians and Gynecologists. *The Obstetrician-Gynecologist and Primary-Preventive Health Care.* Washington, DC: American College of Obstetricians and Gynecologists, 1993.
American College of Physicians. Guidelines. In: Eddy DM, ed. *Common Screening Tests.* Philadelphia, Pa: American College of Physicians; 1991:402-403.
Canadian Task Force on the Periodic Health Examination. Periodic health examination: 2. 1993 update. Lowering the blood total cholesterol level to prevent coronary heart disease. *Can Med Assoc J.* 1993;148:521-535.

Ch. 30. Cholesterol — Adults/Older Adults — SCREENING

**Figure 30-1. Primary Prevention in Adults Without Evidence of CHD: Initial Classification Based on Total Cholesterol and HDL-Cholesterol**

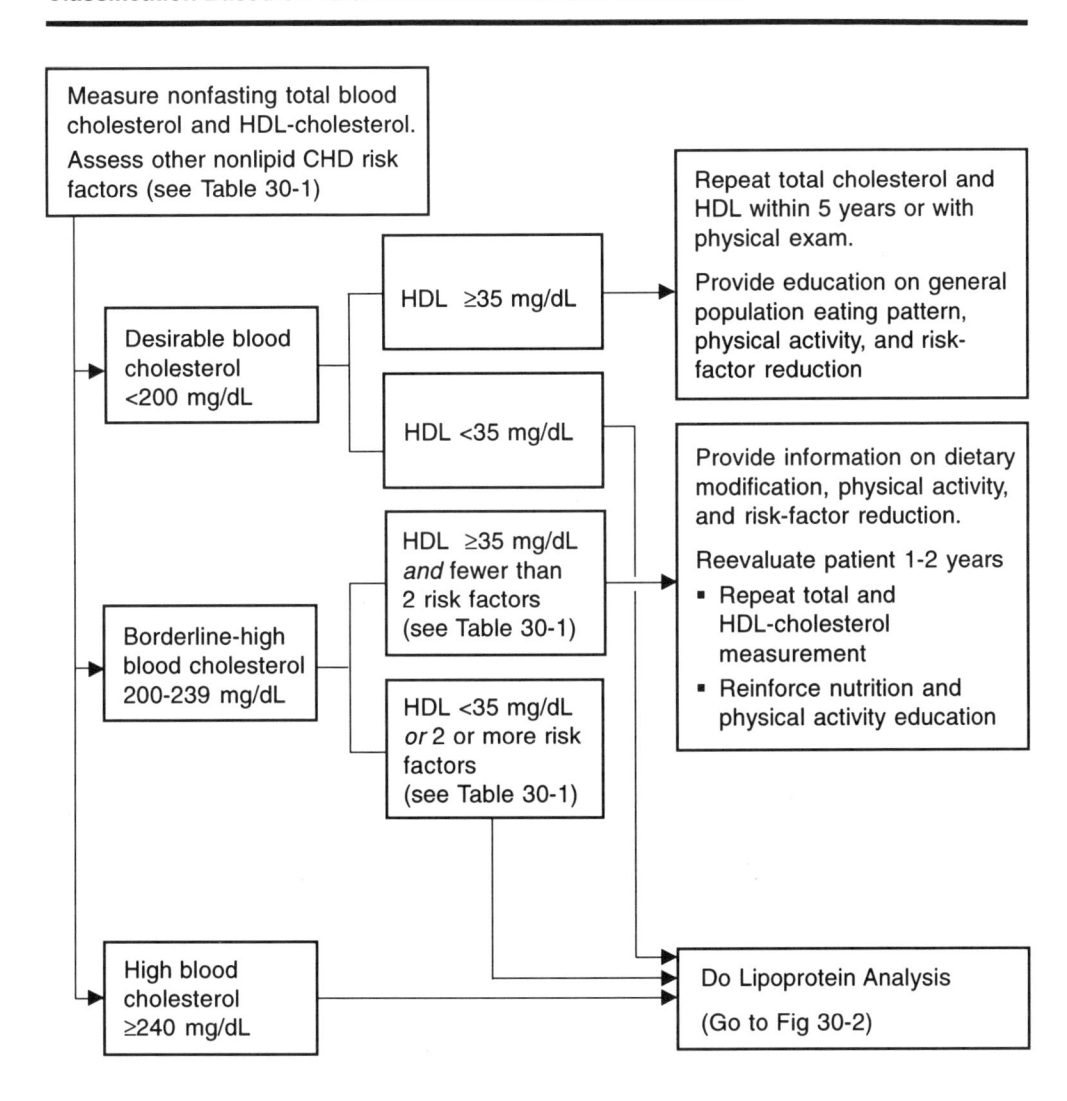

```
┌─────────────────────────────┐
│ Measure nonfasting total    │
│ blood cholesterol and       │
│ HDL-cholesterol.            │
│ Assess other nonlipid CHD   │      ┌──────────────────────────────┐
│ risk factors (see Table     │      │ Repeat total cholesterol and │
│ 30-1)                       │      │ HDL within 5 years or with   │
└─────────────────────────────┘      │ physical exam.               │
         │                           │                              │
         │          ┌─────────────┐  │ Provide education on general │
         │       ┌──│ HDL ≥35     │──▶│ population eating pattern,   │
         │       │  │ mg/dL       │  │ physical activity, and risk- │
  ┌──────────┐   │  └─────────────┘  │ factor reduction             │
  │Desirable │───┤                   └──────────────────────────────┘
  │blood     │   │  ┌─────────────┐
  │chol.     │   └──│ HDL <35     │──┐
  │<200 mg/dL│      │ mg/dL       │  │
  └──────────┘      └─────────────┘  │
                                     │  ┌──────────────────────────────┐
                   ┌─────────────────┐│  │ Provide information on       │
                   │ HDL ≥35 mg/dL   ││  │ dietary modification,        │
                ┌──│ and fewer than  │┼─▶│ physical activity, and risk- │
                │  │ 2 risk factors  ││  │ factor reduction.            │
  ┌──────────┐  │  │ (see Table 30-1)││  │                              │
  │Borderline│──┤  └─────────────────┘│  │ Reevaluate patient 1-2 years │
  │-high     │  │                     │  │  • Repeat total and          │
  │blood chol│  │  ┌─────────────────┐│  │    HDL-cholesterol           │
  │200-239   │  │  │ HDL <35 mg/dL   ││  │    measurement               │
  │mg/dL     │  └──│ or 2 or more    ││  │  • Reinforce nutrition and   │
  └──────────┘     │ risk factors    ││  │    physical activity         │
                   │ (see Table 30-1)├┘  │    education                 │
                   └─────────────────┘   └──────────────────────────────┘
                            │
  ┌──────────┐              │
  │High blood│              ▼
  │chol.     │─────▶ ┌──────────────────────────┐
  │≥240 mg/dL│       │ Do Lipoprotein Analysis  │
  └──────────┘       │ (Go to Fig 30-2)         │
                     └──────────────────────────┘
```

Adapted from: National Cholesterol Education Program. *Second Report of the National Cholesterol Education Program Expert Panel on Detection, Evaluation, and Treatment of High Blood Cholesterol in Adults (Adult Treatment Panel II)*. Bethesda, MD: National Institutes of Health, National Heart, Lung, and Blood Institute. USDHHS Pub. No. NIH 93-3095, 1993.

Ch. 30. Cholesterol                                      Adults/Older Adults — SCREENING

**Figure 30-2. Primary Prevention in Adults Without Evidence of CHD: Subsequent Classification Based on LDL-Cholesterol**

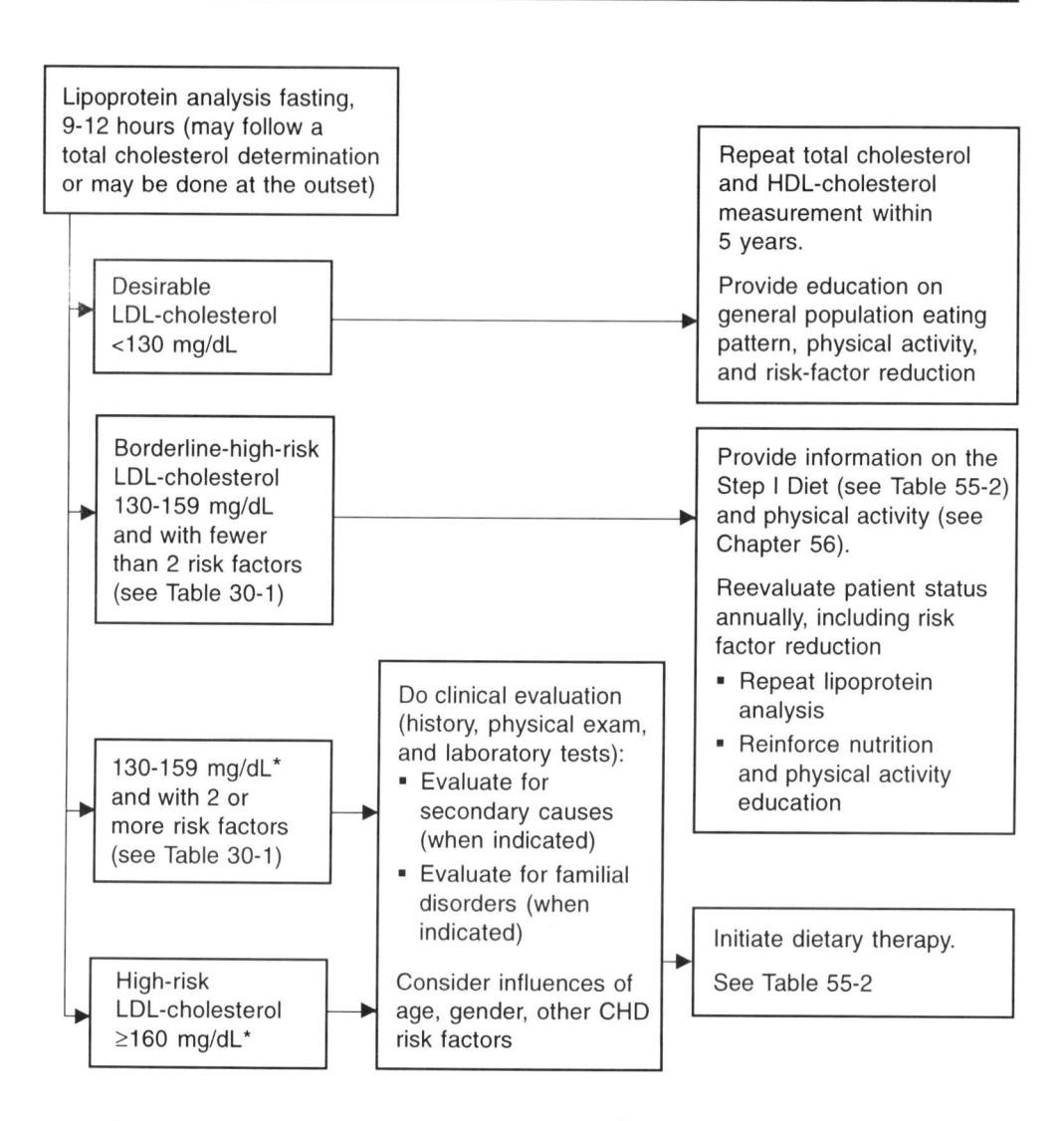

```
┌─────────────────────────────┐
│ Lipoprotein analysis fasting,│
│ 9-12 hours (may follow a    │       ┌─────────────────────────────┐
│ total cholesterol           │       │ Repeat total cholesterol    │
│ determination or may be     │       │ and HDL-cholesterol         │
│ done at the outset)         │       │ measurement within          │
└──────────────┬──────────────┘       │ 5 years.                    │
               │                      │                             │
               │    ┌──────────────┐  │ Provide education on        │
               ├───▶│ Desirable    │  │ general population eating   │
               │    │ LDL-         │─▶│ pattern, physical activity, │
               │    │ cholesterol  │  │ and risk-factor reduction   │
               │    │ <130 mg/dL   │  └─────────────────────────────┘
               │    └──────────────┘
               │    ┌──────────────┐  ┌─────────────────────────────┐
               │    │ Borderline-  │  │ Provide information on the  │
               │    │ high-risk    │  │ Step I Diet (see Table 55-2)│
               ├───▶│ LDL-chol.    │─▶│ and physical activity (see  │
               │    │ 130-159 mg/dL│  │ Chapter 56).                │
               │    │ and with     │  │                             │
               │    │ fewer than 2 │  │ Reevaluate patient status   │
               │    │ risk factors │  │ annually, including risk    │
               │    │(see Tbl 30-1)│  │ factor reduction            │
               │    └──────────────┘  │  ▪ Repeat lipoprotein       │
               │                      │    analysis                 │
               │                      │  ▪ Reinforce nutrition      │
               │    ┌──────────────┐  │    and physical activity    │
               │    │130-159 mg/dL*│  │    education                │
               ├───▶│ and with 2 or│  └─────────────────────────────┘
               │    │ more risk    │
               │    │ factors      │  ┌──────────────────────────┐
               │    │(see Tbl 30-1)│─▶│ Do clinical evaluation   │
               │    └──────────────┘  │ (history, physical exam, │
               │                      │ and laboratory tests):   │
               │                      │  ▪ Evaluate for          │
               │    ┌──────────────┐  │    secondary causes      │
               │    │ High-risk    │  │    (when indicated)      │
               └───▶│ LDL-         │─▶│  ▪ Evaluate for familial │
                    │ cholesterol  │  │    disorders (when       │   ┌──────────────────────┐
                    │ ≥160 mg/dL*  │  │    indicated)            │──▶│ Initiate dietary     │
                    └──────────────┘  │ Consider influences of   │   │ therapy.             │
                                      │ age, gender, other CHD   │   │ See Table 55-2       │
                                      │ risk factors             │   └──────────────────────┘
                                      └──────────────────────────┘
```

*On the basis of average of two determinations. If the first two LDL-cholesterol tests differ by more than 30 mg/dL, a third test should be obtained within 1-8 weeks and the average value of 3 tests used.

Adapted from: National Cholesterol Education Program. *Second Report of the National Cholesterol Education Program Expert Panel on Detection, Evaluation, and Treatment of High Blood Cholesterol in Adults (Adult Treatment Panel II).* Bethesda, MD: National Institutes of Health, National Heart, Lung, and Blood Institute. USDHHS Pub. No. NIH 93-3095, 1993.

Ch. 30. Cholesterol                                    Adults/Older Adults — SCREENING

**Figure 30-3. Secondary Prevention in Adults With Evidence of CHD: Classification Based on LDL-Cholesterol**

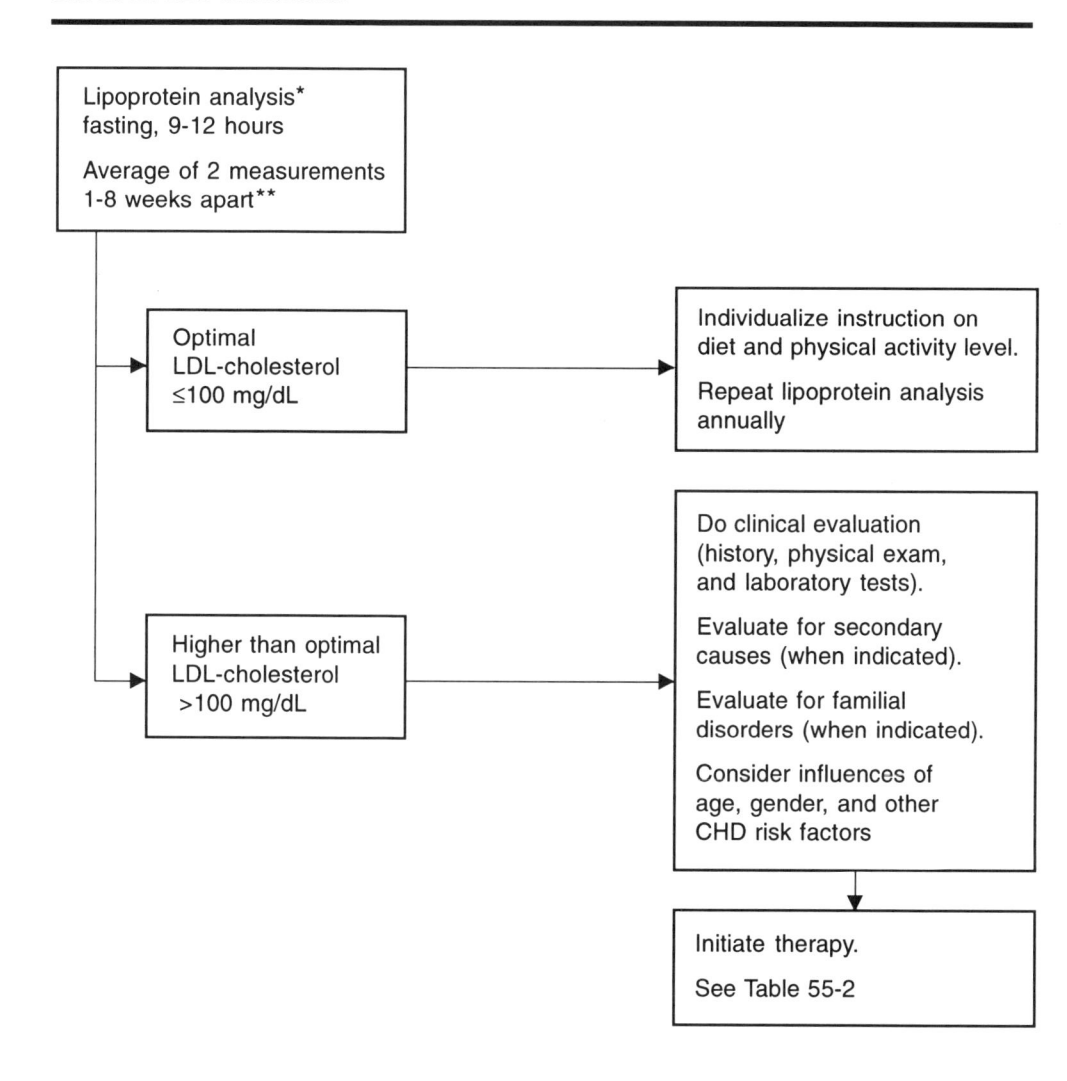

```
┌─────────────────────────┐
│ Lipoprotein analysis*   │
│ fasting, 9-12 hours     │
│                         │
│ Average of 2 measurements│
│ 1-8 weeks apart**       │
└─────────────────────────┘
      │
      │         ┌──────────────────┐          ┌──────────────────────────────┐
      │         │ Optimal          │          │ Individualize instruction on │
      ├────────▶│ LDL-cholesterol  │─────────▶│ diet and physical activity   │
      │         │ ≤100 mg/dL       │          │ level.                       │
      │         └──────────────────┘          │ Repeat lipoprotein analysis  │
      │                                       │ annually                     │
      │                                       └──────────────────────────────┘
      │
      │                                       ┌──────────────────────────────┐
      │                                       │ Do clinical evaluation       │
      │                                       │ (history, physical exam,     │
      │                                       │ and laboratory tests).       │
      │         ┌──────────────────┐          │ Evaluate for secondary       │
      │         │ Higher than optimal│        │ causes (when indicated).     │
      └────────▶│ LDL-cholesterol   │────────▶│ Evaluate for familial        │
                │ >100 mg/dL        │         │ disorders (when indicated).  │
                └──────────────────┘          │ Consider influences of       │
                                              │ age, gender, and other       │
                                              │ CHD risk factors             │
                                              └──────────────────────────────┘
                                                           │
                                                           ▼
                                              ┌──────────────────────────────┐
                                              │ Initiate therapy.            │
                                              │ See Table 55-2               │
                                              └──────────────────────────────┘
```

*Lipoprotein analysis should be performed when the patient is not in the recovery phase from an acute coronary or other medical event that would lower the patient's usual LDL-cholesterol level.

**If the first two LDL-cholesterol tests differ by more than 30 mg/dL, a third test should be obtained within 1-8 weeks and the average value of the three tests used.

Adapted from: National Cholesterol Education Program. *Second Report of the National Cholesterol Education Program Expert Panel on Detection, Evaluation, and Treatment of High Blood Cholesterol in Adults (Adult Treatment Panel II)*. Bethesda, MD: National Institutes of Health, National Heart, Lung, and Blood Institute. USDHHS Pub. No. NIH 93-3095, 1993.

Expert Panel on Detection, Evaluation, and Treatment of High Blood Cholesterol in Adults. Summary of the second report of the National Cholesterol Education Program (NCEP) Expert Panel on Detection, Evaluation, and Treatment of High Blood Cholesterol in Adults (Adult Treatment Panel II). *JAMA*. 1993;269:3015-3023.

Greenland P, Bowley NL, Meiklejohn B, Doane KL, Sparks CE. Blood cholesterol concentration: Fingerstick plasma vs venous serum sampling. *Clin Chem*. 1990;36:628-630.

National Cholesterol Education Program. Second Report of the National Cholesterol Education Program Expert Panel on Detection, Evaluation, and Treatment of High Blood Cholesterol in Adults (Adult Treatment Panel II). Bethesda, Md: National Heart, Lung, and Blood Institute. 1993.

National Cholesterol Education Program. *Report of the Expert Panel on Population Strategies for Blood Cholesterol Reduction*. Bethesda, Md: National Institutes of Health, National Heart, Lung, and Blood Institute; 1990. US Dept of Health and Human Services, Public Health Service, publication NIH 90-3046.

NIH Consensus Development Panel on Triglyceride, High-Density Lipoprotein, and Coronary Heart Disease. Triglyceride, high-density lipoprotein, and coronary heart disease. *JAMA*. 1993;269:505-510.

Sampos CT, Cleeman JI, Carroll MD, et al. Prevalence of high blood cholesterol among US adults: an update based on guidelines from the second report of the National Cholesterol Education Program Adult Treatment Panel. *JAMA*. 1993;269:3009-3014.

US Preventive Services Task Force. Screening for high blood cholesterol. In: *Guide to Clinical Preventive Services*. Baltimore, Md: Williams & Wilkins; 1989:chap 2.

## Adults/Older Adults — SCREENING

# ■—31. Cognitive and Functional Impairment—■

Cognitive impairment is common among older individuals, with prevalence increasing with age. Between 5% and 10% of those older than 65 years and up to 47% of those over 85 years of age suffer from some degree of dementia. The most common causes (Alzheimer's disease and vascular infarctions) are largely untreatable. Roughly 10% to 15% of cases of cognitive impairment in the older adult are due to treatable causes, such as hypothyroidism and drug intoxications. Dementia, particularly in its early stages, can be difficult for the clinician to detect. Only about half of patients with dementia are detected through routine history and physical examination by primary care physicians. In its most extreme forms, dementia can impair virtually all important functions of life. Early intervention in cases of treatable dementia can arrest or reverse cognitive defects. For untreatable cases, accurate assessment of cognitive function can be of value in counseling patients and family members and in planning support services.

Functional impairment in the older adult can have several different causes, including cognitive, physical, social, and psychological disorders. Approximately 2% to 8% of community-dwelling elderly suffer from impairments of activities of daily living (ADLs)—basic activities such as dressing, bathing, and eating. As many of 25% of community-dwelling older adults may suffer from functional impairment in carrying out instrumental activities of daily living (IADLs)—advanced but necessary functions of life, such as using transportation, going shopping, or handling finances. Clinicians may underestimate (by up to 50%) the amount of impairment patients experience in daily living.

**Recommendations of Major Authorities**

- **American Academy of Family Physicians** and **U.S. Preventive Services Task Force**—Routine screening tests for dementia are not recommended for elderly individuals with no evidence of cognitive impairment. Providers should, however, periodically inquire into the functional status of elderly patients at home and at work, and they should remain alert to changes in performance with age.

- **American College of Physicians**—Functional assessment screening by the clinician is useful for evaluating the health status of elderly patients and determining their needs for in-home assistance, home health services, or institutional placement. In the acute-care setting, functional assessment in selected patients facilitates discharge planning and is essential in patients over 75 years of age. Primary care providers should incorporate into the routine medical management of older adults procedures for measuring functional deficits and identifying dependency needs. Employing a comprehensive screening instrument followed by targeted screening instruments can be useful in systematically assessing functional deficits that otherwise might be overlooked by conventional examination methods.

- **Canadian Task Force on the Periodic Health Examination**—As part of the periodic health examination for patients over 65 years of age, the health care professional should inquire about sensory, psychological, and locomotor function as well as ADLs. There is insufficient evidence to include routine screening for cognitive impairment in or exclude it from the periodic health examination of people over 65 years of age.

- **Society of General Internal Medicine**—The evaluation of each outpatient over the age of 65 years should include a formal review of IADLs. This should be repeated on all home-dwelling individuals over the age of 65 years at least once every 3 years. Among patients over the age of 75 years, patients over the age of 65 years in hospitals or nursing homes, and patients who have problems in performing IADLs, evaluation of mental status and basic ADLs should be performed. It is important to assess mental status periodically in any elderly patient, because it affects diagnosis, choice of and ability to comply with interventions, and prognosis.

## Basics of Cognitive and Functional Impairment Screening

### *Cognitive Impairment*

1. Effective screening for cognitive impairment requires assessment of multiple aspects of mental functioning, including orientation, short-term memory, receptive and expressive language ability, attention, and visual-spatial ability.

2. Orientation can be rapidly assessed by asking the patient to give the day of the week, the month, the year, and location. Short-term memory can be rapidly assessed by asking the patient to repeat a seven-digit number or recall three objects. Language ability can be rapidly assessed by asking the patient to name simple objects, repeat a phrase, or write a sentence. Attention can be rapidly assessed by asking the patient to count backward from 100 to 65 by subtracting 7, or to name the months of the year in reverse order. Visual-spatial ability can be rapidly assessed by asking the patient to draw a complex figure, such as the face of a clock or a three-dimensional cube.

3. Use of a short, standardized screening instrument can accomplish this basic assessment and provide a baseline for assessing changes in cognitive function in the future. No single screening instrument best addresses all areas of cognition nor is appropriate for all patients. The most widely used and studied brief screening instrument is the Mini-Mental State Examination (Table 31-1).

4. Any assessment of cognitive functioning must take into consideration the patient's level and clarity of consciousness (Is the patient delirious?), affective state (Is the patient depressed?), effects of medications and drugs (Is the patient intoxicated?), level of education and baseline intelligence (Would the patient have understood as a young person?), and native language (Is the patient fluent in English?).

5. Patients with indications of cognitive impairment should be considered for referral to a specialist for more definitive evaluation before the diagnosis of dementia is made and treatment begun.

Ch. 31. Cognitive and Functional Impairment           Adults/Older Adults — SCREENING

### Table 31-1. Mini-Mental State Examination

| Maximum Score | Patient's Score | Questions |
|---|---|---|
| 5 | | "What is the (year) (season) (date) (day) (month)?" |
| 5 | | "Where are we?" Name of (state) (county) (city or town) (place, such as hospital or clinic) (specific location, such as floor or room) |
| 3 | | The examiner names three unrelated objects clearly and slowly, then asks the patient to name all three of them. The patient's response is used for scoring. The examiner repeats them until patient learns all of them, if possible. |
| 5 | | "Begin with 100 and count backwards by subtracting 7." Stop at 65. (5 responses). |
| 3 | | If the patient learned the three objects above, ask the patient to recall them now. |
| 2 | | The examiner shows the patient two simple objects, such as a wrist watch and pencil, and asks the patient to name them. |
| 1 | | "Repeat the phrase, 'No ifs, ands or buts.'" |
| 3 | | The examiner gives the patient a piece of blank paper and asks him or her to follow the three-step command: "Take the paper in your right hand, fold it in half, and put it on the floor." |
| 1 | | On a blank piece of paper the examiner prints the command "Close your eyes," in letters large enough for the patient to see clearly, then asks the patient to read it and follow the command. |
| 1 | | "Make up and write a sentence about anything." This sentence must contain a noun and verb. |
| 1 | | The examiner gives the patient a blank piece of paper and asks him or her to draw this symbol. All 10 angles must be present and 2 must intersect. |
| Total Possible=30 | Patient's Total= | If total score is 23 or below, further evaluation may be indicated. |

Instructions: Score one point for each correct response within each question or activity.

Adapted from: Folstein MF, Folstein SE, McHugh PR. "Mini-mental state": a practical method for grading the cognitive state of patients for the clinician. *J Psychiatr Res*. 1975;12:189-98. Used with kind permission from Pergamon Press, Ltd., Oxford, UK, and the authors; copyright © 1975.

## Functional Impairment

1. Assessment of functional impairment can be performed by a variety of methods, including observation of the patient in the home; observation of the patient in the office; questioning of the patient or family, or both; and use of brief, structured questionnaires. Within the limits of time and resources, a variety of methods of assessment should be used.

2. Structured questions should be used to supplement, not replace, clinical observation and more extensive forms of assessment.

3. IADLs can be briefly evaluated by using the following five structured questions:

   - Can you get to places outside of walking distance without help? (For example, travel alone on buses, taxis, or drive a car.)

   - Can you go shopping for groceries or clothes without help? (This assumes that the patient has transportation.)

   - Can you prepare your own meals without help? (For example, plan and cook full meals without help.)

   - Can you do your housework without help?

   - Can you handle your own money without help? (For example, write checks, pay bills.)

   Adapted from: Fillenbaum GG. Screening the elderly: a brief instrumental activities of daily living measure. *Journal of the American Geriatrics Society*. 1985;33:698-706. Reproduced with permission of the American Geriatrics Society; copyright © 1985.

4. ADLs can be briefly assessed using the following six structured questions:

   - Do you bathe yourself without help?

   - Do you dress yourself without help?

   - Do you use the toilet without help?

   - Do you move in and out of bed or a chair without help?

   - Do you have any trouble controlling your bladder or your bowels?

   - Do you feed yourself without help?

   Adapted from: Katz S, Ford AB, Moskowitz RW, Jackson BA, Jaffe MW, Cleveland MA. The index of ADL: a standardized measure of biological and psychosocial function. *Journal of the American Medical Association*. 1963;185:914-919. Reproduced by permission of the American Medical Association; copyright © 1963.

5. Any identified impairments in function should be investigated for etiology (physical, psychological, environmental) and possible means of treatment or amelioration (in-home support services, speech and language therapy, physical and occupational therapy).

**Patient Resources**

*Memory and Aging: Alzheimer's Disease and Related Disorders*, and many other materials. Alzheimer's Association, 919 N Michigan Ave., Suite 1000, Chicago, IL 60611; 1-800 272-3900.

*Memory Loss: What's Normal, What's Not.* American Academy of Family Physicians, 8880 Ward Parkway, Kansas City, MO 64114; 1-800 944-0000.

*Where Did I Put My Keys?* (videotape). American Association of Retired Persons, Fulfillment Services, 601 E St. NW, Washington, DC 20049; (202) 434-2534.

*Age Page—Senility: Myth or Madness*; *Age Page—Confusion and Memory Loss in Old Age: It's Not What You Think.* National Institute on Aging, Bldg 31, Rm 5C27, Bethesda, MD 20892; (301) 496-1752.

**Provider Resources**

*Older Voices* (trainer's manual, resource materials for communication problems of older persons). American Speech-Language-Hearing Association, 10801 Rockville Pike, Rockville, MD 20852; (301) 897-5700.

**Selected References**

American Academy of Family Physicians, Commission on Public Health and Scientific Affairs. *Age Charts for Periodic Health Examination*. Kansas City, Mo: American Academy of Family Physicians; 1993.
American College of Physicians, Health and Public Policy Committee. Comprehensive functional assessment for elderly patients. *Ann Intern Med*. 1988;109:70-72.
Canadian Task Force on the Periodic Health Examination. The periodic health examination. *Can Med Assoc J*. 1979;121:1193-1254.
Canadian Task Force on the Periodic Health Examination. Periodic Health Examination Monograph. Hull, Quebec: Ministry of Supply and Services. 1980.
Canadian Task Force on the Periodic Health Examination. Periodic health examination: 1. 1991 update: screening for cognitive impairment in the elderly. *Can Med Assoc J*. 1991;144:425-431.
Fillenbaum GG. Screening the elderly: a brief instrumental activities of daily living measure. *J Amer Geriatr Soc*. 1985;33:698-706.
Folstein MF, Folstein SE, McHugh PR. "Mini-mental state": a practical method for grading the cognitive state of patients for the clinician. *J Psychiatr Res*. 1975;12:189-98.
Katz S, Ford AB, Moskowitz RW, Jackson BA, Jaffe MW, Cleveland MA. The index of ADL: a standardized measure of biological and psychosocial function. *JAMA*. 1963;185:914-919.
National Institutes of Health, Consensus Development Panel. Differential diagnosis of dementing diseases. *JAMA*. 1987;258:3411-3416.

Patterson CJ. Detecting cognitive impairment in the elderly. In: Goldbloom RB, Lawrence RS. *Preventing Disease: Beyond the Rhetoric*. New York, NY: Springer-Verlag; 1990:chap 18.

Pfeiffer E. A short portable mental status questionnaire for the assessment of organic brain deficit in elderly patients. *J Amer Geriatr Soc*. 1975;23:433-441.

Siu AL. Screening for dementia and investigating its causes. *Ann Intern Med*. 1991;115:122-132.

Siu AL, Reubens DB, Hays RD. Hierarchical measures of physical function in ambulatory geriatrics. *J Amer Geriatr Soc*. 1990;38:1113-1119.

Rubenstein LV, Calkins DR, Greenfield S, et al. Health status assessment for elderly patients: report of the Task Force on Health Assessment, Society of General Internal Medicine. *J Amer Geriatr Soc*. 1988;37:562-569.

US Preventive Services Task Force. Screening for dementia. In: *Guide to Clinical Preventive Services*. Baltimore, Md: Williams & Wilkins; 1989:chap 42.

## Adults/Older Adults — SCREENING

# 32. Depression

Major depressive episodes are common in adults, affecting over 6 million Americans and costing over $16 billion yearly. Depression affects all ages, genders, and races. See Table 32-1 for a list of risk factors for major depression.

Between 3% and 8% of primary care patients meet criteria for major depression, and many patients with depressive disorders are seen only by nonpsychiatric providers. Research has shown that up to 50% of depressed patients seen in primary care are not recognized as having this disorder. Patients with major depressive disorders have a great deal of functional impairment, resulting in lost time on the job, decreased job performance, and decreased family and social functioning. Effective medical treatments are available for major depression.

**Recommendations of Major Authorities**

- **American Academy of Family Physicians** and **U.S. Preventive Services Task Force**—The performance of routine screening tests for depression in asymptomatic individuals is not recommended. Clinicians should, however, maintain an especially high index of suspicion for depressive symptoms in adolescents and young adults, individuals with a family or personal history of depression, those with chronic illnesses, and those who have or perceive they have experienced a recent loss.

**Table 32-1. Risk Factors for Depression**

| |
|---|
| Prior episode(s) of depression |
| Family history of depressive disorder |
| Prior suicide attempt(s) |
| Female gender |
| Age of onset <40 years |
| Postpartum period |
| Medical comorbidity |
| Lack of social support |
| Stressful life events |
| Personal history of sexual abuse |
| Current substance abuse |

From: Agency for Health Care Policy and Research, Depression Guideline Panel. *Depression in Primary Care: Detection, Diagnosis, and Treatment.* Rockville, MD: U.S. Department of Health and Human Services, Public Health Service. In press. Technical Report 5.

- **American College of Physicians**—Elderly patients should undergo functional assessment screening, including measures of emotional status.

- **American College of Obstetricians and Gynecologists**—All women should receive age-specific psychosocial evaluations to detect depression and other problems.

- **Canadian Task Force on the Periodic Health Examination**—There is fair evidence to exclude the use of depression detection tests from the periodic health examination of asymptomatic people.

## Basics of Depression Screening

1. The diagnostic criteria for a major depressive episode, as defined in the *Diagnostic and Statistical Manual of Mental Disorders* (DSM-III-R), are given in Table 32-2. Because the essential feature is either depressed mood or loss of pleasure in usual activities for at least 2 weeks, these symptoms should be elicited first in history-taking.

2. Some of the features of depression in elderly individuals may be confused with dementia, resulting in what has been called pseudodementia due to depression. The clinician should keep in mind that disorientation, memory loss, and distractibility in the elderly may be signs of depression rather than dementia.

**Table 32-2. Criteria for Major Depressive Disorder**

| At least 5 of the following symptoms are present during the same period; depressed mood or loss of interest or pleasure must be present. Symptoms are present most of the day, nearly daily for at least 2 weeks. |
| --- |
| Depressed mood (can be irritable in children and adolescents) most of the day, nearly every day |
| Markedly diminished interest or pleasure in almost all activities most of the day, nearly every day (as indicated either by subjective account or observation by others of apathy most of the time) |
| Significant weight loss or gain |
| Insomnia or hypersomnia |
| Psychomotor agitation or retardation |
| Fatigue (loss of energy) |
| Feelings of worthlessness (guilt) |
| Impaired concentration (indecisiveness) |
| Recurrent thoughts of death or suicide |

From: American Psychiatric Association. *Diagnostic and Statistical Manual of Mental Disorders, Third Edition, Revised*. Washington, DC: American Psychiatric Association; 1987. Reproduced by permission of the publisher; copyright © 1987.

3. Basic steps in detecting depression in primary care include:

- Maintaining a high index of suspicion, especially with patients who have risk factors.

- Using the clinical interview or a written questionnaire (see item 4 below).

- Eliciting additional information by questioning family or caretakers (with patient consent).

- Identifying (and treating, if present) other possible causes for mood disorders, such as medical illness, medications, or substance abuse.

- Making the diagnosis of major depressive disorder and proceeding to treatment or referral if no other causes for the mood changes are found (or if the depression continues after they are treated).

4. Several short self-report questionnaires for depression have been evaluated and found to be useful in primary care settings (Coulehan et al, 1989). These include the Short Beck Depression Inventory (BDI), the Zung Self-Rating Depression Scale (SDS), and the Center for Epidemiologic Studies Depression Scale (CES-D). The CES-D is given in Table 32-3. Self-report questionnaires are helpful in finding patients with depressive symptoms, but they are not diagnostic instruments. Many patients with mild depression that does not meet diagnostic criteria for a major depressive episode will be identified with these questionnaires. If a patient scores above the cut point on a questionnaire, the clinical interview should be used to elicit the criterion symptoms of a major depressive episode. Because self-report questionnaires are very sensitive to depressive symptoms, they can also be used appropriately to exclude major depression in patients who score below the cut points.

**Patient Resources**

*Depression Is a Treatable Illness: A Patient's Guide.* Agency for Health Care Policy and Research Publications Clearinghouse, PO Box 8547, Silver Spring, MD 20907; 1-800 358-9295.

*Depression: What You Need to Know*; *If You're Over 65 and Feeling Depressed*; *Helping the Depressed Person Get Treatment*; *What to Do When a Friend is Depressed*; *La Depresion—Existen Tratamientos Eficaces*; and many other materials. DEPRESSION Awareness, Recognition, and Treatment (D/ART) Public Education Campaign, 5600 Fishers Lane, Rm 14C-02, Rockville, MD 20857; 1-800 421-4211.

Many types of materials are available from National Mental Health Association, 1021 Prince St., Alexandria, VA 22314; 1-800 969-6642.

Ch. 32. Depression                                            Adults/Older Adults — SCREENING

Table 32-3. Center for Epidemiologic Studies Depression Scale

| DURING THE PAST WEEK | RARELY or NONE of the time. (Less than 1 day) | SOME or a LITTLE of the time. (1-2 days) | OCCASIONALLY or a MODERATE amount of the time. (3-4 days) | MOST or ALL of the time. (5-7 days) |
|---|---|---|---|---|
| 1. I was bothered by things that don't usually bother me. | 0 | 1 | 2 | 3 |
| 2. I did not feel like eating; my appetite was poor. | 0 | 1 | 2 | 3 |
| 3. I felt that I could not shake off the blues even with the help of my family or friends. | 0 | 1 | 2 | 3 |
| 4. I felt that I was just as good as other people. | 3 | 2 | 1 | 0 |
| 5. I had trouble keeping my mind on what I was doing. | 0 | 1 | 2 | 3 |
| 6. I felt depressed. | 0 | 1 | 2 | 3 |
| 7. I felt everything I did was an effort. | 0 | 1 | 2 | 3 |
| 8. I felt hopeful about the future. | 3 | 2 | 1 | 0 |
| 9. I thought my life had been a failure. | 0 | 1 | 2 | 3 |
| 10. I felt fearful. | 0 | 1 | 2 | 3 |
| 11. My sleep was restless. | 0 | 1 | 2 | 3 |
| 12. I was happy. | 3 | 2 | 1 | 0 |
| 13. I talked less than usual. | 0 | 1 | 2 | 3 |
| 14. I felt lonely. | 0 | 1 | 2 | 3 |
| 15. People were unfriendly. | 0 | 1 | 2 | 3 |
| 16. I enjoyed life. | 3 | 2 | 1 | 0 |
| 17. I had crying spells. | 0 | 1 | 2 | 3 |
| 18. I felt sad. | 0 | 1 | 2 | 3 |
| 19. I felt that people disliked me. | 0 | 1 | 2 | 3 |
| 20. I could not get "going". | 0 | 1 | 2 | 3 |

Interpretation: A total score of 22 or higher is indicative of depression when this scale is used in primary care.

From: Radloff LS. The CES-D Scale: a self-report depression scale for research in the general population. *Appl Psychol Meas.* 1977;1:385-401. Copyright © 1977, West Publishing Company/Applied Psychological Measurement, Inc. Reproduced by permission.

## Provider Resources

*Depression in Primary Care: Detection and Diagnosis* (vol. 1; AHCPR publication 93-0550); *Treatment of Major Depression* (vol. 2; AHCPR publication 93-0551); *Diagnosis and Treatment* (Quick Reference Guide for Clinicians; AHCPR publication 93-0552). Agency for Health Care Policy and Research Publications Clearinghouse, PO Box 8547, Silver Spring, MD 20907; 1-800 358-9295.

*Depression in Women* (American College of Obstetricians and Gynecologists Technical Bulletin). ACOG Resource Center, 409 12th St. SW, Washington, DC 20024-2188; 1-800 762-2264.

*Diagnosis and Treatment of Depression in Late Life* (NIH Consensus Development Conference, November 4-6, 1991; NIH Consensus Statements vol 9, no. 3). NIH Consensus Clearing House, PO Box 2577, Kensington, MD 20891, 1-800 644-6627.

## Selected References

Agency for Health Care Policy and Research, Depression Guideline Panel. *Depression in Primary Care: Detection, Diagnosis, and Treatment.* Rockville, Md: US Dept of Health and Human Services, Public Health Service. In press. Technical Report 5.

American Academy of Family Physicians, Commission on Public Health and Scientific Affairs. *Age Charts for Periodic Examination.* Kansas City, Mo: American Academy of Family Physicians; 1993.

American College of Obstetricians and Gynecologists. *Depression in Women.* Washington, DC: American College of Obstetricians and Gynecologists. In press. ACOG Technical Bulletin.

American College of Obstetricians and Gynecologists. *The Obstetrician-Gynecologist and Primary-Preventive Health Care.* Washington, DC: American College of Obstetricians and Gynecologists; 1993.

American College of Physicians, Health and Public Policy Committee. Comprehensive functional assessment for elderly patients. *Ann Intern Med.* 1988;109:70-72.

American Psychiatric Association. *Diagnostic and Statistical Manual of Mental Disorders.* 3rd ed., rev. Washington, DC: American Psychiatric Association; 1987.

Beck AT, Rial WY, Rickels K. Short form of depression inventory: cross validation. *Psychological Reports.* 1974;34:1184-1186.

Canadian Task Force on the Periodic Health Examination. Periodic health examination: 2. 1990 update: early detection of depression and prevention of suicide. *Can Med Assoc J.* 1990;142:1233-1238.

Coulehan JL, Schulberg HC, Block MR. The efficiency of depression questionnaires for case-finding in primary medical care. *J Gen Intern Med.* 1989;4:542-7.

Kamerow DB, Pincus HA, Macdonald DI. Alcohol abuse, other drug abuse, and mental disorders in medical practice: prevalence, costs, recognition, and treatment. *JAMA.* 1986;255:2054-2057.

Radloff LS. The CES-D Scale: a self-report depression scale for research in the general population. *Appl Psychol Meas.* 1977;1:385-401.

US Preventive Services Task Force. Screening for depression. In: *Guide to Clinical Preventive Services.* Baltimore, Md: Williams & Wilkins; 1989:chap 44.

Wells KB, Stewart A, Hays RD, et al. The functioning and well-being of depressed patients: results from the Medical Outcomes Study. *JAMA.* 1989;4:7-13.

Zung WWK. A self-rating depression scale. *Arch Gen Psychiatry.* 1965;12:63-70.

# Adults/Older Adults — SCREENING

## 33. Fecal Occult Blood

There will be approximately 149,000 new cases of colorectal cancer and 56,000 deaths caused by it in 1994. On average, clinically diagnosed colorectal cancer deprives its victims of 6 to 7 years of life. Principal risk factors for colorectal cancer include a history of one of the familial polyposis syndromes, familial cancer syndromes, colorectal cancer in first-degree relatives, or a personal history of ulcerative colitis, adenomatous polyps, or endometrial, ovarian, or breast cancer. If detected at an early stage, colorectal cancer can be successfully treated with surgery.

Malignancies and, to a lesser extent, polyps bleed intermittently. This bleeding can be detected by tests that identify occult blood or breakdown products of blood in fecal material. Recent evidence indicates that the sensitivity of commonly used fecal occult blood tests for detecting colorectal cancer in low-risk, asymptomatic patients may be as low as 25%. (Rehydration of dried samples before testing can increase sensitivity, at the cost of producing more false-positive results.) The predictive value of a positive fecal occult blood test for colorectal cancer in general populations is only 5% to 10%. Thus, up to 75% of cancers will be missed and up to 20 patients will undergo workups that will be negative for every case of colorectal cancer detected by fecal occult blood testing.

Until recently, no studies had shown decreased mortality as a result of fecal occult blood testing. In 1993, however, Mandel et al found that yearly fecal occult blood testing using rehydrated stool specimens decreased mortality from colorectal cancer by about one third. In that study, guaiac-impregnated paper slides were used to test for fecal blood.

For information about other methods of screening for colorectal cancer, refer to chapters 29 and 40.

### Recommendations of Major Authorities

- **American Academy of Family Physicians (AAFP), Canadian Task Force on the Periodic Health Examination**, and **U.S. Preventive Services Task Force (USPSTF)**—There is insufficient evidence to recommend either initiating or terminating the routine provision of fecal occult blood testing in low-risk, asymptomatic individuals (see above). These recommendations are currently under review. **AAFP** and **USPSTF** recommend that it may be clinically prudent to offer screening, including fecal occult blood testing, to individuals 50 years of age or older who are at increased risk for disease.

- **American Cancer Society (ACS), American College of Physicians (ACP), American Gastroenterological Association, American Society for Gastrointestinal Endoscopy**, and **National Cancer Institute (NCI)**—Annual fecal occult blood testing should be done for all asymptomatic individuals without known risk factors beginning at 50 years of age. **ACP** recommends annual fecal occult blood testing beginning at 40 years of age for individuals at high risk for disease. **ACS** and **NCI** recommend that special surveillance be considered for individuals at high risk for disease, without specifically designating fecal occult blood testing.

- **American College of Obstetricians and Gynecologists**—Fecal occult blood testing should be done for all women 40 years of age and older as part of their periodic health examination.

## Basics of Fecal Occult Blood Screening

1. Many tests are available for detecting fecal occult blood. These are of three basic types: guaiac-impregnated cards and other carriers that detect the peroxidase-like activity of hemoglobin (Hemoccult®); quantitative tests based on the conversion of heme to fluorescent porphyrins (HemoQuant®); and immunoassay tests for human hemoglobin. Currently only the first two types are routinely used in practice. Guaiac-based tests have the disadvantage of giving false-negative and false-positive results because of a number of dietary factors, and thus are more accurate in patients on a special diet (see Table 33-1). Guaiac-based tests have the advantages of being relatively easy for patients and clinicians to use, and they are relatively specific for lower gastrointestinal tract bleeding. The quantitative porphyrin tests are not affected by dietary factors and are potentially more sensitive, depending on the cut point designated for a positive result. Recent evidence indicates, however, that at matched levels of specificity, the quantitative porphyrin tests are not significantly more sensitive than guaiac-based tests. Quantitative porphyrin tests have the potential disadvantages of not being specific for lower gastrointestinal bleeding and of requiring interpretation by a laboratory.

2. Stool samples should not be collected if hematuria or obvious rectal bleeding, such as from hemorrhoids, is present. Women should be instructed to avoid collecting stool samples during and just after a menstrual period.

### Table 33-1. Diet for Patients Using Guaiac-Based Tests

| | |
|---|---|
| Foods permissible to eat | Well-cooked pork, poultry, and fish |
| | Any cooked fruits and vegetables |
| | High fiber grains (e.g., whole wheat bread, bran cereal, popcorn) |
| Foods, drugs, and vitamins to avoid | Red meat (beef, lamb), including processed meats and liver |
| | Any raw fruits and vegetables (especially melons, radishes, turnips and horseradish) |
| | Excess amounts of vitamin C-enriched foods, such as citrus fruits and juices, or vitamin C tablets in excess of 250 mg per day |
| | Aspirin and nonsteroidal anti-inflammatory drugs for 7 days before and during the testing period |
| If patients have trouble with adherence, these items may be included | Moderate amounts of these raw fruits and vegetables: apples, apricots, bananas, celery, lettuce, oranges, peaches, pears, plums, raisins, raspberries, strawberries, tomatoes |
| | Moderate amounts of alcoholic beverages |

Adapted from: SmithKline Diagnostics. *Product Instructions for Hemoccult® Sensa® Screening Test.* San Jose, CA: SmithKline Diagnostics, Inc; 1988. Reproduced by permission of the publisher; copyright © 1988.

3. If possible, medications that cause gastric irritation and bleeding should be avoided for at least 48 hours prior to and during the testing period. These include: aspirin, nonsteroidal anti-inflammatory drugs, corticosteroids, anticoagulants, reserpine, antimetabolites, chemotherapeutic agents, and alcohol in excess. Avoidance of aspirin and nonsteroidal anti-inflammatory drugs for 7 days is recommended by the manufacturer of Hemoccult®. When using guaiac-based tests, patient adherence to the dietary guidelines in Table 33-1 for at least 48 hours prior to and during the testing period can help avoid false-positive and false-negative results. Despite reports in earlier years, dietary iron does not cause false-positive tests. Application of antiseptic preparations containing iodine to the anal area should be avoided immediately before and during the testing period to prevent false-positive results.

4. When guaiac-impregnated cards are used, two separate samples from different sections of three consecutive bowel movements should be collected using the supplied applicator and applied as thin smears to the cards. Patients should be instructed to return samples as soon as possible for processing. Optimally, processing of the cards should occur within 6 days, but definitely not after 14 days. Rehydration of the samples with a drop of water before application of the developer increases sensitivity by approximately 30% to 40%, but it also decreases specificity by 2% to 3%, leading to significantly more false-positive results. For this reason, authorities disagree about the use of rehydration. A positive result on even one sample qualifies the entire test as positive. Cards and developer should be stored at room temperature and protected from heat and light.

5. If patients are asked to return samples through the mail, special U.S. Postal Service-approved envelopes should be used, not standard paper envelopes.

6. Because of the intermittent nature of bleeding by colorectal cancer, malignancy cannot be conclusively ruled out by repeat fecal occult blood testing. Follow-up of positive fecal occult blood screening requires diagnostic procedures (e.g., sigmoidoscopy, colonoscopy, barium enema).

## Patient Resources

*What You Need to Know about Cancer of the Colon and Rectum.* Office of Cancer Communications, National Cancer Institute, Bethesda, MD 20892; 1-800 4-CANCER.

## Selected References

Ahlquist DA, Wieand HS, Moertal CG, et al. Accuracy of fecal occult blood screening for colorectal neoplasia. *JAMA.* 1993;269:1262-1267.

American Academy of Family Physicians, Commission on Public Health and Scientific Affairs. *Age Charts for Periodic Health Examination.* Kansas City, Mo: American Academy of Family Physicians; 1993.

American College of Obstetricians and Gynecologists. *The Obstetrician-Gynecologist and Primary-Preventive Health Care.* Washington, DC: American College of Obstetricians and Gynecologists, 1993.

American College of Physicians. Guidelines. In: Eddy DM, ed. *Common Screening Tests.* Philadelphia, Pa: American College of Physicians; 1991:415-416.

Boring CC, Squires TS, Tong T, Montgomery S. Cancer Statistics, 1994. *CA.* 1994;4:7-26.

Canadian Task Force on the Periodic Health Examination. The periodic health examination: 2. 1989 update. *Can Med Assoc J.* 1989;141:4-16.

Eddy DM. Screening for colorectal cancer. *Ann Intern Med.* 1990;113:373-384.

Fleischer DE, Goldberg SB, Browing TH, et al. Detection and surveillance of colorectal cancer. *JAMA.* 1989;261:580-585.

Gnauck R, Macrae FA, Fleisher M. How to perform the fecal occult blood test. *CA.* 1984;34:134-7.

Kewenter J, Bjork S, Haglind E, Smith L, Svanvik J, Ahren C. Screening and rescreening for colorectal cancer: a controlled trial of fecal occult blood testing in 27,700 subjects. *Cancer.* 1988;62:645-651.

Knight KK, Fielding JE, Battista RN. Occult blood screening for colorectal cancer. *JAMA.* 1989;261:587-593.

Levin B, Murphy GP. Revision in American Cancer Society recommendations for the early detection of colorectal cancer. *CA.* 1992;42:296-299.

Mandel JS, Bond JH, Church TR, et al. Reducing mortality from colorectal cancer by screening for fecal occult blood. *N Engl J Med.* 1993;328:1365-71.

McCrae FA, St John JB, Caligiore P, Taylor LS, Legge JW. Optimal dietary conditions for Hemoccult® testing. *Gastroenterology.* 1982;82:899-903.

Pye G, Thomas WM, Hardcastle JD. Comparison of coloscreen self-test and Haemoccult faecal occult blood tests in the detection of colorectal cancer in symptomatic patients. *Br J Surg.* 1990;77:630-31.

Ransohoff DF, Lang CA: Screening for Colorectal Cancer. *N Engl J Med.* 1991;325:37-41.

Selby JV, Friedman GD, Quesenberry CP, Weiss NS. Effect of fecal occult blood testing on mortality from colorectal cancer: a case-control study. *Ann Intern Med.* 1993;118:1-6.

Selby JV. How should we screen for colorectal cancer? *JAMA.* 1993;269:1294-1296.

Smart CR, Chu K, Conley V, Henson DE, Pommerenke F, Srivastova S. Cancer Screening and Early Detection. In: Holland JF, Frei III EF Bast Sr. RC, Kufe DW, Morton DL, Weichselbaum RR, eds. *Cancer Medicine*, 3rd ed. Vol 1. Philadelphia: Lea and Febiger, 1993:408-431.

SmithKline Diagnostics. *Product Instructions for Hemoccult® Sensa® Screening Test.* San Jose, Ca: SmithKline Diagnostics, Inc; 1988.

US Preventive Services Task Force. Screening for colorectal cancer. In: *Guide to Clinical Preventive Services.* Baltimore, Md: Williams & Wilkins, 1989:chap 7.

Walter SD, Frommer DJ, Cook RJ. The estimation of sensitivity and specificity in colorectal cancer screening methods. *Cancer Detect Prev.* 1991;15:465-469.

Winawer SJ, Schottenfeld D, Flehinger BJ. Colorectal cancer screening. *JNCI.* 1991;83:243-253.

## Adults/Older Adults — SCREENING

# 34. Hearing

Hearing loss increases in prevalence with age and is very common in older adults. Approximately one fourth of adults aged 65 to 74 years and one half of adults 85 years and older report some degree of hearing loss. Hearing loss, particularly when it develops late in life and is progressive in nature, can compromise the ability to perform many important activities, such as using the telephone, driving, and shopping. It also may lead to social withdrawal, depression, and exacerbation of coexisting psychiatric problems. Some older people with hearing loss also have cognitive impairment, and there is evidence that improvement of hearing may contribute to improvement in cognitive ability. Many types of hearing loss can be improved with the use of hearing aids; however, only 10% to 15% of patients who could benefit from a hearing aid actually use one.

See Chapter 6 for information about hearing screening for children and adolescents.

**Recommendations of Major Authorities**

- **American Academy of Family Physicians** and **U.S. Preventive Services Task Force**—Hearing screening is not necessary for asymptomatic adults under 65, except for those who are exposed regularly to excessive noise (e.g., in recreational or occupational settings). Screening of workers for noise-induced hearing loss should be performed in the context of existing worksite programs and occupational medicine guidelines. Elderly patients should be periodically evaluated regarding their hearing, counseled regarding the availability of hearing aids, and referred appropriately for any abnormalities. The optimal frequency of hearing assessment should be determined by clinical discretion. It is unclear that benefits are sufficient to justify the substantial cost of audiometric screening of the nearly 30 million Americans over age 65. A more practical but unproven strategy might include a careful historical evaluation of hearing in older individuals, a simple otoscopic examination for cerumen and other findings, and patient education regarding the availability of efficacious hearing aid devices.

- **American College of Obstetricians and Gynecologists**—Women 65 years and older should be evaluated for hearing loss.

- **American Speech-Language-Hearing Association**—Considerable debate concerning the efficacy of selected screening protocols for older adults has taken place in recent years, and it remains to be seen whether the choice of protocol actually influences compliance with the follow-up recommendations. The clinician may choose to use a hearing handicap questionnaire, pure-tone audiometry, or both. The rationale for using a questionnaire and pure-tone audiometry in combination is that compliance with audiologic recommendations is often greater when individuals perceive their hearing loss to be a handicap. Selection of the protocol should take into consideration cost, compliance data for the particular population, and the specificity, sensitivity, and predictive values of screening. Equipment used should be appropriately calibrated, and self-assessment scales must be reliable. Compliance-improving strategies (e.g., educational materials) should be an integral part of any screening program and appropriate follow-up services should be available.

- **Canadian Task Force on the Periodic Health Examination**—There is fair justification for looking for hearing loss in a periodic health examination of adults. Further study is warranted if adults report being hard of hearing or fail to respond to the normal spoken voice; have a medical or family history placing them at high risk for hearing loss (e.g., family history of hearing loss, occupational history of exposure to noise, pursuit of noisy leisure activities, or history of recurring ear problems).

**Basics of Hearing Screening**

1. All older adult patients should be questioned about signs of hearing loss. Because patients may not be fully aware of impairment, family members also should be questioned, if possible.

2. A screening questionnaire may be used to screen for communication problems and social and emotional handicaps stemming from hearing loss. Questionnaires may be filled out by the patient or administered by staff. One type of standardized questionnaire for this purpose is presented in Table 34-1. This instrument has been shown to have sensitivity and specificity values in the 60% to 80% range—values almost as high as those attained by pure-tone audiometry screening. Some authorities recommend audiologic referral for patients scoring 10 or higher on this questionnaire. Screening questionnaires have the advantage of identifying patients who perceive hearing loss to be a problem and who, therefore, may be particularly motivated to use a hearing aid. Some authorities recommend using both a questionnaire and pure-tone testing for screening. This may modestly improve sensitivity and specificity.

3. Pure-tone screening can be administered using either a standard pure-tone audiometer or a hand-held audioscope (an otoscope that emits tones of calibrated frequencies and intensities). With either method, the environment in which screening is administered should be as quiet as possible. Frequencies used should be within the speech range. There is disagreement about the sound intensity that should be used in screening. Following are two examples of suggested screening protocols:

   - Pure tones are presented at 25 dB at 1000, 2000, and 4000 Hz. Failure to respond to any one frequency in either ear at 25 dB constitutes a "fail." For adults under 65, this may be the preferred protocol. The majority of those over 65 years of age screened with this protocol, however, may fail. Because of this, some authorities recommend using a 40 dB tone at 4000 Hz.

   - Pure tones are presented at 25 and 40 dB at 1000, 2000, and 4000 Hz (optional). Failure to respond to the 40 dB signal at any one frequency in either ear constitutes a "fail." Inability to hear any one frequency at 25 dB places an individual "at risk" for hearing loss. A referral for audiologic assessment may be appropriate if the person reports being handicapped by their hearing loss. Persons who fail the screening should be monitored annually to determine whether their hearing loss is progressive.

4. Simple physical examination procedures for hearing screening, such as the whispered voice and finger rub tests, are not recommended by major authorities. Although they are fairly accurate crude hearing tests, they are insensitive to disorders of central auditory processing and speech understanding.

**Table 34-1. Hearing Handicap Inventory in the Elderly Screening Questionnaire**

Instructions: Check one answer for each question. Do not skip a question if you avoid a situation because of a hearing problem. If you use a hearing aid, please answer according to the way you hear without the aid.

| Question | Yes | No | Sometimes |
|---|---|---|---|
| 1. Does a hearing problem cause you to feel embarrassed when you meet new people? | | | |
| 2. Does a hearing problem cause you to feel frustrated when talking to members of your family? | | | |
| 3. Do you have difficulty hearing when someone speaks in a whisper? | | | |
| 4. Do you feel handicapped by a hearing problem? | | | |
| 5. Does a hearing problem cause you difficulty when visiting friends, relatives, or neighbors? | | | |
| 6. Does a hearing problem cause you to attend religious services less often than you would like? | | | |
| 7. Does a hearing problem cause you to have arguments with family members? | | | |
| 8. Does a hearing problem cause you difficulty when listening to TV or radio? | | | |
| 9. Do you feel that any difficulty with your hearing limits or hampers your personal or social life? | | | |
| 10. Does a hearing problem cause you difficulty when in a restaurant with relatives or friends? | | | |

Scoring: No = 0  Sometimes = 2  Yes = 4

Interpretation of Total Scores: 0-8 = no handicap; 10-24 = mild to moderate handicap; 26-40 = severe handicap.

Adapted from: Ventry I, Weinstein B. Identification of elderly people with hearing problems. *Asha.* 1983; 25:37-42. Reproduced by permission of the American Speech and Hearing Association; copyright © 1983.

5. Patients found to have evidence of hearing loss by screening should be considered for referral to a specialist for comprehensive audiologic evaluation, especially if they feel handicapped by the hearing loss. Because approximately 10% of individuals with hearing loss are amenable to medical or surgical treatment, and some patients are incorrectly identified as having hearing loss by screening, patients should not be referred directly to a hearing aid dealer.

6. The primary care clinician should make sure that appropriate follow-up management is provided to all patients referred for audiologic evaluation. Patients may need considerable support and training to use their hearing aids effectively.

## Patient Resources

*Age Page: Hearing and the Elderly.* National Institute on Aging, Bldg 31, RM 5C27, Bethesda, MD 20892; (301) 496-1752.

*Answers to Questions About Noise and Hearing Loss* and *How To Buy a Hearing Aid.* American Speech-Language-Hearing Association, 10801 Rockville Pike, Rockville, MD 20852; 1-800 638-TALK (voice or TTY), (301) 897-8682 (in Maryland).

## Selected References

American Academy of Family Physicians, Commission on Public Health and Scientific Affairs. *Age Charts for Periodic Health Examination.* Kansas City, Mo: American Academy of Family Physicians; 1993.

American College of Obstetricians and Gynecologists. *The Obstetrician-Gynecologist and Primary-Preventive Health Care.* Washington, DC: American College of Obstetricians and Gynecologists, 1993.

American Speech-Language-Hearing Association, Ad Hoc Committee on Hearing Screening in Adults. Considerations in screening adults/older persons for handicapping hearing impairments. *Asha.* 1992;34:81-85.

Bess FH, Lichtenstein MJ, Logan SA, et al. Hearing impairment as a determinant of function in the elderly. *J Am Geriatric Soc.* 1989;37:123-8.

Canadian Task Force on the Periodic Health Examination. *Periodic Health Examination Monograph.* Hull, Quebec: Ministry of Supply and Services Canada; 1980.

Canadian Task Force on the Periodic Health Examination. The periodic health examination: 2. 1984 update. *Can Med Assoc J.* 1984;130:1278-1285.

Gennis V, Garry PJ, Haaland KY, Yeo RA, Goodwin JS. Hearing and cognition in the elderly: new findings and a review of the literature. *Arch Intern Med.* 1991;151:2259-2264.

Havlik RJ. Aging in the Eighties: Impaired senses for sound and light in persons aged 65 years and over: preliminary data from the Supplement on Aging to the National Health Interview Survey: United States; January-June 1984. *Vital and Health Statistics.* 1986;125. Hyattsville, Md: National Center for Health Statistics. US Dept of Health and Human Services publication PHS 86-1250.

Lichtenstein MJ, Bess FH, Logan SA. Screening for impaired hearing in the elderly. *JAMA.* 1988;260:3589-90. Letter.

Macphee GJ, Crowther JA, McAlpine CH. A simple screening test for hearing impairment in elderly patients. *Age Aging.* 1988;17:347-351.

Mulrow CD, Lichtenstein MJ. Screening for hearing impairment in the elderly: rationale and strategy. *J Gen Intern Med.* 1991;6:249-58.

Pappas JJ, Graham SS. *Hearing Aid Dispensing within a Medical Setting.* Alexandria, Va: American Academy of Otolaryngology—Head and Neck Surgery Foundation; 1990.

Schow R, Nerbonne M. Communication screening profile uses with elderly clients. *Ear Hearing.* 1982;3:133-147.

Uhlman RF, Larson EB, Rees TS, Koepsel TD, Duckert LG. Relationship of hearing impairment to dementia and cognitive dysfunction in older adults. *JAMA.* 1989;262:1916-1919.

Uhlmann RF, Rees TS, Psaty BM, Duckert LG. Validity and reliability of auditory screening tests in demented and non-demented older adults. *J Gen Intern Med.* 1980;4:90-96.

US Preventive Services Task Force. Screening for hearing impairment. In: *Guide to Clinical Preventive Services.* Baltimore, Md: Williams & Wilkins; 1989:chap 33.

Ventry I, Weinstein B. Identification of elderly people with hearing problems. *Asha.* 1983;25:37-42.

# Adults/Older Adults — SCREENING

# 35. Mammography

Breast cancer is the most common type of cancer in women and the second leading cause of cancer death in American women (after lung cancer). There will be an estimated 182,000 new cases and 46,000 deaths in 1994. The average lifetime risk for a woman in the United States of developing breast cancer is approximately 1 in 9. Breast cancer mortality increases with age, with first deaths occurring at approximately 30 years of age. Mortality from breast cancer does not plateau, even in extreme old age. Aside from age, the next strongest risk factor is a family history of breast cancer in a first-degree relative (sister or mother). Very modest increases in risk are also associated with nulliparity, first pregnancy after 30 years of age, menarche before 12 years of age, menopause after 50 years of age, postmenopausal obesity, some types of benign breast disease, high socioeconomic status, and a personal history of ovarian or endometrial cancer.

Mortality from breast cancer is strongly influenced by stage at detection. The 5-year survival rate is 93% for women found to have localized disease. The 5-year survival rate for women with distant spread is only 18%. African-American women have somewhat lower survival rates than white women at every stage of diagnosis. Mammography is the most effective means of early detection for breast cancer, with sensitivity estimates of 70% to 90% and specificity estimates of 90% to 95%. Although mammography can detect small tumors in younger women, there has been controversy about whether mammography screening actually reduces mortality in women less than 50 years of age.

Well-maintained, modern mammography equipment is very safe, using very low levels of radiation. Screening does, however, carry the added risk of morbidity from unnecessary biopsies performed to follow up false-positive mammograms.

For information about clinical breast examination to detect breast cancer, refer to chapter 29.

**Recommendations of Major Authorities**

- For women 50 and older: All major authorities, including **American Academy of Family Physicians**, **American Cancer Society**, **American College of Obstetricians and Gynecologists**, **American College of Physicians**, **Canadian Task Force on the Periodic Health Examination**, and **U.S. Preventive Services Task Force (USPSTF)**—Routine mammography screening is recommended. Yearly screening is recommended by all these authorities, with the exception of **USPSTF**, which recommends a frequency of 1 to 2 years. **American Geriatrics Society** recommends that women over 65 years of age receive mammograms at least every two or three years until at least 85 years of age. **National Cancer Institute** states that experts agree that routine mammography and clinical breast examination screening every 1 to 2 years can reduce breast cancer mortality by about one-third in women aged 50 and over.

- For women under 50: **American Cancer Society** and **American College of Obstetricians and Gynecologists**—Women 40-49 years of age should receive screening mammograms every 1 to 2 years. **National Cancer Institute** states that experts do not agree on the role of routine screening mammography for women aged 40 to 49.

*High-Risk Women*

- **American Academy of Family Physicians and American College of Obstetricians and Gynecologists**—Women with a family history of premenopausally diagnosed breast cancer in a first-degree relative should have mammography regularly beginning at 35 years of age.

- **American College of Physicians**—Women 40 years of age and older who have a family history of breast cancer or who are otherwise at increased risk should have annual mammography.

- **Canadian Task Force on the Periodic Health Examination** and **U.S. Preventive Services Task Force**—Physicians may elect to recommend mammography starting at age 35 for women at high risk, especially those whose first-degree relatives have had breast cancer diagnosed before menopause.

## Basics of Mammography Screening

1. Clinicians should clearly communicate the importance of mammograms. Patients often report as a major reason for not getting a mammogram the fact that they simply did not know they needed one. It is important that women understand the need for regular mammograms, not just one.

2. Pamphlets, videotapes, and other media should be used to educate and motivate patients to obtain mammography.

3. Because cost can be a significant barrier for patients in obtaining mammography, the clinician should be knowledgeable about low-cost, high-quality mammography facilities available in the community and should make referrals to these facilities as needed.

4. The patient should wear pants or a skirt, since she will have to undress from the waist up. She should be instructed not to use deodorants, powders, or other topical applications on the breasts or in underarm areas as these may cause artifacts on the mammogram.

5. Because of potential perimenstrual breast tenderness, it is preferable to schedule mammography at other times in the patient's menstrual cycle.

6. Mild discomfort is common during the performance of a mammogram. The patient should be instructed to tell the technician if discomfort becomes unacceptable.

7. Clinicians should verify that mammography facilities use only dedicated mammography equipment that meets minimum safety and image-quality standards. Facilities that receive Medicare reimbursement must use equipment that complies with minimum standards for patient safety. The American College of Radiology provides certification for compliance with minimum standards for image quality. As of October 1, 1994, all U.S. mammography facilities will have to be certified by the Food and Drug Administration (FDA) as providing quality mammography. Certification requirements will cover personnel, equipment, radiation exposure, quality assurance programs, and record keeping and

reporting. Further information on this program is available from FDA Center for Devices and Radiological Health, Office of Training and Assistance, Division of Mammography Quality and Radiation Programs, HFZ-240, 5600 Fishers Lane, Rockville, MD 20857.

8. Clinicians should establish a tracking system to make sure that mammograms that are ordered are actually performed, that results return in a timely fashion, and that patients who are not seen frequently can be called or contacted by letter about the importance of getting mammograms and other needed preventive care. Patients should be encouraged to keep track of and prompt their own mammograms through use of a patient-held record form or card.

9. Any palpable breast lump, even with a normal mammogram, requires a careful evaluation, including possible biopsy.

## Patient Resources

*Breast Cancer: Steps to Finding Breast Lumps Early*. American Academy of Family Physicians, 8880 Ward Parkway, Kansas City, MO 64114-2797; 1-800 944-0000.

*Mammography*. American College of Obstetricians and Gynecologists, 409 12th Street SW., Washington, DC 20024; 1-800 762-2264.

*What You Need To Know About Breast Cancer*; *A Mammogram Once a Year for Life*; *Smart Advice for Women 40 and Over: Have a Mammogram*, and many other materials. Office of Cancer Communications, National Cancer Institute, Bldg 31, Rm 10A24, Bethesda, MD 20892; 1-800 4-CANCER.

## Provider Resources

*Mammography Awareness Kit*. Office of Cancer Communications, National Cancer Institute, Bldg 31, Rm 10A24, Bethesda, MD 20892; 1-800 4-CANCER.

*Educating Older Women About Mammography: A Guide For Program Planners and Volunteer Leaders*. American Association of Retired Persons, 1909 K Street NW., Washington, DC 20049; (202) 434-2277.

*The Health Professional and Cancer Prevention and Detection*. American Cancer Society, 1559 Clifton Rd. NE, Atlanta, GA 30329-4251; 1-800 ACS-2345.

## Selected References

American Academy of Family Physicians, Commission on Public Health and Scientific Affairs. *Age Charts for Periodic Health Examination*. Kansas City, Mo: American Academy of Family Physicians; 1993.

American Cancer Society. *Summary of American Cancer Society Recommendations for the Early Detection of Cancer in Asymptomatic People*. Atlanta, Ga: American Cancer Society; 1992.

American College of Obstetricians and Gynecologists. *The Obstetrician-Gynecologist and Primary-Preventive Health Care*. Washington, DC: American College of Obstetricians and Gynecologists, 1993.

American College of Physicians. Guidelines. In: Eddy DM, ed. *Common Screening Tests*. Philadelphia, Pa: American College of Physicians; 1991:411-412.

American Geriatrics Society, Clinical Practice Committee. Screening for breast cancer in elderly women. *J Amer Geriatr Soc*. 1989;37:883-884.

Canadian Task Force on the Periodic Health Examination. The periodic health examination: 2. 1985 update. *Can Med Assoc J*. 1986;134:724-727.

Eddy DM. Screening for breast cancer. In: Eddy DM, ed. *Common Screening Tests*. Philadelphia, Pa: American College of Physicians; 1991:chap 9.

Smart CR, Chu K, Conley V, Henson DE, Pommerenke F, Srivastova S. Cancer Screening and Early Detection. In: Holland JF, Frei EF, Bast RC, Kufe DW, Morton DL, Weichselbaum RR, eds. *Cancer Medicine*, 3rd ed. Vol 1. Philadelphia: Lea and Febiger, 1993:408-431.

US Preventive Services Task Force. Screening for breast cancer. In: *Guide to Clinical Preventive Services*. Baltimore, Md: Williams & Wilkins; 1989:chap 6.

## Adults/Older Adults — SCREENING

# 36. Papanicolaou Smear

Approximately 15,000 cases of invasive cervical cancer will be diagnosed and 4600 women will die of cervical cancer in the United States in 1994. Risk factors for cervical cancer include early age at first intercourse, having multiple sexual partners, and smoking. Rates for carcinoma in situ reach a peak for both black and white women between 20 and 30 years of age. After the age of 25, however, the incidence of invasive cancer in black women increases dramatically with age while in white women the incidence rises more slowly. Over 25% of invasive cervical cancers occur in women older than 65, and 40% to 50% of all women who die from cervical cancer are over 65 years of age.

The effectiveness of early detection through Papanicolaou (Pap) smear testing and early treatment has been impressive, resulting in a marked decrease in mortality from cervical cancer. The incidence of invasive cervical cancer has been estimated to have been decreased 70% by screening. However, a large proportion of women, particularly elderly black women and middle-aged poor women, have not had regular Pap smears. In some areas, as many as 75% of women over 65 have not had a Pap smear within the previous five years.

Depending on the technique used, Pap testing has a sensitivity of 50% to 90% and a specificity of 90% to 99%. A large proportion of false-negative pap smears are thought to be due to poor technique in performance (as many as half of all false negatives) and inadequate laboratory interpretation. Because of the long lead time from development of precancerous changes to invasive carcinoma (8 to 9 years by some estimates), almost all precancerous or early stage malignancies initially missed can still be detected by repeat testing.

### Recommendations of Major Authorities

- **American Academy of Family Physicians**—Women who are sexually active or (if the sexual history is thought to be unreliable) are 18 years of age or older should have annual Pap tests. After a woman has had three or more consecutive satisfactory normal annual examinations, the Pap test may be performed at the discretion of the physician and the patient, but not less frequently than every 3 years.

- **American Cancer Society, American College of Obstetricians and Gynecologists**, and **National Cancer Institute**—All women should begin having annual Pap tests at the onset of sexual activity or at 18 years of age, whichever occurs first. After a woman has had three or more consecutive satisfactory normal annual examinations, the Pap test may be performed less frequently at the discretion of the patient and clinician.

- **American College of Physicians**—Sexually active women between 25 and 65 years of age should be screened with a Pap smear every 3 years. Women 66 to 75 years of age who have not been screened within the 10 years prior to age 66 should be screened every 3 years. Women at increased risk for cervical cancer should be screened every 2 years. Initial screening tests may be done as frequently as annually for two or three examinations to ensure diagnostic accuracy.

- **Canadian Task Force on the Periodic Health Examination**—There is fair justification for including a Pap smear as part of the periodic health examination. The optimum age and frequency at which these smears should be taken is not known, but since the incidence of cervical cancer is positively associated with early age of sexual activity and multiplicity of sexual partners, smears should probably be taken at least annually in women in these high-risk groups. For those not in high-risk groups, an initial smear should be taken soon after a woman begins sexual activity, then another 1 year later, then every 3 years until about 15 years after first intercourse, then every 5 years until age 60.

- **U.S. Preventive Services Task Force**— All women who are or have been sexually active should have regular Pap tests. Testing should begin at the age when the woman first engages in sexual intercourse. Adolescents whose sexual history is thought to be unreliable should be presumed to be sexually active at age 18. Pap tests are appropriately performed at an interval of 1 to 3 years, to be recommended by the clinician based on the presence of risk factors (e.g., early onset of sexual intercourse, history of multiple sexual partners, low socioeconomic status). Pap smears may be discontinued at age 65, but only if the provider can document previous Pap screening in which smears have been consistently normal.

## Basics of Pap Smear Screening

1. It is important that the performance of a Pap smear not be an unpleasant or painful experience for the patient. Clinicians should be sure to clearly explain the importance of the procedure and the steps in carrying it out.

2. Patients should be instructed not to douche on the day of the examination. A Pap smear should not be performed if the patient has significant menstrual flow or obvious inflammation.

3. The Pap smear should be performed before the bimanual examination and before obtaining culture specimens. In general, the speculum should not be lubricated with anything except water, as contamination of Pap smear specimens with lubrication jelly tends to obscure cellular detail. Use of a small amount of lubricating jelly may be necessary for speculum insertion in some older patients.

4. The cervix and vagina should be completely visualized before collection of the specimen. Excess cervical mucus should be gently removed with a swab.

5. The gold standard for the adequacy of a Pap smear has traditionally been the presence of endocervical cells in the sample. This is because 90% of cervical cancers develop at the junction of the squamous epithelium of the vagina and the columnar epithelium of the endocervix (located at the external os in young women and inside the endocervical canal in older women). Studies differ on whether the presence of endocervical cells actually improves detection rates of abnormalities, but the presence of endocervical cells remains widely accepted as a standard of adequacy for Pap smears.

6. A variety of implements have been used to obtain Pap smear samples, including simple cotton swabs, wooden and plastic spatulas, and endocervical and combined endocervical-exocervical brushes. The best sensitivity (defined as presence of endocervical cells) is

obtained by using both a spatula (preferably Ayer's type) and an endocervical brush. The spatula should be used first because of the bleeding commonly caused by the endocervical brush and the susceptibility of endocervical cells to drying effects.

7. The spatula should be firmly, yet gently rotated circumferentially around the os at least one complete turn, to obtain a 360° sample. The specimen should be promptly transferred to a slide. Patients who have been exposed to DES should also have smears taken circumferentially with a spatula from the upper two thirds of the vagina. In obtaining the endocervical sample, the brush should be inserted into the os no deeper than the length of the bristled section. It should be rotated 360° (avoiding excessive rotation), and then the specimen transferred by rolling on a slide.

8. Specimens should be uniformly applied to the slides without clumping. Fixation should be performed promptly, and care must be taken to minimize air drying of the specimens. If one slide is used for both specimens, it is important to collect, transfer, and fix the endocervical sample as quickly as possible. The use of two separate slides can help avoid prolonged air exposure of the spatula specimen while the endocervical specimen is being collected. This does, however, double the amount of work for the cytotechnologist. The use of a combined endocervical-exocervical brush requires the collection and fixation of only a single specimen (thus decreasing the risk of air drying), but it has been shown to be somewhat less sensitive than using a spatula and an endocervical brush.

9. Providers should inquire about the quality control of laboratories to which specimens are sent. Laboratories should be certified by the American Society of Cytologists or the College of American Pathologists, or both. Many authorities recommend that laboratories use the new Bethesda System developed by a National Cancer Institute consensus conference for reporting results (see Table 36-1). The Bethesda System standardizes classification categories and provides for reporting on aspects of the sample not addressed in traditional Pap smear reports, such as adequacy and hormonal effects. In the Bethesda System, human papillomavirus (HPV) infection is classified as a low-grade squamous intraepithelial lesion; both moderate and severe dysplasia are classified as high-grade squamous intraepithelial lesions. There is some concern, not substantiated by research, that these classifications may lead to excess colposcopic exams for HPV infection and moderate dysplasia. The National Workshop on Screening for Cancer of the Cervix has issued guidelines for Pap smear reporting and follow-up in Canada (Miller et al., 1991).

10. Only about 60% of women with abnormal Pap smears return for follow-up. Clinicians should establish a tracking system to make sure that Pap smears are performed regularly, that results return in a timely fashion, that patients with abnormal results are contacted, and that women who are not seen frequently are called or contacted by letter about the importance of getting Pap smears and other needed preventive care. Patients should be encouraged to keep track of and prompt their own Pap smears through use of a patient-held record form or card.

**Table 36-1. The Revised Bethesda System for Reporting Cervical and/or Vaginal Cytologic Diagnoses**

Adequacy of the specimen
  Satisfactory for evaluation
  Satisfactory for evaluation but limited by . . . (specify reason)
  Unsatisfactory for evaluation . . . (specify reason)

General categorization (optional)
  Within normal limits
  Benign cellular changes: See descriptive diagnosis
  Epithelial cell abnormality: See descriptive diagnosis

Descriptive diagnoses
  Benign cellular changes
    Infection
      *Trichomonas vaginalis*
      Fungal organisms morphologically consistent with *Candida* spp
      Predominance of coccobacilli consistent with shift in vaginal flora
      Bacteria morphologically consistent with *Actinomyces* spp
      Cellular changes associated with Herpes simplex virus
      Other
    Reactive changes
      Reactive cellular changes associated with:
        Inflammation (includes typical repair)
        Atrophy with inflammation ("atrophic vaginalis")
        Radiation
        Intrauterine contraceptive device (IUD)
        Other
  Epithelial cell abnormalities
    Squamous cell
      Atypical squamous cells of undetermined significance: Qualify*
      Low-grade squamous intraepithelial lesion encompassing:
        HPV**, mild dysplasia/CIN 1
      High-grade squamous intraepithelial lesion encompassing:
        Moderate and severe dysplasia, CIS/CIN 2 and CIN 3
      Squamous cell carcinoma
    Glandular cell
      Endometrial cells, cytologically benign, in post-menopausal women
      Atypical glandular cells of undetermined significance: Qualify*
      Endocervical adenocarcinoma
      Endometrial adenocarcinoma
      Extrauterine adenocarcinoma
      Adenocarcinoma, NOS
  Other malignant neoplasms: Specify
  Hormonal evaluation (applies to vaginal smears only)
    Hormonal pattern compatible with age and history
    Hormonal pattern incompatible with age and history: Specify
    Hormonal evaluation not possible due to: Specify

**Table 36-1. The Revised Bethesda System for Reporting Cervical and/or Vaginal Cytologic Diagnoses—Continued**

*Atypical squamous or glandular cells of undetermined significance should be further qualified as to whether a reactive or a premalignant/malignant process is favored.

**Cellular changes of human papillomavirus (HPV)—previously termed koilocytosis, koilocytotic atypia, or condylomatous atypia—are included in the category of low grade squamous intraepithelial lesion.

From: National Cancer Institute Workshop. The revised Bethesda system for reporting cervical and/or vaginal cytologic diagnoses; report of the 1991 Bethesda workshop. *Acta Cytol.* 1992;36:273-275. Reproduced by permission of Science Printers and Publishers, Inc.; copyright © 1992.

## Patient Resources

*The Pap Test.* American College of Obstetricians and Gynecologists, 409 12th St. SW, Washington DC 20024; 1-800 762-2264.

## Provider Resources

*Cervical Cytology: Evaluation and Management of Abnormalities.* American College of Obstetricians and Gynecologists, 409 12th St. SW, Washington, DC 20024; 1-800 762-2264. Technical Bulletin 183.

## Selected References

American Cancer Society. *Summary of American Cancer Society Recommendations for the Early Detection of Cancer in Asymptomatic People.* Atlanta, Ga: American Cancer Society; 1992.

American College of Obstetricians and Gynecologists. *The Obstetrician-Gynecologist and Primary-Preventive Health Care.* Washington, DC: American College of Obstetricians and Gynecologists. 1993.

American College of Physicians. Guidelines. In: Eddy DM, ed. *Common Screening Tests.* Philadelphia, Pa: American College of Physicians; 1991:413-414.

Boon ME, de Graaff Guilloud JC, Rietveld WJ. Analysis of five sampling methods for the preparation of cervical smears. *Acta Cytol.* 1989;33:843-848.

Canadian Task Force on the Periodic Health Examination. *Periodic Health Examination Monograph.* Hull, Quebec: Minister of Supply and Services Canada; 1980.

Crouse BS, Elliott BA, Nesin N. Clinical follow-up of cervical sampling with the Ayre spatula and Zelsmyr cytobrush. *Arch Fam Med.* 1993;2:145-148.

Eddy DM. Screening for cervical cancer. In: Eddy DM, ed. *Common Screening Tests.* Philadelphia, Pa: American College of Physicians; 1991:chap 10.

Herbst AL. The Bethesda System for cervical/vaginal cytologic diagnoses: a note of caution. *Obstet Gynecol.* 1990;449-450.

Lai-Goldman M, Nieberg RK, Mulcahy D, Wiesmeier. The cytobrush for evaluating routine cervicovaginal-endocervical smears. *J Repro Med.* 1990;35;959-963.

McCord ML, Stovall TG, Meric JL, Summitt RL, Coleman SA. Cervical cytology: a randomized comparison of four sampling methods. *Am J Obstet Gynecol.* 1992;166:1772-1779.

Mandelblatt J, Gogaul I, Wistreich M. Gynecological care of elderly women: another look at Papanicolaou testing. *JAMA.* 1986;256:367-371.

Miller AB, Anderson G, Brisson J, et al. Report of a national workshop on screening for cancer of the cervix. *Can Med Assoc J.* 1991;145:1301-1325.

National Cancer Institute Workshop. The 1988 Bethesda System for reporting cervical/vaginal cytologic diagnoses. *JAMA*. 1989;262:931-934.

National Cancer Institute Workshop. The revised Bethesda System for reporting cervical/vaginal cytologic diagnoses: report of the 1991 Bethesda workshop. *Acta Cytol*. 1992;36:273-275.

Neinstein JS, Church J, Akiyoshi T. Comparison of cytobrush with cervix-brush for endocervical cytologic sampling. *J Adoles Health*. 1992;13:520-523.

Ruffin MT, Van Noord GR. Improving the yield of endocervical elements in a Pap smear with the use of the cytology brush. *Fam Med*. 1991;23:365-369.

Schumann JL, O'Connor DM, Covell JL, Greening SE. Pap smear collection devices: technical, clinical, diagnostic, and legal considerations associated with their use. *Diagn Cytopathol*. 1992;8:492-502.

Smart CR, Chu K, Conley V, Henson DE, Pommerenke F, Srivastova S. Cancer Screening and Early Detection. In: Holland JF, Frei EF, Bast RC, Kufe DW, Morton DL, Weichselbaum RR, eds. *Cancer Medicine*, 3rd ed. Vol.1. Philadelphia: Lea and Febiger, 1993;408-431.

US Preventive Services Task Force. Screening for cervical cancer. In: *Guide to Clinical Preventive Services*. Baltimore, Md: Williams & Wilkins; 1989:chap 8.

# Adults/Older Adults — SCREENING

## 37. Plasma Glucose

It is estimated that 13 million Americans suffer from diabetes mellitus (DM). Approximately half are undiagnosed. DM is the seventh leading cause of death in the United States. Insulin-dependent (Type I) DM accounts for approximately 5% of all diabetics. Type I diabetics have an absolute insulin deficiency and require insulin for survival. Onset of Type I DM has a bimodal presentation, with the largest peak in childhood and a smaller peak in early adulthood. These individuals tend to present symptomatically and are usually diagnosed soon after the onset of the disease. Noninsulin-dependent (Type II) DM accounts for approximately 95% of all diabetics. Type II diabetics have a relative insulin deficiency. As such, onset of their disease is insidious. They can be relatively symptom-free for years prior to diagnosis. Risk factors for Type II DM include advancing age (over age 40 years), obesity, family history, and a history of gestational DM.

Although the prevalence of DM in the United States is approximately 5.2% of the population, certain ethnic groups, including Hispanics, African Americans, and Native Americans, have significantly higher prevalence rates. Diabetic complications are varied and serious. DM accounts for 30% of all end-stage renal disease, and it is the leading cause of blindness in adults. Other complications include neuropathy, cardiovascular disease, and peripheral vascular disease.

Screening can identify occult cases of Type II DM. The most accurate method of screening is measurement of plasma glucose. Measurement of urine glucose has been used in the past but is much less accurate and no longer recommended. Evidence is limited that early treatment of asymptomatic patients decreases long-term complications of DM. There is evidence, however, that weight reduction, exercise, and diet change are beneficial in primary and secondary prevention of Type II DM. Most authorities recommend screening only for people with an increased risk of developing DM.

Screening and treatment for gestational DM is an important aspect of prenatal care, but like other aspects of prenatal care is beyond the scope of this book.

**Recommendations of Major Authorities**

- **American Academy of Family Physicians, American College of Obstetricians and Gynecologists**, and **U.S. Preventive Services Task Force**—Fasting plasma glucose levels should be periodically measured in patients who are at high risk due to marked obesity, a family history of DM, or a personal history of gestational DM. General screening of the asymptomatic, nonpregnant adult population is not recommended.

- **American College of Physicians**—Screening for DM in healthy asymptomatic individuals is not recommended. Screening is reasonable in obese adults over the age of 40 years if a diagnosis of DM would motivate weight loss. Screening may also be indicated for women planning to become pregnant who are at increased risk of DM and in other people with one or more of the following risk factors: history of DM in a first-degree relative, age over 50 years, weight more than 25% over ideal body weight, personal history of gestational DM, and membership in an ethnic group with a high prevalence of DM.

- **American Diabetes Association**—Screening for DM every 3 years is recommended for adults with one or more of the following risk factors: history of DM in a first-degree relative; more than 20% over ideal body weight; Native American, Hispanic, or African-American heritage; age 40 years or over; previously identified impaired glucose tolerance; hypertension, hypercholesterolemia, or hyperlipidemia; personal history of gestational DM or of one or more infants weighing more than 9 lb at birth.

- **Canadian Task Force on the Periodic Health Examination**—Urine testing for glucose and fasting or postprandial blood glucose tests should not be a routine part of the periodic health examination. Screening is appropriate for nonpregnant asymptomatic adults with one or more of the following risk factors: family history of DM, personal history of hyperglycemia associated with pregnancy, and evidence of circulatory dysfunction or frank vascular impairment.

## Basics of Plasma Glucose Screening

1. Measurement of fasting plasma glucose is the principal method of screening in nonpregnant, asymptomatic adults.

2. Patients should be instructed not to take food or beverage (other than water) for at least 3 hours before the blood sample is collected. It is most convenient to perform the procedure in the morning, when patients will have fasted overnight. A venous blood sample is more accurate, but capillary samples may be more practical for office-based screening purposes.

3. A fasting plasma glucose level lower than 115 mg/dL should be considered normal. A fasting blood glucose level greater than 140 mg/dL should be considered elevated. Most authorities recommend further testing of patients with fasting plasma glucose levels of 115 mg/dL or more (see Table 37-1 for American Diabetes Association diagnostic criteria).

4. If a fasting sample is not available, random blood glucose levels can also be used in screening for DM. A random blood glucose level in excess of 200 mg/dL should be considered elevated and an indicator for further assessment.

## Patient Resources

*Diagnosis: Diabetes* and other materials are available from American Diabetes Association, 1660 Duke Street, Alexandria, VA 22314; (703) 549-1500.

## Table 37-1. Criteria for Diagnosing Diabetes in Non-Pregnant Adults

| | |
|---|---|
| Conditions that must be met in order to make a diagnosis of diabetes. Any one is sufficient. | Unequivocal elevation of plasma glucose (≥200 mg/dL) and classic symptoms of diabetes, including polydipsia, polyuria, polyphagia, and weight loss |
| | Fasting plasma glucose ≥140 mg/dL on two occasions |
| | Fasting plasma glucose <140 mg/dL and two oral glucose tolerance tests, each with both the 2-hour plasma glucose and one intervening value ≥200 mg/dL after a 75-g oral glucose load |
| Criteria for the diagnosis of impaired glucose tolerance | Fasting plasma glucose <140 mg/dL, and a 2-hour plasma glucose ≥140 but <200 mg/dL, with one intervening value ≥200 mg/dL, after a 75-g oral glucose load |

From: American Diabetes Association. Office guide to diagnosis and classification of diabetes mellitus and other categories of glucose intolerance. *Diabetes Care.* 1993;16:4. Reproduced by permission of the American Diabetes Association; copyright © 1993.

## Selected References

American Academy of Family Physicians, Commission on Public Health and Scientific Affairs. *Age Charts for Periodic Health Examination.* Kansas City, Mo: American Academy of Family Physicians; 1993.

American College of Obstetricians and Gynecologists. The Obstetrician-Gynecologist and Primary-Preventive Health Care. Washington, DC: American College of Obstetricians and Gynecologists. 1993.

American College of Physicians. Guidelines. In: Eddy DM, ed. *Common Screening Tests.* Philadelphia, Pa: American College of Physicians; 1991:404-405.

American Diabetes Association. Office guide to diagnosis and classification of diabetes mellitus and other categories of glucose intolerance. *Diabetes Care.* 1993;16:4.

American Diabetes Association. Position statement: Screening for diabetes. *Diabetes Care.* 1993;16:7-9.

Canadian Task Force on the Periodic Health Examination. The periodic health examination 1979. *Can Med Assoc J.* 1979; 121:1194-532.

Eriksson KF, Lindgarde F. Prevention of type 2 (noninsulin-dependent) diabetes mellitus by diet and physical exercise. *Diabetologia.* 1991;34:891-898.

Gerken KM, Van Lente E. Effectiveness of screening for diabetes. *Arch Pathol Lab Med.* 1990;114:201-3.

Howard BV, Abbott WGH, Swinburn BA. Evaluation of metabolic effects of substitution of complex carbohydrates for saturated fat in individuals with obesity and NIDDM. *Diabetes Care.* 1991;14:786-795.

Manson JE, Nathan DM, Krolewski AS, Stampfer MJ, Willett WC, Hennekens CH. A prospective study of exercise and incidence of diabetes among US male physicians. *JAMA.* 1992;268:63-67.

Manson JE, Rimm EB, Stampfer MJ, et al. Physical activity and incidence of noninsulin-dependent diabetes mellitus in women. *Lancet.* 1991;338:774-778.

Marshall JA, Hamman RF, Baxter J. High-fat, low-carbohydrate diet and the etiology of noninsulin-dependent diabetes mellitus: The San Luis Valley diabetes study. *Am J Epidemiol.* 1991;134:590-603.

Schwartz MK. The role of the laboratory in the prevention and detection of chronic disease. *Clin Chem.* 1992; 38:1539-1546.

Singer DE, Samet JH, Coley CM, Nathan DM. Screening for diabetes mellitus. *Ann Intern Med.* 1988;109:639-649.

US Preventive Services Task Force. Screening for diabetes mellitus. In: *Guide to Clinical Preventive Services.* Baltimore, Md: Williams & Wilkins, 1989:chap 16.

World Health Organization Expert Committee on Diabetes Mellitus. *Third Report on Diabetes Mellitus.* Geneva, Switzerland: World Health Organization, 1985. WHO Technical Report Series 727.

## Adults/Older Adults — SCREENING

# 38. Prostate-Specific Antigen

Prostate cancer is the leading cause of cancer in men (excluding skin cancer) in the United States, with an estimated 200,000 new cases in 1994. The second leading cause of death from cancer in men, prostate cancer will cause an estimated 38,000 deaths in the United States in 1994. Risk factors for prostate cancer include African-American race, increasing age, and (perhaps) increased dietary fat intake. Although prostate cancer is common, its course is extremely variable. Some prostate cancers grow rapidly, metastasize, and quickly lead to death. Many other prostate cancers, however, are clinically silent and found only incidentally at autopsy. One study found only one death from prostate cancer for every 380 men found to have histologic evidence of the disease at autopsy. It is estimated that at least 30% of elderly men die with prostate cancer that has never become clinically apparent.

Prostate-specific antigen (PSA) is a glycoprotein that is specific to the prostate but not to prostate cancer. Thus, it is produced by all types of prostate tissue, whether normal, hyperplastic, or malignant. PSA screening has a sensitivity for prostate cancer of 70% to 90%. Because it has a low specificity (38% to 59%), however, the predictive value of a positive PSA test is in the range of 20% to 30%. Thus, many men with benign prostatic hyperplasia will have an elevated PSA level, and some men with prostate cancer will have PSA tests in the normal range.

Whether to screen asymptomatic men for prostate cancer with PSA is controversial. Unlike with Pap smears and mammograms, there are no data indicating that PSA screening decreases mortality from prostate cancer. Although PSA testing is FDA-approved for monitoring patients with prostate cancer, it is not currently approved as a screening test for detecting early prostate cancer. Further, although both the incidence of prostate cancer and the rate of radical prostatectomy for prostate cancer treatment have increased markedly in recent years, mortality rates for this disease have not declined. Definitive evidence is lacking that treatments such as radical prostatectomy are superior to "watchful waiting" for localized prostate cancer.

See chapter 29 for information on the use of the rectal examination to screen for prostate cancer.

**Recommendations of Major Authorities**

- **American Academy of Family Physicians, Canadian Task Force on the Periodic Health Examination, National Cancer Institute**, and **U.S. Preventive Services Task Force**—PSA testing is not recommended for routine screening in asymptomatic men.

- **American Cancer Society (ACS)**, and **American Urological Association (AUA)**—Annual PSA testing is recommended for all men aged 50 years and older. **AUA** recommends discontinuing screening at age 70. **AUA** also recommends annual testing for men aged 40 and over who have a family history of prostate cancer and for men who have had a vasectomy at least 20 years previously or who had their vasectomy at age 40 years or older. **ACS** recommends discontinuing annual screening when the patient's life expectancy is less than 10 years. **ACS** also recommends screening patients less than age 50 who are in high-risk groups.

**Basics of Prostate-Specific Antigen Screening**

1. Many experts recommend that men 50 years of age and over receive individualized counseling about the known risks and possible benefits of PSA testing. Patients should be informed that:

    - The possible benefit from PSA screening is decreased mortality from prostate cancer that is discovered early, although there are no data to show that PSA testing decreases mortality from prostate cancer.

    - Up to 70% of men with PSA levels greater than 4 ng/mL will not have prostate cancer and thus will have undergone the expense and discomfort of transrectal ultrasound, biopsies, or both, for no benefit.

    - Prostate cancer treatments have serious side effects that can include impotence, incontinence, and (in 1% to 2% of patients) surgical mortality. Radical prostatectomy, radiation therapy, or both in combination have not been proven to be superior to watchful waiting for localized disease.

2. PSA levels need not be drawn before rectal examination. An early concern about PSA testing was that PSA results would be falsely elevated by the compression of the prostate that occurs with a digital rectal examination. This is the case with another prostate tumor marker, prostatic acid phosphatase. A recent study, however, has reported that the digital rectal examination has little effect on PSA levels.

3. Although there is debate about the upper limits of normal for PSA testing, manufacturers recommend using 4.0 ng/mL for monoclonal PSA tests and 2.5 ng/mL for polyclonal PSA results. Some authorities recommend varying the strategy for follow-up of a positive PSA depending on the degree of elevation. Thus, patients with levels of 10 ng/mL or more may all get a biopsy to determine if cancer is present, but those with levels greater than 4 and less than 10 ng/mL may first receive a rectal examination, a transrectal ultrasound of the prostate, or both to help determine whether a biopsy is needed. Because of the poor predictive value of the PSA test alone, most authorities recommending the test advocate combining it with other modalities, such as digital rectal examination or transrectal ultrasound.

4. Three methods have been proposed recently to improve the accuracy of PSA testing. These are still under study, and none has been incorporated into the recommendations of major authorities.

    - *Calculation of the ratio of the PSA level to the volume of the prostate*: Because malignant tissue produces a higher level of PSA per unit weight than does normal or hypertrophied prostate tissue, PSA density has been proposed as a more accurate marker for cancer.

- *Measurement of serial PSA levels and calculation of the rate of change of PSA*: One study found that PSA values that increased at least 0.75 ng/mL per year were more specific for cancer than was a single value of 4 ng/mL or greater.

- *Adjustment of the PSA level for increasing age*: A PSA of 5 ng/mL may be more significant in a 50-year-old, for example, than in a 70-year-old.

## Patient Resources

*Prostate Disease: What Every Man Over 40 Should Know*, and other patient materials on prostate cancer and PSA testing. Prostate Health Council. American Foundation for Urologic Disease, 1120 N Charles St., Suite 401, Baltimore, MD 21202; 1-800 242-2383.

The prostate puzzle. *Consumer Reports*. 1993;58(7):459-465.

## Selected References

American Cancer Society. *Summary of American Cancer Society Recommendations for the Early Detection of Cancer in Asymptomatic People*. Atlanta, Ga: American Cancer Society; 1992.

American Urological Association. *Early Detection of Prostate Cancer and Use of Transrectal Ultrasound*. Baltimore, Md: American Urological Association; 1992.

Benson MC, Whang IS, Olsson CA, et al. The use of prostate-specific antigen density to enhance the predictive value of intermediate levels of serum prostate-specific antigen. *J Urol*. 1992;147:817-21.

Canadian Task Force on the Periodic Health Examination. Periodic health examination: 3. 1991 update. Secondary prevention of prostate cancer. *Can Med Assoc J*. 1991;145:15-30.

Carter HB, Pearson JD, Metter EJ, et al. Longitudinal evaluation of prostate-specific antigen levels in men with and without prostate disease. *JAMA*. 1992;267:2215-20.

Catalona WJ, Smith DS, Ratliff TL. Measurement of prostate-specific antigen in serum as a screening test for prostate cancer. *N Engl J Med*. 1991;324:1156-61.

Crawford ED, Schutz MJ, Clejan S. The effect of digital rectal examination on prostate-specific antigen levels. *JAMA*. 1992;267:2227-2228.

Fleming C, Wasson JH, Albertsen PC, Barry MJ, Wennberg JE. A decision analysis of alternative treatment strategies for clinically localized prostate cancer. *JAMA*. 1993;269:2650-2658.

Kramer BS, Brown ML, Prorok PC, Potosky AL, Hohagan JK. Prostate cancer screening: what we know and what we need to know. *Ann Intern Med*. 1993: 119:914-923.

Littrup PJ, Lee F, Mettlin C. Prostate cancer screening: current trends and future implications. *CA*. 1992;42:198-212.

Lu-Yao GL, McLerran D, Wasson J, Wennberg JE. An assessment of radical prostatectomy: time trends, geographic variation, and outcomes. *JAMA*. 1993;269:2633-2636.

Stuart ME, Handley MA, Thompson RS, Conger M, Timlin D. Clinical practice and new technology: prostate-specific antigen (PSA). *HMO Practice*. 1993;6(4):5-11.

## Adults/Older Adults — SCREENING

# 39. Sexually Transmitted Diseases and HIV Infection

Sexually transmitted diseases (STDs) are among the most common and harmful communicable diseases. Chlamydia, gonorrhea, and syphilis are easily treated when diagnosed early. Left undetected, however, all three conditions can lead to serious complications. Human immunodeficiency virus (HIV) infection is the biggest public health problem of the late twentieth century. Although HIV infection has no cure, early diagnosis and treatment can delay the onset of acquired immunodeficiency syndrome (AIDS) and can help those infected avoid transmitting the disease to others. Groups at particularly high risk for STDs and HIV infection include sexually active individuals under age 25, those who have multiple sexual partners, those with prior history of an STD, those who practice anal intercourse, prostitutes and their sex partners, users of illicit drugs, and inmates of detention centers.

Prevention and control of STDs and HIV infection depend on four major activities: 1) educating those at risk about means of reducing transmission; 2) detecting untreated cases, both symptomatic and asymptomatic; 3) effectively diagnosing, counseling, and treating infected individuals; and 4) evaluating, counseling, and treating the sex partners of infected individuals. Screening—along with early diagnosis, counseling, and treatment—plays an essential role in STD and HIV prevention.

Refer to the following chapters for related information: chapters 22 and 58, STD and HIV prevention counseling in adolescents and adults; chapters 14 and 47, hepatitis B immunization and prophylaxis in children/adolescents and adults; and chapters 24 and 60, counseling on preventing unintended pregnancy in adolescents and adults. Screening for and treatment of STDs during pregnancy is also an important component of prenatal care, which is beyond the scope of this book.

## ■ Syphilis ■

The reported incidence of all stages of syphilis increased dramatically from 1985 (28.5 cases per 100,000 population) to 1990 (54.3 per 100,000). It then decreased to 45.3 cases per 100,000 in 1992. Congenital syphilis increased from 1985 (7 per 100,000 live births) to 1990 (91.8 per 100,000 live births), peaked in 1991 (107.2 per 100,000 live births), and then decreased in 1992 (94.3 per 100,000 live births). Over 30,000 new cases of primary and secondary syphilis occur annually, and the prevalence of HIV infection among syphilis-infected individuals is increasing.

The usual presentation of primary syphilis is a single painless ulcer or chancre on the genitalia. The ulcer usually heals on its own, even without antibiotic therapy. These manifestations, however, may not occur at all, or they may be overlooked. If the condition goes unnoticed or untreated in the primary stage, most patients progress to secondary syphilis, often manifested as a skin rash. This resolves with or without treatment; untreated patients then enter the latent stage. About one third of untreated patients with latent syphilis will progress to neurosyphilis or other late complications such as gummatous lesions of bone, tissue, and skin, as well as cardiovascular problems (aortic valve lesions and aneurysms). Neurosyphilis can occur at any point in the course of untreated syphilis and may consist of meningitis, meningovascular lesions, psychiatric illnesses, and tabes dorsalis. Early diagnosis and treatment can prevent these grave complications.

### Recommendations of Major Authorities

- Most major authorities, including **American Academy of Family Physicians (AAFP)**, **American College of Obstetricians and Gynecologists**, **American College of Physicians (ACP)**, **American Medical Association (AMA)**, **Centers for Disease Control and Prevention**, and **U.S. Preventive Services Task Force (USPSTF)**—Syphilis screening should be performed on individuals at high risk of developing syphilis, sexual partners of known syphilis cases, and individuals with multiple sexual partners—especially in areas where syphilis prevalence is high. **ACP** also recommends that male homosexuals be routinely screened; **AAFP** and **USPSTF** also suggest screening prostitutes. **American Academy of Pediatrics** and **AMA** recommend periodic screening for syphilis in sexually active adolescents.

### Basics of Syphilis Screening

1. Because the causative agent of syphilis cannot be cultured, screening relies on serology. A nontreponemal test—usually either the Venereal Disease Research Laboratory (VDRL) test or the Rapid Plasma Reagin (RPR) test—is recommended for initial screening.

2. Occasionally, uninfected individuals may have reactive tests. If a sample is RPR- or VDRL-reactive, a treponemal test, such as the Fluorescent Treponemal Antibody Absorption (FTA-ABS) Test, should be obtained to confirm the diagnosis. It is very uncommon for an individual to test falsely reactive to both treponemal and nontreponemal tests. Some causes of falsely reactive syphilis serologies are listed in Table 39-1.

3. Early in the course of syphilis, serology may be nonreactive. As many as 25% of all cases of primary syphilis may have nonreactive RPR and VDRL tests. If a patient is a recent contact of an individual who has documented syphilis (or is suspected to have primary syphilis), he or she should be treated, even if serologic tests are nonreactive.

4. RPR and VDRL test titers correlate with disease activity, usually becoming nonreactive after therapy; however, even in untreated patients, they can revert to nonreactive after many years. FTA-ABS tests usually remain reactive for life. A reactive FTA-ABS may not necessarily indicate the need for therapy if the patient was adequately treated for syphilis previously. If a patient tests reactive, an accurate history and thorough search for previous syphilis tests or treatment are essential to determine the duration of infection and to plan appropriate therapy.

5. Patients with known exposure to syphilis and those with proven or suspected infection should be screened for other STDs; counseled to practice safer sex, including using latex condoms; and advised to seek HIV counseling and testing.

Ch. 39. STDs and HIV Infection                    Adults/Older Adults — SCREENING

Table 39-1. Conditions That May Cause Falsely Reactive Syphilis Tests

| Falsely Reactive RPR and VDRL | Falsely Reactive FTA-ABS |
|---|---|
| Viral infections<br>  Measles<br>  Chicken pox<br>  Infectious mononucleosis<br>  Viral hepatitis | Infections<br>  Infectious mononucleosis<br>  Lyme disease<br>  Malaria<br>  Leptospirosis |
| Non-viral infections<br>  Tuberculosis<br>  Scarlet fever<br>  Chancroid<br>  Pneumococcal pneumonia | Other<br>  Systemic lupus erythematosus |
| Other<br>  Pregnancy<br>  Injection drug use<br>  Connective tissue diseases (including<br>    sytemic lupus erythematosus)<br>  Malignancy | |

Adapted from: Larson SA. Syphilis. *Clinics in Laboratory Medicine.* 1989;9(3):545-557. Used with permission of W.B. Saunders Company; copyright © 1989.

## ■ Chlamydia and Gonorrhea ■

Chlamydia is the most common sexually transmitted disease in the United States, causing an estimated 4 million infections in 1992. Gonorrhea is the second leading cause of sexually transmitted disease, with an estimated 1.1 million infections in 1992. These two organisms usually cause urethritis in men and cervicitis in women. The clinical presentation is usually swifter and more dramatic for gonococcal infection, but the two conditions cannot be distinguished solely by history and physical findings. Often the two organisms are transmitted together and must be treated simultaneously. Usual symptoms in men include penile discharge and dysuria. Occasionally these infections can lead to epididymitis. Women may experience vaginal discharge and symptoms of pelvic inflammatory disease (PID). PID can result in infertility. Unlike chlamydia, gonorrhea may also cause pharyngitis, proctitis, and a disseminated infection involving dermatitis, tenosynovitis, and arthritis; and, rarely, it may cause meningitis and endocarditis. Both chlamydia and gonorrhea may cause only subtle symptoms, or they may occur entirely without symptoms, particularly in females. Screening to detect asymptomatic carriers is, therefore, important for preventing complicated infections and for controlling the spread of infection in the community.

### Recommendations of Major Authorities

■ All major authorities, including **American Academy of Family Physicians, American Academy of Pediatricians, American College of Obstetricians and Gynecologists, American Medical Association, Canadian Task Force on the Periodic Health Examination, Centers for**

Disease Control and Prevention, and U.S. Preventive Services Task Force—Asymptomatic individuals attending STD, family planning, or adolescent health clinics should be screened for chlamydia and gonorrhea. Those who have multiple sexual partners and sexually active individuals less than 20 years of age should also be screened. Prostitutes and individuals with a history of STDs should also be screened. Recent sexual partners of individuals with a documented gonococcal or chlamydial infection should be tested and treated.

### Basics of Chlamydia and Gonorrhea Screening

1. Because chlamydia and gonorrhea cause similar symptoms and often occur simultaneously, diagnostic and screening tests for the two infections are usually performed together.

2. Specimens should be collected from the urethra in males and from the endocervix in females. In women who have had a hysterectomy, urethral specimens should be obtained. If spontaneous discharge from the urethra or cervix is apparent, diagnostic studies including a Gram stain should be performed.

3. *Gonorrhea:* Gonorrhea culture remains the gold standard for screening and diagnosis of gonococcal infections. For routine screening and diagnosis of males, however, the Gram-stained smear is nearly as specific and sensitive as the culture; it may be the preferred method, because results can be obtained immediately. Specimen collection and inoculation for gonorrhea culture should be performed as follows:

    - *For male patients:* The patient should refrain from urinating for at least 2 hours prior to testing to minimize the possibility of a false-negative test. An adequate sample can often be obtained by milking the penis from the base of the shaft to the glans, expressing exudate and collecting it with a swab. If there is no exudate, a small calcium alginate or dacron swab should be inserted into the urethral meatus, advanced into the canal 2 to 3 cm, and gently rotated.

    - *For female patients:* Unless urethral samples are anticipated, the patient should void prior to the examination. The specimen is obtained by gently inserting a calcium alginate or dacron swab into the endocervical canal and rotating. A bimanual and rectal examination should also be performed, with careful attention to signs of PID: cervical motion tenderness, fundal or adnexal tenderness, masses. Any endocervical discharge should be sampled for microscopic examination.

    - Once the specimen is collected, the swab should be Z-streaked onto a Thayer-Martin (chocolate agar) or Martin-Lewis plate that has been brought to room temperature.

    - Inoculated culture plates should be transported to the laboratory in a candle jar or other $CO_2$-enriched environment.

4. *Chlamydia:* Both culture and nonculture methods are available to detect chlamydial infection. All of the available methods frequently give false-negative results. Nonculture antigen detection methods are somewhat less sensitive and specific than culture but have

the advantages of being more economical and less demanding technically. Therefore, nonculture tests are most appropriate for screening purposes.

The objective of good specimen collection for detection of chlamydial infection is to obtain columnar epithelial cells from the endocervix or the urethra. Specimens should be collected as follows:

- *Endocervical specimens:* Specimens for chlamydia tests should be taken **after** any specimens for Gram stain, gonorrhea culture, and Papanicolaou smear are taken. Before a specimen for a chlamydia test is taken, all secretions and discharge from the cervical os should be removed with a sponge or a proctology or other large swab. The appropriate swab (see below) or endocervical brush is inserted 1 to 2 cm into the endocervical canal (past the squamocolumnar junction). The swab is rotated against the wall of the endocervical canal several times during a 10- to 30-second period, then withdrawn without touching any vaginal surfaces and placed in the appropriate transport medium (culture, EIA, or DNA probe testing) or used to prepare a slide for direct fluorescent antibody testing (DFA).

- *Urethral specimens:* It is preferable to delay taking specimens until at least 2 hours after the patient has voided. Specimens for chlamydia tests should be taken **after** any specimens for Gram stain or gonorrhea culture are taken. The appropriate urogenital swab is gently inserted into the urethra (1 to 2 cm in females, 2 to 4 cm in males). The swab is rotated in one direction for at least one revolution for approximately 5 seconds, then withdrawn and placed in the appropriate transport medium (culture, EIA, or DNA probe testing) or used to prepare a slide for DFA testing.

- *Swabs to use for chlamydia screening:*

    For **nonculture chlamydia tests**, use the swab supplied or specified by the manufacturer of the test.

    For **culture specimens**, swabs with plastic or wire shafts are usually satisfactory. Swab tips can be made of cotton, rayon, dacron, or calcium alginate, although certain manufacturers' lots of calcium alginate swabs have been shown to be toxic for chlamydia. Swabs with wooden shafts should not be used, because the wood may contain substances that are toxic to chlamydia. As part of routine quality control, samples of each lot of swabs that are used to collect specimens for chlamydia isolation should be screened for possible toxicity to chlamydia, regardless of the composition of the swabs. Labs offering chlamydia culture services should provide clinicians with prescreened swabs.

- *Specimen transport:* The specimen should be inserted into chlamydia transport medium and the tip broken off to leave it immersed in the medium. The container should be sealed and transported to the laboratory. If specimens cannot be processed within 24 hours, they should be frozen at -70°C. For nonculture tests, follow the manufacturer's instructions.

# Ch. 39. STDs and HIV Infection — Adults/Older Adults — SCREENING

5. Negative culture or nonculture screening tests do not completely rule out infection. Patients who have had sexual contact with a person having a documented gonorrhea or chlamydial infection should be treated as soon as cultures are performed and before results are reported back. Also, a second test may be used to confirm a positive nonculture test for chlamydia if a false-positive would have adverse consequences.

6. Some authorities have recently recommended using dipstick urinalysis to screen young males for chlamydia and gonorrhea infection. See chapter 10 for further information on this issue.

7. In areas with a high prevalence of syphilis, all patients with gonorrhea or chlamydia should have a serologic test for syphilis and should be offered confidential counseling and testing for HIV infection.

8. All recent sexual contacts of patients with gonorrhea or chlamydia should be tested and treated.

## ■ HIV Infection ■

As of June 30, 1993, 315,390 cases of AIDS have been reported in the United States since the illness was first described. A total of 194,334 deaths from AIDS have been reported over the same time period. Seroprevalence studies show that HIV infection is present in 0.2% to 8.9% of patients visiting emergency departments and 0.1% to 7.8% of admissions to acute-care hospitals. Certain high-risk groups, such as injection drug users and prostitutes, have higher rates of HIV infection.

Many HIV-infected individuals are unaware of their status, since the characteristic symptoms of AIDS usually do not develop until years after infection. Early knowledge of HIV infection allows infected individuals to seek early treatment, which has been shown to delay the onset of AIDS, and to change high-risk behavior. Counseling and screening are, therefore, essential strategies for preventing the spread of HIV infection and the progression of symptoms. Screening high-risk individuals may be useful even when their test results are negative. The related counseling may change their behavior and thus may keep them free of disease.

### Recommendations of Major Authorities

- All major authorities, including **American Academy of Family Physicians**, **American College of Obstetricians and Gynecologists**, **American Medical Association (AMA)**, **Centers for Disease Control and Prevention (CDC)**, and **U.S. Preventive Services Task Force**—HIV screening should be offered to patients with another STD; homosexual and bisexual men; past or present injection drug users; individuals with a history of prostitution or multiple sexual partners; women whose past (or present) sexual partners are HIV-infected or injection drug users, or both; patients with a history of blood transfusion between 1978 and 1985; and individuals born in or with long-term residence in a community where HIV is prevalent. **AMA** also recommends offering testing and counseling to high-risk individuals receiving family planning services or undergoing surgery. **CDC** recommends that health facilities with an HIV seroprevalence rate of at least 1% or an AIDS diagnosis rate of 1 or more per 1000 discharges should consider a policy of routine counseling and voluntary HIV testing for patients aged 15 to 54 years.

## Basics of HIV Screening

1. Serologic studies for the presence of antibodies to HIV-1 are the standard method of screening for HIV disease.

2. Enzyme immunoassay (EIA) is the most widely used screening test for HIV-1 infection. Because any screening test can result in a false-positive reaction, it is necessary to validate positive results by confirmatory testing. This is usually accomplished using Western blot tests.

3. A single serum or plasma specimen is tested first by EIA. If the test result is positive (reactive), multiple samples from the initial specimen are retested. If at least two of three retests are reactive, the specimen is considered repeatedly reactive and must be verified with a supplemental test such as the Western blot.

4. The percentage of repeatedly reactive samples found positive with additional, more specific, tests varies according to the true antibody prevalence in the tested population. It has been estimated that when properly performed, the average specificity of EIA tests is >99.8%. In populations with a low prevalence of HIV-1 infections, the positive predictive value remains low (8-10%) despite this high level of specificity. The problem of low positive predictive value is addressed by the further testing of the repeatedly reactive EIAs with supplemental tests such as the Western blot, yielding positive predictive values approaching 100% for the complete testing algorithm.

   Western blot tests may be interpreted as positive, negative, or indeterminate. In low-risk populations, it is estimated that the false-positive rate of combined EIA and Western blot testing is less than 1 in $10^5$. Indeterminate Western blot patterns, which can occur in up to 15% of samples tested, require careful interpretation. Current experience suggests that indeterminate Western blot patterns that are persistent for 6 months or more indicate a lack of HIV infection. Persons presenting with indeterminate Western blots should be counseled that they should continue to be monitored for their band pattern by Western blot for at least 6 months. If no additional bands develop by that time and the patient has not engaged in any high-risk behavior, he or she can be considered negative for HIV-1 infection and so advised.

5. After infection with HIV-1, antibodies to the virus develop. The interval between infection and seroconversion is called the "window" period. Although there have been reports of delayed antibody response to HIV-1 infection, 95% or more of infected persons seroconvert within 6 months. Individuals who test negative should be reminded that, despite their negative test, they may be infected. They should be counseled to stop all high-risk behaviors and return for retesting in 6 months, or earlier, to make sure they have not converted to a positive test. Patients who continue practicing high-risk behavior should be counseled and retested periodically.

6. HIV culture and polymerase chain reaction (PCR) testing are currently not used for screening.

7. HIV screening must always include pre- and post-test counseling. Individualized client-centered counseling is recommended. Specially trained clinicians or counselors should provide clients with accurate, clear, understandable information regarding HIV testing at both pre- and post-test counseling sessions. Table 39-2 includes guidelines for information that should be provided in pre- and post-test counseling sessions. Also see chapter 58 for information about HIV counseling.

### Table 39-2. Pre- and Post-Test Information for HIV Testing

Counseling should include a review of the risk factors for acquiring HIV infection along with a focused and tailored risk assessment.

Counselors should review strategies for HIV prevention and assist the client in developing a plan to reduce his/her risk of HIV infection or transmission.

Clients should understand the difference between a positive test for antibodies to HIV and clinical AIDS. The median duration between development of HIV antibodies and onset of clinical disease is approximately 10 years. Detection of antibodies can occur at any time between development of antibodies and clinical disease.

All clients must be informed that a negative antibody test does not conclusively exclude the possibility of HIV infection. Typically, it takes 3 to 6 months following infection before the test (ELISA) reliably detects HIV antibodies; it is important to inform the client that a false-negative test may occur during this early period.

The importance of post-test counseling should be stressed. At the completion of the initial post-test counseling session, the counselor should assess the client's need for additional sessions.

Retesting every 6 to 12 months should be recommended to high-risk patients, particularly if they continue to engage in high-risk behavior.

Adapted from: Centers for Disease Control and Prevention. Recommendations for HIV testing services for inpatients and outpatients in acute-care hospital settings and technical guidance on HIV counseling. *MMWR*. 1993;42:1-17.

## Patient Resources

*AIDS: How to Reduce Your Risk of Catching It*. American Academy of Family Physicians, 8880 Ward Parkway, Kansas City, MO 64114-2797; 1-800 944-0000.

*How to Prevent STDs, Genital Herpes, Gonorrhea and Chlamydial Infections, Pelvic Inflammatory Disease*. American College of Obstetricians and Gynecologists, 409 12th Street SW., Washington, DC 20024; 1-800 762-2264.

*HIV and AIDS*. American Red Cross; to order, contact local Red Cross chapter or American Red Cross Office of HIV-AIDS Education; (202) 973-6000.

*Condoms and Sexually Transmitted Diseases...Especially AIDS*. National AIDS Information Clearinghouse, PO Box 6003, Rockville, MD 20849; 1-800 458-5231; a Spanish version is available from the National AIDS Information Hot Line; 1-800 344-SIDA (Spanish speaking).

*Women, AIDS, and Drug Use Annotated Client Education Directory.* NOVA Research Co., 4600 East-West Highway, Suite 700, Bethesda, MD 20814; (301) 986-1891.

*Surgeon General's Report to the American Public on HIV Infection and AIDS* and many other materials. CDC National AIDS Information Hot Line; 1-800 342-AIDS (English speaking); 1-800 344-SIDA (Spanish speaking); 1-800 AIDS-TTY (hearing impaired). All phone calls are confidential.

National STD Hotline; 1-800 227-8922. All phone calls are confidential.

**Provider Resources**

*HIV Infection and Physician Emotions* (videotape and discussion guide). American Academy of Family Physicians, 8880 Ward Parkway, Kansas City, MO 64114-2797; 1-800 944-0000.

*The Practitioner's Handbook for the Management of STDs.* Sciences Center for Educational Resources, Distribution, University of Washington, SB-56, Seattle, WA 98195; (206) 545-1186.

**Selected References**

American Academy of Family Physicians, Commission on Public Health and Scientific Affairs. *Age Charts for Periodic Health Examination.* Kansas City, Mo: American Academy of Family Physicians; 1993.
American College of Obstetricians and Gynecologists. *The Obstetrician-Gynecologist and Primary-Preventive Health Care.* Washington, DC: American College of Obstetricians and Gynecologists. 1993.
American Medical Association. *Guidelines for Adolescent Preventive Services (GAPS).* Chicago, Ill: American Medical Association; 1992.
Centers for Disease Control. CDC Public health service guidelines for counseling and antibody testing to prevent HIV infection and AIDS. *MMWR.* 1987;36:509-515.
Centers for Disease Control. Sexually transmitted diseases treatment guidelines. *MMWR.* 1989;38(S-8):1-43.
Centers for Disease Control. CDC estimates of HIV prevalence and projected AIDS cases: summary of a workshop, October 31-November 1, 1989. *MMWR.* 1990;39:110-112,117-119.
Centers for Disease Control. Primary and secondary syphilis—United States, 1981-1990. *MMWR.* 1991;40:314-323.
Centers for Disease Control and Prevention. Recommendations for HIV testing services for inpatients and outpatients in acute-care hospital settings and technical guidance on HIV counseling. *MMWR.* 1993;42:1-17.
Centers for Disease Control and Prevention. Recommendations for the prevention and management of *Chlamydia trachomatis* infections. *MMWR* 1993;42(RR-12):1-39.
Hardy AM. AIDS knowledge and attitudes for January-March 1991: provisional data from the National Health Interview Survey. *Advance Data.* August 21, 1992:216.
Higgins DL, Galavotti C, O'Reilly KR, et al. Evidence for the effects of HIV antibody counseling and testing on risk behaviors. *JAMA.* 1991;266:2419-2429.
Hook EW, Marra CM. Acquired syphilis in adults. *N Engl J Med.* 1992;326:1060-1069.

Larson SA. Syphilis. *Clinics in Laboratory Medicine.* 1989;9:545-557.

Sellors JW, et al. Effectiveness and efficiency of selective vs universal screening for chlamydia infection in sexually active young women. Arch Intern Med 1992;152:1837-1844.

Swango PA, Kleinman DV, Konzelman JL. HIV and periodontal health. *J Am Dent Assoc* 1991;122:49-54.

US Preventive Services Task Force. Screening for syphilis, Screening for gonorrhea, Screening for infection with human immunodeficiency virus, Screening for chlamydial infection, Screening for genital herpes simplex, Counseling to prevent human immunodeficiency virus and other sexually transmitted diseases. In: *Guide to Clinical Preventive Services.* Baltimore, Md: Williams & Wilkins; 1989:chaps 22-26, 53.

## Adults/Older Adults — SCREENING

# 40. Sigmoidoscopy

Colorectal cancer is the second leading cause of death from cancer in the United States, afflicting people mainly over the age of 40 years. Of the three widely used methods of screening for colorectal cancer (digital rectal examination and fecal occult blood testing being the other two), examination using a sigmoidoscope is the most specific and sensitive. Because it enables the examiner to perform a biopsy during the procedure, the specificity of sigmoidoscopy approaches 100%. Sensitivity is largely determined by the skill of the examiner and the length of the instrument. Approximately 30% of colorectal cancers are within reach of the 25-cm rigid sigmoidoscope. The 35-cm flexible sigmoidoscope can reach 45% to 50% of cancers, and the 60-cm flexible sigmoidoscope can reach 50% to 60%. Screening with sigmoidoscopy has been limited by costs, patient and provider noncompliance, and controversy about effectiveness. Patient compliance problems have been somewhat diminished by the advent of the more comfortable flexible instruments. The 35-cm sigmoidoscope is particularly well-accepted by patients, and the 60-cm sigmoidoscope is relatively well-accepted. The controversy about effectiveness has revolved around a lack of evidence that screening with sigmoidoscopy decreases mortality from colorectal cancer. Two recently published case-control studies (Selby et al., 1992, and Newcomb et al., 1992) have demonstrated significant decreases in risk (59% and 79%, respectively) of death from colorectal cancer for screened patients. In the Selby study, significant benefit was suggested from rigid sigmoidoscopy screening performed as infrequently as every 10 years.

For information about colorectal cancer and about other methods of screening for it, refer to chapters 29 and 33.

**Recommendations of Major Authorities**

*Normal Risk*

- **American Academy of Family Physicians, Canadian Task Force on the Periodic Health Examination,** and **U.S. Preventive Services Task Force (USPSTF)**—There is insufficient evidence to recommend either initiating or terminating the provision of sigmoidoscopy screening for low-risk, asymptomatic individuals. This recommendation is currently under review by **USPSTF.**

- **American Cancer Society, American College of Obstetricians and Gynecologists, American College of Physicians (ACP), American Gastroenterological Association, American Society for Gastrointestinal Endoscopy,** and **National Cancer Institute**—Patients at normal risk should be screened with sigmoidoscopy every 3 to 5 years beginning at 50 years of age. **ACP** has stated that performance of an air-contrast barium enema every 5 years is an acceptable alternative to sigmoidoscopy.

## Ch. 40. Sigmoidoscopy — Adults/Older Adults — SCREENING

*Increased Risk*

- **All major authorities**—Patients at increased risk of colorectal cancer should receive more frequent screening. What constitutes increased risk and the nature and frequency of recommended screening differs slightly among the authorities.

- **American Academy of Family Physicians** and **U.S. Preventive Services Task Force**—It may be clinically prudent to offer screening to individuals aged 50 and older who have a first-degree relative with colorectal cancer; a personal history of endometrial, ovarian, or breast cancer; or a previous diagnosis of inflammatory bowel disease, adenomatous polyps, or colorectal cancer. Periodic colonoscopy is recommended for all people with a family history of familial polyposis or cancer family syndrome.

- **American Cancer Society**—For patients having a first-degree relative with a history of colorectal cancer at 55 years of age or younger, the entire colon and rectum should be examined with colonoscopy or air-contrast barium enema every 5 years beginning at 35 to 40 years of age. Members of families with a history of familial adenomatous polyposis should receive earlier screening utilizing flexible sigmoidoscopy. Members of families with a history of hereditary nonpolyposis colorectal cancer require earlier and more intense surveillance utilizing colonoscopy. Individuals with inflammatory bowel disease are at exceptionally high risk and require individualized treatment. Patients under the age of 55 years with a first-degree family member with a history of colorectal cancer are at increased risk and may need earlier and more frequent examinations. People with a history of breast, ovarian, or endometrial cancer are at some increased risk but should follow screening recommendations for normal-risk patients.

- **American College of Obstetricians and Gynecologists**—Colonoscopy should be a part of primary preventive care for individuals with a personal history of inflammatory bowel disease or colonic polyps, or a family history of familial polyposis coli, colorectal cancer, or cancer family syndrome.

- **American College of Physicians**—Individuals 40 years and older who have familial polyposis, inflammatory bowel disease, or a history of colon cancer in a first-degree relative should be screened with air-contrast barium enema or colonoscopy every 3 to 5 years.

- **American Gastroenterological Association** and **American Society for Gastrointestinal Endoscopy**—Individuals with a first-degree relative with a history of colon cancer should have colonoscopy performed every 5 years beginning at age 40 years, especially if the relative developed cancer before age 60 years. Women undergoing irradiation for gynecologic cancer should have flexible sigmoidoscopy every 3 years after diagnosis and beginning radiation therapy. Women with previous gynecologic or breast cancer should have flexible sigmoidoscopy every 3 to 5 years after diagnosis. Patients with left-sided ulcerative colitis for over 15 years and patients with universal colitis for over 8 years should have colonoscopy with multiple biopsies every 1 to 2 years. Patients with a family history of familial polyposis and associated syndromes should have flexible sigmoidoscopy annually from age 10 to 12 years to age 40 years, and every 3 years thereafter. Patients with a family history of hereditary nonpolyposis colorectal cancer should have colonoscopy every 2 years beginning at age 25 years, or at an age 5 years younger than the age of the earliest colon cancer diagnosis in the family.

- **Canadian Task Force on the Periodic Health Examination**—Periodic colonoscopy should be included in the clinical management of patients with a history of colorectal cancer, adenomatous polyps, or ulcerative colitis of 10 years duration. Periodic sigmoidoscopy among family members of patients with familial polyposis, who are at highest risk for colonic cancer, should begin at an early age and should be followed by periodic colonoscopy after 30 years of age.

- **National Cancer Institute**—The physician should identify for special surveillance high-risk patients, including those with a strong family history of colon cancer or with a personal history of adenomas, colon cancer, or inflammatory bowel disease.

**Basics of Sigmoidoscopy Screening**

1. Sigmoidoscopy is a rather complex procedure that requires considerable technical training and practice. It is beyond the scope of this book to fully explain the performance of this procedure; only very basic aspects will be addressed.

2. *Sigmoidoscope type*: Most authorities recommend use of a flexible sigmoidoscope (preferably 60 cm in length) rather than a rigid sigmoidoscope, because of better patient acceptance and ability to visualize lesions higher in the sigmoid colon.

3. *Training*: Sigmoidoscopy should be performed only by or under the supervision of a trained examiner. Training should be obtained from an experienced endoscopist. Training may consist of diagnostic instruction with audiovisual materials, endoscopic models, and photo atlases, followed by patient demonstrations and successful completion of a number of supervised examinations.

4. *Patient preparation*: Proper bowel preparation is essential for performance of an adequate screening examination. Recommendations for bowel preparation differ somewhat. The minimum preparation consists of two enemas a few hours before examination.

5. *Instrument cleaning:* Proper instrument cleaning is essential for patient safety and maintenance of equipment. The instrument should be promptly cleaned and inspected after use to remove organic materials. A 2% aqueous glutaraldehyde-based disinfectant should be used to clean instruments between procedures. Exposure times of 20 to 30 minutes are recommended to achieve high-level disinfection. Other agents, such as povidone-iodine solution, alcohol, surgical scrubs, phenolics, quaternary ammonium compounds, and water, have not been found to be acceptable for disinfecting sigmoidoscopes. The safety and efficacy of automatic endoscope washers have not been established. The same individual(s) in the office should consistently perform the decontamination to ensure quality. Endoscopes should be air-dried and stored in a hanging position to diminish bacterial contamination.

6. *Maintenance of Competence*: Clinicians should perform sigmoidoscopy routinely in order to maintain their competence. Performance of only occasional procedures may lead to missed or inappropriate diagnoses or a high rate of complications, or both.

7. *Follow-up of Abnormal Results*: All authorities agree that patients found to have adenomatous polyps of 1 cm or larger need colonoscopic examination of the entire colon. Approximately 10% of individuals screened will have small tubular adenomas less than 1 cm in diameter. Controversy exists about whether patients with these lesions need colonoscopic follow-up in view of their low potential for malignancy.

## Patient Resources

*Cancer of the Colon and Rectum—Research Report*; *What You Need to Know About Cancer of the Colon and Rectum*. Office of Cancer Communications, National Cancer Institute, Bldg 31, Rm 10A24, Bethesda, MD 20892; 1-800 4-CANCER.

*Colonoscopy: Questions and Answers*; *Polyps of the Colon and Rectum: Questions and Answers*. American Society of Colon and Rectal Surgeons, 800 E Northwest Highway, Suite 1080, Palatine, IL 60067; (708) 359-9184.

## Selected References

American Academy of Family Physicians, Commission on Public Health and Scientific Affairs. *Age Charts for Periodic Health Examination*. Kansas City, Mo: American Academy of Family Physicians; 1993.

American College of Obstetricians and Gynecologists. *The Obstetrician-Gynecologist and Primary-Preventive Health Care*. Washington, DC: American College of Obstetricians and Gynecologists; 1993.

American College of Physicians, Health and Public Policy Committee. Clinical competence in the use of flexible sigmoidoscopy for screening purposes. *Ann Intern Med*. 1987;107:589-591.

American College of Physicians. Guidelines. In: Eddy DM, ed. *Common Screening Tests*. Philadelphia, Pa: American College of Physicians; 1991:415-416.

Canadian Task Force on the Periodic Health Examination. The periodic health examination: 2. 1989 update. *Can Med Assoc J*. 1989;141:4-16.

Eddy DM. Screening for colorectal cancer. *Ann Intern Med*. 1990;113:373-384.

Fleischer DE, Goldberg SB, Browning TH, et al. Detection and surveillance of colorectal cancer. *JAMA*. 1989;261:580-585.

Gorse GJ, Messner RL. Infection control practices in gastrointestinal endoscopy in the United States: a national survey. *Infect Control Hosp Epidem*iol. 1991;12:289-296.

Levin B, Murphy GP. Revision in American Cancer Society recommendations for the early detection of colorectal cancer. *CA*. 1992;42:296-299.

Smart CR, Chu K, Conley V, Henson DE, Pommerenke F, Srivastova S. Cancer Screening and Early Detection. In: Holland JF, Frei EF III, Bast RC Sr, Kufe DW, Morton DL, Weichselbaum RR, eds. *Cancer Medicine*. vol 1. 3rd ed. Philadelphia, Pa: Lea & Febiger; 1993:408-431.

Newcomb PA, Norfleet RG, Storer B, Surawicz, Marcus PM. Screening sigmoidoscopy and colorectal cancer mortality. *JNCI*. 1992;84:1572-1575.

Ransohoff DF, Lang CA. Sigmoidoscopic screening in the 1990s. *JAMA*. 1993;269:1278-1281.

Selby JV, Friedman GD. Sigmoidoscopy in the periodic examination of asymptomatic adults. *JAMA*. 1989;261:595-601.

Selby JV, Friedman GD, Quesenberry CP, Weiss NS. A case-control study of screening sigmoidoscopy and mortality from colorectal cancer. *N Engl J Med*. 1992;326:653-657.

US Preventive Services Task Force. Screening for colorectal cancer. In: *Guide to Clinical Preventive Services*. Baltimore, Md: Williams & Wilkins; 1989:chap 7.

Wigton RS, Bland LL, Monsour H, Nicolas JA. Procedural skills of practicing gastroenterologists. *Ann Int Med*. 1990;113:540-46.

# Adults/Older Adults — SCREENING

## 41. Thyroid Function

Thyroid dysfunction affects 1% to 4% of the adult population in the United States. Hypothyroidism occurs with an annual incidence of 0.08%; the incidence of hyperthyroidism is estimated to be 0.05% per year. Both forms of thyroid dysfunction are more common in women, older adults, and individuals with a family history of thyroid disease. Laboratory evidence of hypothyroidism occurs in up to 10% of women and 2% of men aged 60 years and older. Other risk factors for thyroid hypofunction include prior autoimmune conditions, history of head or neck surgery or radiation exposure, Down Syndrome, and the postpartum state. Most affected persons develop typical symptoms shortly after the onset of thyroid dysfunction. Lethargy, weight gain, confusion, cold intolerance, constipation, alopecia, dyspnea, myalgias, and paresthesias are common features of hypothyroidism. Restlessness, emotional lability, insomnia, heat intolerance, dyspnea, palpitations, ophthalmopathy, diarrhea, muscle atrophy, weakness, tremors, and tachycardia are symptoms of hyperthyroidism. Some individuals, particularly older adults, experience an insidious onset of thyroid disease, with atypical symptoms that often go unrecognized or symptoms that are confused with normal aging. For example, individuals with apathetic hyperthyroidism may present with depression, weight loss, congestive heart failure, or atrial fibrillation. Studies suggest that some patients with subclinical disease or mild alterations in thyroid function tests may benefit from early treatment if they are identified through screening. For this reason, some authorities recommend screening of certain high-risk populations for thyroid dysfunction.

Chapters 8 and 29 provide information about screening for congenital hypothyroidism and thyroid cancer, respectively.

### Recommendations of Major Authorities

A number of authorities have recommended screening for high-risk populations:

- **American Academy of Family Physicians** and **U.S. Preventive Services Task Force**—Routine screening for thyroid disorders is not warranted in asymptomatic adults. It may be clinically prudent to screen populations at increased risk, such as older individuals, especially women.

- **American College of Obstetricians and Gynecologists**—Thyroid-stimulating hormone (TSH) levels should be obtained every 3 to 5 years from all women aged 65 and older and from younger women with an autoimmune condition or strong family history of thyroid disease.

- **American College of Physicians**—Routine screening for thyroid disease is not indicated in asymptomatic individuals nor in patients admitted to the hospital for acute medical or psychiatric illnesses; testing may be indicated to identify unsuspected disease in women over 50 years of age who have general symptoms that could be caused by thyroid disease.

- **American Thyroid Association**—Tests of thyroid function should not be a part of multiphasic screening for patients who are not suspected of having thyroid disease except in certain high-risk populations. Suspect populations include individuals with a strong family history of thyroid disease; elderly patients; postpartum women 4 to 8 weeks after delivery; and patients with autoimmune diseases.

- **Canadian Task Force on the Periodic Physical Examination**—Routine screening of the general population for hyperthyroidism is not indicated; postmenopausal women should be examined for clinical evidence of hypothyroidism.

## Basics of Thyroid Function Screening

1. Just as there is controversy over which high-risk populations should be screened for thyroid dysfunction, there is also disagreement over which tests should be used for screening purposes. Many authorities now recommend performing a TSH level using a "sensitive" TSH assay as the initial screen, and obtaining a free thyroxine ($FT_4$) or free thyroxine index ($FT_4I$) level only if the TSH level is abnormal. In unselected populations, these TSH assays have sensitivities of 85% to 95% and specificities of 90% to 96% for thyroid dysfunction. Total thyroxine ($TT_4$) and $FT_4I$ levels, while less expensive, are less sensitive and less specific than the "sensitive" TSH assays.

2. An elevated TSH value (greater than 7 mU/L) and a suppressed $FT_4$ level (less than 0.8 ng/dL) suggest primary thyroid failure, which necessitates therapy. (Normal values may vary with each laboratory.) It is not clear whether asymptomatic patients with an elevated TSH but a normal $FT_4$ or $FT_4I$ will benefit from treatment. Some evidence suggests that thyroid replacement may diminish the potential for developing long-term complications of subclinical thyroid hypofunction. As only a small number of these individuals go on to develop overt disease, some authorities recommend serial testing of these patients rather than immediate replacement therapy.

3. A depressed TSH level (less than 0.4 mU/L) usually indicates the presence of an elevated serum thyroxine ($T_4$) level. This is not always the case, however. If clinical findings of hyperthyroidism are present and the $T_4$ is normal, serum total triiodothyronine ($TT_3$) should be measured, as the patient may have a $T_3$ thyrotoxicosis. In the absence of clinical findings, many authorities recommend following the patient closely and deferring treatment until symptoms develop.

4. The clinician should be aware that medications and clinical conditions can affect the interpretation of thyroid screening tests. TSH levels may be depressed in euthyroid patients taking large doses of glucocorticoids or dopamine. Also, the TSH level may be misleading in the presence of pituitary or hypothalamic hypothyroidism and during changes in thyroid status that occur in subacute thyroiditis or after treatment for hyperthyroidism. In these cases, measurement of the $FT_4$ is preferred. Phenytoin, carbamazepine, and rifampin can depress $TT_4$ levels. The effect of drugs on reported $FT_4$ levels varies with the laboratory method used. Increased levels of thyroid binding globulin (TBG), resulting in elevated $TT_4$ levels, may occur with pregnancy, oral contraceptive or estrogen use, acute or chronic active hepatitis, acute intermittent porphyria, and certain inherited traits. Patients with cirrhosis, nephrotic syndrome, severe illness, and those

using testosterone or corticosteroids may have slightly reduced $TT_4$ levels because of diminished TBG. Severe illnesses, such as those requiring treatment in an intensive-care unit, can also affect the production, secretion, distribution, and metabolism of thyroid hormone.

## Selected References

American Academy of Family Physicians, Commission on Public Health and Scientific Affairs. *Age Charts for Periodic Health Examination*. Kansas City, Mo: American Academy of Family Physicians; 1993.

American College of Obstetricians and Gynecologists. *The Obstetrician-Gynecologist and Primary-Preventive Health Care*. Washington, D.C.: American College of Obstetricians and Gynecologists; 1993.

American College of Physicians. Guidelines. In: Eddy DM, ed. *Common Screening Tests*. Philadelphia, Pa: American College of Physicians; 1991:406-408.

Becker DV, Bigos ST, Gaitan E, et al. Optimal use of blood tests for assessment of thyroid function. *JAMA*. 1993;269:2736-2737.

Canadian Task Force on the Periodic Health Examination. The periodic health examination. *Can Med Assoc J*. 1979;121:1194-254.

de los Santos ET, Starich GH, Mazzaferri EL. Sensitivity, specificity, and cost-effectiveness of the sensitive thyrotropin assay in the diagnosis of thyroid disease in ambulatory patients. *Arch Intern Med*. 1989;149:526-532.

Hay ID, Bayer MF, Kaplan MM, Klee GG, Larsen PR, Spencer CA. American Thyroid Association assessment of free thyroid hormone and thyrotropin measurements and guidelines for future clinical assays. *Clin Chem*. 1991;37:2002-2008.

Helfand M, Crapo LM. Screening for thyroid disease. *Ann Intern Med*. 1990;112:840-849.

Sawin CT, Geller A, Kaplan MM, Bacharach P, Wilson PWF, Hershman JM. Low serum thyrotropin (thyroid-stimulating hormone) in older persons without hyperthyroidism. *Arch Intern Med*. 1991;151:165-168.

Sawin CT. Thyroid dysfunction in older persons. *Advances Intern Med*. 1991;37:223-248.

Staub JJ, Althaus BU, Engler H, et al. Spectrum of subclinical and overt hypothyroidism: effect on thyrotropin, prolactin, and thyroid reserve, and metabolic impact on peripheral target tissues. *Am J Med*. 1992;92:631-642.

Surks MI, Chopra IJ, Mariash CN, Nicoloff JT, Solomon DH. American Thyroid Association guidelines for use of laboratory tests in thyroid disorders. *JAMA*. 1990;263:1529-1532.

US Preventive Services Task Force. Screening for thyroid disease. In: *Guide to Clinical Preventive Services*. Baltimore, Md: Williams & Wilkins; 1989:chap 17.

# Adults/Older Adults — SCREENING

## 42. Tuberculosis
### (Including Prophylaxis and BCG Vaccination)

In 1991, 26,283 new cases of active tuberculosis (TB) were reported in the United States. That is the largest number of cases since 1981 and almost 10,000 cases more than could have been anticipated based on incidence trends in the early 1980s. Another 10 million Americans have latent TB infections. Factors contributing to the increase in TB include adverse social and economic conditions, the HIV epidemic, immigration of individuals with TB infection, and clinician and patient noncompliance with recommended screening and treatment regimens. Efforts to control the spread of TB have also been confounded by the emergence of strains of *Mycobacterium tuberculosis* resistant to multiple drugs. In April 1991, as many as 33% of all positive TB cultures in New York City were resistant to one or more anti-TB drugs.

TB control in the United States depends on screening populations at high risk and providing preventive therapy to those who are most likely to develop active disease. Groups at high risk for TB include: 1) medically underserved low-income populations, including racial and ethnic minority groups (African-American, Hispanic, American Indian, and Alaskan native heritage); 2) foreign-born individuals from countries of high prevalence (African, Asian, and Latin American nations); 3) domestic or occupational contacts of infectious TB cases; 4) alcoholics and injection drug users; 5) residents and staff of acute and long-term facilities (such as hospitals, nursing homes, and correctional and mental health institutions); and 6) individuals with chronic disease. Some of the conditions and chronic diseases that predispose patients to developing active TB include HIV infection, diabetes mellitus, end-stage renal disease, and hematologic and reticuloendothelial diseases; history of intestinal bypass or gastrectomy, chronic malabsorption syndromes, silicosis, cancers of the upper gastrointestinal tract or oropharynx, prolonged steroid use, and immunosuppressive therapy; and being 10% or more below desirable body weight.

Prophylaxis with isoniazid is very effective in preventing the onset of clinical disease. When taken for 12 months, isoniazid has been shown to reduce the incidence of clinical TB infection by 54% to 88%. Efficacy is directly related to the length of prophylaxis and the extent of patient compliance with the prophylaxis regimen. The effectiveness of BCG vaccination is considerably less certain, with effectiveness rates that vary from 0% to 76% in major trials.

Chapter 9 provides information on TB screening, preventive therapy, and BCG immunization in children and adolescents.

**Recommendations of Major Authorities**

*Screening*

- All major authorities, including **American Academy of Family Physicians, American College of Obstetricians and Gynecologists, American Thoracic Society, Canadian Task Force**

Ch. 42. Tuberculosis                                            Adults/Older Adults — SCREENING

on the Periodic Health Examination, Centers for Disease Control and Prevention, and U.S. Preventive Services Task Force—Tuberculin skin testing should be performed on all individuals at high risk. Frequency of testing is not specified.

*Prophylaxis*

- **American Thoracic Society (ATS), Centers for Disease Control and Prevention (CDC), and U.S. Preventive Services Task Force**—Adults with a reactive skin test and no evidence of active disease should be considered for preventive therapy with isoniazid. **ATS** and **CDC** also recommend that anergic patients recently exposed to an active TB case or from populations where the prevalence of TB is greater than 10% (injection drug users, homeless individuals, migrant laborers, and first-generation immigrants from Asia, Africa, or Latin America) should be considered for isoniazid prophylaxis even when their skin test is negative.

*BCG Vaccination*

- **American Thoracic Society, Centers for Disease Control and Prevention**, and **U.S. Preventive Services Task Force**—Vaccination with BCG is not recommended for adults in the United States.

- **Canadian Task Force on the Periodic Health Examination (CTFPHE)**—BCG vaccination should be offered to tuberculin-negative adults who have household or occupational exposure to a person with TB in communities or groups in which the infection rate is high.

**Basics of Tuberculosis Screening, Prophylaxis, and BCG Vaccination**

*Screening*

1. The Mantoux test should be used when possible. Multiple-puncture tests are not sufficiently sensitive or specific for screening purposes. Any reaction to a multiple puncture test should be confirmed by a standard Mantoux test unless vesiculation occurs, in which case the patient should be considered a candidate for preventive therapy without a Mantoux test.

2. For the Mantoux test, 0.1 mL of purified protein derivative (PPD) containing 5 tuberculin units (TU) is administered on the volar or dorsal surface of the forearm by intradermal injection using a disposable tuberculin syringe. The bevel of the needle should face upward and the injection should produce a pale, discrete 6-mm to 10-mm weal on the skin.

3. The test should be read 48 to 72 hours after placement by palpating the margin of induration and measuring the diameter transverse to the long axis of the forearm. It may be helpful to outline the margin of induration with a ballpoint pen. Erythema surrounding the induration should not be considered in evaluating test results. Providers should always record the actual millimeters of induration. Simply recording "positive" or "negative" is not precise enough and may lead to improper treatment.

4. Absence of tuberculin reaction does not exclude a diagnosis of TB infection, especially when symptoms suggest active disease. Induration of less than 5 mm may occur early in

the course of TB infection or in individuals with altered immune function. Anergy testing with at least two other delayed-type hypersensitivity skin tests (i.e., Candida, mumps, or tetanus toxoid) should be conducted in conjunction with PPD testing in adults with decreased cell-mediated immune function (including those with HIV infection).

5. Reactions to PPD may wane with age and can be restored by repeat testing. Because of this "booster effect," patients (particularly those over 55) who undergo repeat testing may be falsely classified as new converters and unnecessarily treated with isoniazid. Some authorities advise initial screening of adults in institutional and hospital settings using a two-step PPD testing procedure. If the first Mantoux test is negative, a second test should be done 1 to 2 weeks later. Reaction to the "booster" test usually indicates old—not new—TB infection. CDC recommends this two-step procedure for the initial screening of residents and employees of long-term care facilities, such as nursing homes, adult foster-care homes, and board and care homes.

6. Adverse reactions to TB skin testing are very uncommon. Reactions described include pain, fever, ulceration, vesiculation, and regional adenopathy. Because of the potential for adverse reactions, it is not advisable to retest patients with documented history of a positive Mantoux test.

7. BCG vaccination can cause false-positive Mantoux reactions, but this decreases with time and rarely causes reactions of 15 mm or greater. In general, BCG-vaccinated persons with positive Mantoux tests should be considered to have true infection with *M. tuberculosis* and given appropriate follow-up care.

8. Live vaccines, such as MMR and OPV, may interfere with reponse to the Mantoux test. TB testing may be administered either concurrently with these vaccines or 4 to 6 weeks afterwards.

## *Prophylaxis*

1. *Indications:* CDC has issued recommendations for preventive therapy in previously untreated adults without evidence of active TB. These are presented in Table 42-1. Certain anergic patients should be considered for preventive therapy regardless of their skin test reaction. These include adults who have had close contact with an infectious case of TB in the past 3 months and those who are members of populations in which the prevalence of TB is greater than 10%—including injection drug users, homeless individuals, migrant laborers, and those born in Asia, Africa, or Latin America.

2. *Dosage and Administration*: Preventive therapy should be initiated with isoniazid. The correct daily dosage of isoniazid for adults is 5 mg/kg to a maximum of 300 mg, given orally once daily. For noncompliant adult patients, isoniazid may be administered by a health professional on a twice-weekly schedule of 15 mg/kg per dose to a maximum of 900 mg. By insuring that patients take appropriate doses, this form of directly observed therapy may help reduce the emergence of newly resistant strains. In general, isoniazid prophylaxis should be continued for at least 6 months up to a maximum of 12 months.

Patients who are HIV-positive or have evidence of prior untreated TB on chest X-ray should receive isoniazid prophylaxis for 12 months. Patients who have had contact with infectious TB known to be resistant to isoniazid should be considered for preventive therapy with rifampin (600 mg by mouth daily for 1 year).

3. *Precautions:* Contraindications to isoniazid prophylaxis include acute or active liver disease of any etiology, history of previous completion of isoniazid preventive therapy, or previous adverse reaction to isoniazid. For adults over 35 years of age there is a 10% to 20% incidence of mild isoniazid-induced liver function test abnormalities. Adults over age 35 years should have baseline and periodic transaminase (ALT or AST) levels tested during the course of therapy. If the transaminase test exceeds 3 to 5 times the upper limit of the laboratory normal range, discontinuation of isoniazid should be considered. Individuals who use alcohol daily or in whom chronic liver disease is suspected should also be monitored closely for isoniazid-induced hepatitis. Supplementation with pyridoxine (vitamin $B_6$, 50 mg by mouth daily) may be helpful in preventing neuropathy in certain patients on isoniazid, such as those with diabetes, uremia, alcoholism, and malnutrition. Pregnant women who are candidates for preventive treatment should delay therapy until after delivery. If it is likely that the woman has been recently infected, therapy may be instituted after completion of the first trimester of pregnancy.

**Table 42-1. Criteria for Determining Need for Preventive Therapy by Category and Age Group**

| Category | Age Groups (Years) <35 | ≥35 |
|---|---|---|
| With risk factor* | Treat at all ages if reaction to 5 TU purified protein derivative ≥10 mm (or ≥5 mm and recent TB contact, HIV-infected, or has radiographic evidence of old TB) | |
| Without risk factor High-incidence group** | Treat if PPD ≥10 mm | Do not treat |
| Without risk factor Low-incidence group | Treat if PPD ≥15 mm*** | Do not treat |

*Risk factors include HIV infection, recent (within past three months) contact with infectious person, abnormal chest radiograph, injection drug abuse, certain medical risk factors, and recent skin-test conversion. Recent converters are those who have had an increase of ≥10 mm in PPD reaction within 2 years, or an increase of ≥15 mm for adults ≥35 years old. Medical risk factors include: HIV infection, diabetes, end-stage renal disease, hematologic and reticuloendothelial diseases, history of intestinal bypass or gastrectomy, chronic malabsorption syndromes, silicosis, cancers of the upper gastrointestinal tract or oropharynx, prolonged steroid use, immunosuppressive therapy, and being 10% or more below ideal body weight.

**High-incidence groups include foreign-born persons, medically underserved low-income populations, and residents of long-term care facilities.

***Lower or higher cut points may be used for identifying positive reactions, depending upon the relative prevalence of *M. tuberculosis* infection and nonspecific cross-reactivity in the population.

From: Centers for Disease Control. The use of preventive therapy for tuberculosis infection in the United States: recommendations of the Advisory Committee for the Elimination of Tuberculosis. *MMWR.* 1990;39:(RR-8)9-12.

4. *Adverse Reactions:* Patients should be monitored monthly for signs and symptoms of adverse reactions while on isoniazid. These include drug fever or rash, hypersensitivity reactions, peripheral neuritis, and hepatitis. The signs and symptoms of hepatitis include loss of appetite, nausea, vomiting, persistent dark urine, jaundice, fever, and abdominal tenderness—especially in the right upper quadrant. Patients concurrently taking other medications should be monitored for potential drug interactions.

## *BCG Vaccination*

1. *Indications:* BCG vaccination is not recommended for adults in the United States. CTFPHE recommends BCG vaccination for tuberculin-negative contacts of active TB cases in Canadian communities in which the infection rate is high.

2. *Dosage and Administration:* The Tice® strain is the only BCG preparation currently available in North America. The dosage and administration is the same for adults as for children (see chapter 9 for details).

3. *Precautions:* BCG vaccine should not be given to individuals who may be immunocompromised or immunosuppressed, including those with known or suspected HIV infection.

4. *Adverse Reactions:* Side effects occur in 1% to 10% of vaccinated individuals and may include severe or prolonged ulceration at the vaccination site, lymphadenitis, and lupus vulgaris.

## Patient Resources

*Facts About the TB Skin Test*; *Facts About Tuberculosis.* American Lung Association, 1740 Broadway, New York, NY 10019-4373; (212) 315-8700.

*TB: Get the Facts*; *Tuberculosis: Connection between TB and HIV.* Centers for Disease Control and Prevention, Attn: Information Services Office, 1600 Clifton Road NE, Atlanta, GA 30333; (404) 639-1819.

## Provider Resources

*Core Curriculum on Tuberculosis.* American Thoracic Society/Centers for Disease Control. Division of Tuberculosis Elimination, National Center for Prevention Services, Centers for Disease Control and Prevention, 1600 Clifton Road, Mailstop E-10, Atlanta, GA 30333; (404) 639-2508.

*Initial Therapy for TB in the Era of Multiple Drug Resistance*; *Mantoux Tuberculin Skin Testing* (videotape). Centers for Disease Control and Prevention, Attn: Information Services, 1600 Clifton Road NE, Atlanta, GA 30333; (404) 639-1819.

## Selected References

American Academy of Family Physicians, Commission on Public Health and Scientific Affairs. *Age Charts for Periodic Health Examination*. Kansas City, Mo: American Academy of Family Physicians; 1993.

American College of Obstetricians and Gynecologists. *The Obstetrician-Gynecologist and Primary-Preventive Health Care*. Washington, DC: American College of Obstetricians and Gynecologists; 1993.

American Thoracic Society. Control of tuberculosis in the United States. *Amer Rev Respir Dis*. 1992;146:1623-1633.

American Thoracic Society/Centers for Disease Control. Diagnostic standards and classification of tuberculosis. *Am Rev Respir Dis*. 1990;142:725-35.

Canadian Task Force on the Periodic Health Examination. The periodic health examination 1979. *Can Med Assoc J*. 1979;121:1194-254.

Centers for Disease Control. *Control of Tuberculosis in Correctional Facilities-A Guide for Health Care Workers*. Atlanta, Ga: Centers for Disease Control; 1992.

Centers for Disease Control. Guidelines for preventing the transmission of tuberculosis in health-care settings, with special focus on HIV-related issues. *MMWR*. 1990;39(RR-17):1-29.

Centers for Disease Control. Prevention and control of tuberculosis in facilities providing long-term care to the elderly: recommendations of the Advisory Committee for Elimination of Tuberculosis. *MMWR*. 1990;39(RR-10):7-20.

Centers for Disease Control. Prevention and control of tuberculosis in U.S. communities with at-risk minority populations and prevention and control of tuberculosis among homeless persons: recommendations of the Advisory Council for Elimination of Tuberculosis. *MMWR*. 1992;41(RR-5):1-23.

Centers for Disease Control. Purified protein derivative (PPD) tuberculin anergy and HIV infection: guidelines for anergy testing and management of anergic persons at risk of tuberculosis. *MMWR*. 1991;40(RR-5):27-33.

Centers for Disease Control. Screening for tuberculosis and tuberculous infection in high-risk populations: recommendations of the Advisory Committee for Elimination of Tuberculosis. *MMWR*. 1990;39(RR-8):1-7.

Centers for Disease Control. Use of BCG vaccines in the control of tuberculosis: a joint statement by the Advisory Committee for Immunization Practices and the Advisory Committee for Elimination of Tuberculosis. *MMWR*. 1988;37:663-664, 669-675.

Centers for Disease Control. The use of preventive therapy for tuberculous infection in the United States: recommendations of the Advisory Committee for the Elimination of Tuberculosis. *MMWR*. 1990;39(RR-8):9-12.

Frieden TR, Sterling T, Pablos-Mendez A. The emergence of drug-resistant tuberculosis in New York City. *N Engl J Med*. 1993;328:523-6.

Iseman MD, Cohn DL, Sbarbaro JA. Directly observed treatment of tuberculosis: we can't afford not to try it. *N Engl J Med*. 1993;328:576-8.

*Physicians' Desk Reference*. Oradell, NJ: Medical Economics Company; 1993:898-899, 1689-1692.

Pust RE. Tuberculosis in the 1990's: resurgence, regimens, and resources. *South Med J*. 1992;85:584-593.

U.S. Preventive Services Task Force. Screening for tuberculosis. In: *Guide to Clinical Preventive Services*. Baltimore, Md: Williams & Wilkins; 1989:chap 21.

## Adults/Older Adults — SCREENING

# 43. Urinalysis

Examination of urine for signs of occult disease has a long tradition in medical care. The development of modern "dipsticks" that can perform multiple tests in a matter of minutes has made urinalysis inexpensive and quick—perhaps the most convenient of all office-based tests. Most of the abnormalities detected by screening adults with urinalysis, however, are indicative of benign disorders, such as idiopathic proteinuria, or of conditions for which the value of treatment is unclear, such as occult bacteriuria. For this reason, most authorities recommend screening urinalysis only for certain conditions in specific high-risk populations.

Urinalysis is most often recommended to screen for occult bacteriuria. Urinary tract infections are a significant source of disease and morbidity for diabetic women, pregnant women, and older people (particularly women). Table 43-1 shows the prevalence of asymptomatic bacteriuria in selected adult populations and the positive predictive value of nitrite and leukocyte esterase (LE) dipstick tests for detecting asymptomatic bacteriuria in these populations. Positive predictive values are relatively low, except for institutionalized older adults and diabetic women.

Treatment of asymptomatic bacteriuria in institutionalized older adults has not been shown to decrease morbidity or mortality, or even to lead to sustained periods without bacteriuria. There is some evidence that treating elderly women in the community leads to fewer symptomatic infections, but the significance of this for long-term health is unknown. Whether treating diabetic women leads to fewer symptomatic urinary tract infections and decreased long-term morbidity has not been proven, but it is plausible. Treating asymptomatic bacteriuria is of definite proven benefit for pregnant women. For this reason, pregnant women are routinely screened with urine cultures, which are more sensitive and specific than dipstick tests.

Screening has also been advocated to detect occult hematuria, which can be indicative of urinary tract malignancies. These malignancies increase significantly in incidence after the age of 40 and are twice as frequent in men as in women. The sensitivity of dipstick tests for hematuria is good (91% to 100%), but specificity can be as low as 65%. The predictive value of a positive heme dipstick test even in older men has been found to be as low as 0.5% for malignancy, although values as high as 26% have been reported for this population. Unnecessary evaluations for a potential urinary tract malignancy can be harmful. Intravenous pyelograms, for example, can lead to diminished renal function and, rarely, death.

Screening for proteinuria is of little value because most causes are either benign or untreatable. Screening for diabetes with urinalysis is very inaccurate and better accomplished with plasma glucose measurements (see chapter 37). See chapter 10 for a discussion of the use of screening urinalysis in children.

## Recommendations of Major Authorities

- **American Academy of Family Physicians (AAFP), American College of Obstetricians and Gynecologists (ACOG), and U.S. Preventive Services Task Force (USPSTF)**—Dipstick urinalysis for asymptomatic bacteriuria is recommended for patients with diabetes mellitus. **USPSTF** and **AAFP** state that optimal frequency for this screening is left to clinical discretion. **ACOG** designates a schedule of "yearly, as appropriate" for preventive care. All three recommend dipstick urinalysis testing for older adults (60 or 65 years of age and older). **USPSTF** recommendations are currently under review.

- **American College of Physicians**—Urinalysis and urine culture should not be routinely used to screen for asymptomatic bacteriuria.

- **Canadian Task Force on the Periodic Health Examination**—There is fair justification for the recommendation that urinary tract infection not be included among conditions sought in a periodic health examination.

- **All major authorities**—Screening urinalysis is recommended in prenatal care for pregnant women.

## Basics of Urinalysis Screening

1. Early morning urine collected at least 6 hours after previous voiding and 8 hours after fasting is most concentrated and most likely to reveal abnormalities. Women who are menstruating should not undergo routine screening urinalysis.

2. Obtaining a specimen using "clean catch" technique permits a follow-up culture if indicated. Women should clean the vulvar region with lukewarm water, spreading the labia and washing the urethral meatus with a moistened cotton wad or pad several times

**Table 43-1. Prevalence of Asymptomatic Bacteriuria in Adults and Estimated Positive Predictive Values of Nitrite and Leukocyte Esterase Dipstick Tests**

| Population | Estimated Prevalence (%) | Positive Predictive Value (%)* |
|---|---|---|
| Women age <60 years | 3.0 | 8.1 |
| Men age <60 years | 0.3 | 0.8 |
| Women age >60 years in the community | 7.0 | 17.6 |
| Men age >60 years in the community | 2.2 | 6.0 |
| Institutionalized elderly | 22.0 | 44.4 |
| Pregnant women | 5.0 | 13.0 |
| Diabetic women | 15.0 | 33.3 |

*Proportion of those in whom at least one of the two tests is positive that will have bacteriuria.

Adapted from: Pels RJ, Bor DH, Woolhandler S, Himmelstein DU, Lawrence RS. Bacteriuria. In: Goldbloom RB, Lawrence RS, eds. *Preventing Disease: Beyond the Rhetoric*. New York, NY: Springer-Verlag; 1990;chap 8. Used with permission of Springer-Verlag New York and the authors; copyright © 1990.

## Ch. 43. Urinalysis — Adults/Older Adults — SCREENING

from front to back. Each wad or pad should be used only once. The use of soap or disinfectants should be avoided because of possible effects on the sample. Men should draw back their foreskin (if present) and clean the glans and urethral meatus several times with a cotton wad or pad, using each only once.

3. A clean container should be used to collect a sample of urine obtained midstream while the patient urinates into the toilet.

4. Urinalysis should be performed as soon as possible after collection, using any one of the many available types of urine dipsticks. No major authority recommends using urine cultures for routine screening of nonpregnant adults. Specimens that are not examined immediately should be refrigerated.

5. In interpreting the test, the clinician must keep in mind possible causes of false-positive and false-negative results (see Tables 43-2 and 43-3).

## Patient Resources

*Urinary Tract Infection: A Common Problem for Some Women.* American Academy of Family Physicians, 8880 Ward Parkway, Kansas City, MO 64114-2797; 1-800 944-0000.

### Table 43-2. Causes of Inaccurate Nitrite Dipstick Tests

| False Positives | False Negatives |
| --- | --- |
| Specimen contamination | Presence of non-nitrate-reducing organisms (e.g., many non-Enterobacteriaceae species.) |
|  | Presence of occasional organisms that further reduce nitrate to ammonia |
|  | Failure to perform on first morning voided specimen |
|  | Frequent voiding |
|  | Dilute urine |
|  | High specific gravity |
|  | Urine pH <6 |
|  | Presence of urobilinogen |
|  | Large dietary intake of vitamin C |

From: Pels RJ, Bor DH, Woolhandler S, Himmelstein DU, Lawrence RS. Bacteriuria. In: Goldbloom RB, Lawrence RS, eds. *Preventing Disease: Beyond the Rhetoric.* New York, NY: Springer-Verlag; 1990;chap 8. Used with permission of Springer-Verlag New York and the authors; copyright © 1990.

**Table 43-3. Causes of Inaccurate Leukocyte Esterase Dipstick Tests**

| False Positives | False Negatives |
| --- | --- |
| Contamination during collection | Increased specific gravity |
|  | Glycosuria |
|  | Presence of urobilinogen |
|  | Therapy with phenazopyridine hydrochloride, nitrofurantoin, or rifampin |
|  | Large dietary intake of vitamin C |

Note: The use of the LE dipstick to detect the diverse conditions associated with sterile (culture-negative) pyuria is not considered here.

From: Pels RJ, Bor DH, Woolhandler S, Himmelstein DU, Lawrence RS. Bacteriuria. In: Goldbloom RB, Lawrence RS, eds. *Preventing Disease: Beyond the Rhetoric.* New York, NY: Springer-Verlag; 1990;chap 8. Used with permission of Springer-Verlag New York and the authors; copyright © 1990.

## Selected References

American Academy of Family Physicians, Commission on Public Health and Scientific Affairs. *Age Charts for Periodic Health Examination.* Kansas City, Mo: American Academy of Family Physicians; 1993.

American College of Obstetricians and Gynecologists. *The Obstetrician-Gynecologist and Primary-Preventive Health Care.* Washington, DC: American College of Obstetricians and Gynecologists; 1993.

Boscia JA, Kobasa WD, Knight RA, et al. Therapy vs no therapy for bacteriuria in elderly ambulatory nonhospitalized women. *JAMA.* 1987;257:1067-1071.

Canadian Task Force on the Periodic Health Examination. *Periodic Health Examination Monograph.* Hull, Quebec: Minister of Supply and Services Canada; 1980.

Komaroff AL. Urinalysis and urine culture in women with dysuria. In: Sox HC Jr, ed. *Common Diagnostic Tests: Use and Interpretation.* 2nd ed. Philadelphia, Pa: American College of Physicians; 1990:286-301.

Pels RJ, Bor DH, Woolhandler S, Himmelstein DU, Lawrence RS. Bacteriuria. In: Goldbloom RB, Lawrence RS, eds. *Preventing Disease: Beyond the Rhetoric.* New York, NY: Springer-Verlag; 1990:chap 8.

US Preventive Services Task Force. Screening for asymptomatic bacteriuria, hematuria, and proteinuria. In: *Guide to Clinical Preventive Services.* Baltimore, Md: Williams & Wilkins; 1989:chap 27.

Woolhandler S, Pels RJ, Bor DH, Himmelstein DU, Lawrence RS. Hematuria and proteinuria. In: Goldbloom RB, Lawrence RS, eds. *Preventing Disease: Beyond the Rhetoric.* New York, NY: Springer-Verlag; 1990:chap 37.

# Adults/Older Adults — SCREENING

## 44. Vision

Vision loss is common in adults and increases in prevalence with advancing age. Approximately 13% of individuals 65 years of age or older and 28% of those over 85 years of age report some degree of visual impairment. More than 90% of older people require the use of corrective lenses at some time. Common visual disorders affecting adults include cataracts, macular degeneration, glaucoma, and diabetic retinopathy. Visual disorders in older adults frequently lead to trauma from falls, automobile crashes, and other types of unintentional injuries. A substantial number (18% in one study) of hip fractures are attributable to impaired vision. Many older adults are unaware of decreases in their visual acuity, and up to 25% may have incorrect corrective lens prescriptions.

Surgical treatment for cataracts can lead to improved vision and quality of life. Medical and surgical treatment may help prevent visual loss due to glaucoma. Early laser surgical treatment can help prevent visual loss due to diabetic retinopathy and (in some cases) macular degeneration. Visual acuity testing is easily and accurately performed by primary care clinicians. However, glaucoma screening, as usually practiced by primary care clinicians using a Schiotz tonometer, is relatively insensitive and nonspecific. The predictive value of a positive Schiotz test is only about 5%.

### Recommendations of Major Authorities

- **American Academy of Family Physicians** and **U.S. Preventive Services Task Force (USPSTF)**—Vision screening may be appropriate in asymptomatic older individuals. The frequency of this screening should be left to the discretion of the clinician. **USPSTF** recommends examination by an eye specialist beginning at 65 years of age for glaucoma, but does not recommend an optimal frequency.

- **American Academy of Ophthalmology**—A comprehensive eye examination, including screening for visual acuity and glaucoma by an ophthalmologist, should be performed every 3 to 5 years in African Americans aged 20 to 39 years, and regardless of race, every 2 to 4 years in individuals aged 40 to 64 years, and every 1 to 2 years beginning at 65. Diabetic patients, at any age, should have exams at least yearly.

- **American College of Obstetricians and Gynecologists**—Women 65 years of age and older should be evaluated for visual acuity yearly or as appropriate.

- **American Optometric Association**—A comprehensive eye and vision examination is recommended for all adults as follows: ages 20-64, every 1-2 years; ages 65 and over, yearly. Persons at increased risk for eye disease (e.g., with diabetes, hypertension, or any eye disease) should have examinations as recommended by their eye-care professional.

- **Canadian Task Force on the Periodic Health Examination**—Visual acuity testing for asymptomatic adults should be optional. There is poor justification on scientific grounds for inclusion of primary open-angle glaucoma screening in a periodic health examination.

- **National Eye Institute**—A comprehensive eye examination, including screening for visual acuity and glaucoma, should be performed by an eye care professional every 2 years beginning at age 40 years in African Americans and age 60 years in all other individuals. Diabetic patients, at any age, should have yearly exams.

## Basics of Vision Screening

1. Older adults and individuals at high risk should be referred to eye-care professionals for periodic examinations. See Recommendations of Major Authorities.

2. Visual acuity screening should be performed with a standard Snellen wall chart at a distance of 20 feet. A tumbling "E" chart may be used for patients who are not familiar with the Western alphabet. A passing score should be given for each line with a majority of correct responses. Each eye should be tested separately. Corrective lenses should be worn during screening. Patients with significant changes in visual acuity or visual acuity of 20/40 or less using corrective lenses should be referred to an eye-care specialist for further examination.

3. Risk factors for glaucoma include increasing age, family history of glaucoma, African-American race, diabetes mellitus, and myopia. Primary care clinicians should evaluate each patient's risk factors for glaucoma and other ocular problems and refer appropriate patients to eye-care professionals for screening.

4. Loss of vision can begin slowly and go unnoticed for some time, particularly in older adults. Primary care clinicians should encourage patients to seek evaluation at the first sign of vision problems. The use of a standardized, self-administered questionnaire, such as that given in Table 44-1, can help identify individuals needing evaluation of their vision. More extensive questionnaires have been developed (Mangione et al, 1992).

## Patient Resources

*Age-Related Macular Degeneration; Cataracts; Diabetic Retinopathy; Don't Lose Sight of Diabetic Eye Disease; Don't Lose Sight of Glaucoma; Glaucoma.* National Eye Health Education Program, National Institutes of Health, Box 20/20, Bethesda, MD 20892; (301) 496-5248.

*Age Page—Aging and Your Eyes.* National Institute on Aging, Bldg 31, Rm 5C27, Bethesda, MD 20892; (301) 496-1752.

*Your Vision, the Second Fifty Years; Do Adult Vision Problems Cause Reading Problems?* and other publications. American Optometric Association, 243 N. Lindbergh Blvd., St. Louis, MO 63141; (314) 991-4100.

Ch. 44. Vision                                         Adults/Older Adults — SCREENING

### Table 44-1. Visual Impairment Questionnaire

**Does your vision (with glasses if you wear them) make it difficult for you to— (place a check mark next to each question you answer yes)**

_____ Feed yourself?
_____ Recognize your pills or read medication labels?
_____ Dress yourself (find fasteners, button buttons)?
_____ Groom yourself (shave and wash without missing areas)?
_____ Handle your money (make change, write checks)?
_____ Recognize people (nearby, across the street)?
_____ Avoid bumping into objects when moving about in your house?
_____ Find your way around in places outside your own home (stores, shopping malls)?
_____ Read ordinary newsprint?

**Place a check mark next to each visual aid you now use**

_____ Glasses
_____ Contact lenses
_____ Magnifying lenses
_____ Portable lights
_____ Large print books
_____ Writing guides

One or more yes answer(s) indicates the need for further visual acuity testing. Use of one or more visual aid(s) is an indication for review of the patient's last optometric or ophthalmologic examination.

Adapted from: Rubenstein LZ, Lohr KN. *Conceptualization and Measurement of Physiologic Health for Adults.* vol 12: Visual Impairments. Santa Monica, CA: Rand Corporation; 1982. Publication R-2262/12-HHS. Used with permission of Rand Corporation; copyright © 1982.

## Provider Resources

*National Eye Institute Statement on Detection of Glaucoma*; *National Eye Institute Statement on Vision Screening in Adults.* National Eye Health Education Program, National Institutes of Health, Box 20/20, Bethesda, MD 20892; (301) 496-5248.

*Policy Statement: Frequency of Ocular Examinations.* American Academy of Ophthalmology, PO Box 7424, San Francisco, CA 94120; (415) 561-8500.

## Selected References

American Academy of Family Physicians, Commission on Public Health and Scientific Affairs. *Age Charts for Periodic Health Examination.* Kansas City, Mo: American Academy of Family Physicians; 1993.

American Academy of Ophthalmology, Quality of Care Committee. *Comprehensive Adult Eye Examination.* San Francisco, Ca: American Academy of Ophthalmology; 1992.

American Academy of Ophthalmology. *Detection and Control of Diabetic Retinopathy.* San Francisco, Ca: American Academy of Ophthalmology; 1992. Public health note.

Canadian Task Force on the Periodic Health Examination. *Periodic Health Examination Monograph.* Hull, Quebec: Ministry of Supply and Services, Canada; 1980.

Leske MC. The epidemiology of open-angle glaucoma: a review. *Am J Epidemiol.* 1983;118:166-169.

Mangione CM, Phillips RS, Seddon JM, et al. Development of the activities of daily vision scale: a measure of visual functional status. *Med Care*. 1992;30:1111-1126.

Nelson KA. Visual impairment among elderly Americans: statistics in transition. *J Vis Impair Blind*. 1987;81:331-334.

Podgor MJ, Leske MC, Ederer F. Incidence estimates for lens changes, macular changes, open angle glaucoma and diabetic retinopathy. *Am J Epidemiology*. 1983;118:206.

Reuben DB. Visual impairment. In: Beck JC, ed. *Geriatrics Review Syllabus: A Core Curriculum in Geriatric Medicine*. New York, NY: American Geriatrics Society; 1991.

Rubenstein LZ, Lohr KN. *Conceptualization and Measurement of Physiologic Health for Adults*. vol 12: Visual Impairments. Santa Monica, Cal: Rand Corporation; 1982. Publication R-2262/12-HHS.

Winograd CH, Gerety MB. *Geriatric assessment and concepts: visual and hearing assessment*. New York, NY: American Geriatrics Society;1989. Abstract.

US Preventive Services Task Force. Screening for diminished visual acuity. In: *Guide to Clinical Preventive Services*. Baltimore, Md: Williams & Wilkins; 1989:chap 31.

US Preventive Services Task Force. Screening for glaucoma. In: *Guide to Clinical Preventive Services*. Baltimore, Md: Williams & Wilkins; 1989:chap 32.

# Adults/Older Adults — IMMUNIZATION/PROPHYLAXIS

## 45. Aspirin

Seven million Americans have coronary heart disease. Despite recent reductions in major risk factors, heart disease is still the leading cause of death in men and women. In 1991, over 477,000 Americans died from ischemic heart disease. There is evidence from the U.S. Physician's Health Study (a randomized controlled trial) and the Nurses' Health Study (a prospective cohort study) that low-dose aspirin significantly decreases the incidence of first myocardial infarction (MI) in middle-aged men and women. However, these studies did not document a decrease in total cardiovascular mortality with aspirin prophylaxis, and there may be an increased risk of hemorrhagic stroke and sudden death with its use. A smaller British study of aspirin prophylaxis in physicians found no significant reduction in myocardial infarction incidence. The Women's Health Study, a large randomized controlled trial that includes aspirin prophylaxis, is in progress.

Aspirin use for the primary prevention of colon cancer is also being investigated. Observational studies have shown an association between aspirin use and a reduction in the incidence of colon cancer. Although this association is of interest, prospective confirmation (e.g., in a randomized controlled trial) is lacking.

**Recommendations of Major Authorities**

- **American Academy of Family Physicians** and **U.S. Preventive Services Task Force**—Low-dose aspirin therapy should be considered for men aged 40 years and over who are at significantly increased risk for MI and who lack contraindications to the drug. Patients should understand the potential benefits and risks of aspirin therapy before beginning treatment, and they should be encouraged to focus their efforts on modifying such primary risk factors as smoking, elevated cholesterol, and hypertension. This recommendation is currently under review.

- **American Heart Association**—Care should be exercised before beginning a lifelong program of aspirin therapy. The decision to begin taking aspirin should be made only after consultation by each individual with his or her physician. The individual who begins a regular aspirin regimen should be aware of the side effects of the drug and should report symptoms to his or her physician. All risk factors for coronary heart disease and stroke should be determined and a concerted program to reduce those risk factors begun.

- **Canadian Task Force on the Periodic Health Examination**—The evidence is not strong enough to support a recommendation that routine aspirin therapy be used or not be used for the primary prevention of cardiovascular disease in asymptomatic men. The decision on whether to prescribe aspirin should be made on an individual basis after the benefits of decreased risk of ischemic cardiovascular events have been balanced against the potential risks associated with prolonged aspirin use.

## Basics of Aspirin Prophylaxis

1. *Indications:* Patients over 50 years of age with risk factors for coronary heart disease are the group most likely to derive benefit from primary prevention with aspirin. No major authority recommends routine universal aspirin prophylaxis, however. Risks and benefits of aspirin prophylaxis should first be considered and discussed with each patient.

2. *Dosage:* The optimal dosage of aspirin for the primary prevention of heart disease has not been clearly established. The most widely accepted regimens are 325 mg taken by mouth daily or every other day. Dosages above 325 mg daily confer no added protection while increasing the incidence of side effects. It remains to be established whether doses of less than 325 mg every other day confer protection.

3. *Precautions:* Contraindications to regular aspirin use include allergy to aspirin, liver or kidney disease, peptic ulcer disease, and history of gastrointestinal bleeding or a bleeding disorder. Because of the potential increase in risk of hemorrhagic stroke, it is not advisable to use aspirin for prophylaxis in patients with poorly controlled hypertension. Patients using aspirin prophylaxis should inform their surgeon or dentist before undergoing even minor surgical or dental procedures. The tendency to prolonged bleeding can persist for up to 10 days after terminating use of aspirin.

4. *Adverse Reactions:* Side effects of prophylactic aspirin are dose-related. They include gastrointestinal upset and bleeding disorders, such as easy bruising, epistaxis, hematemesis, and melena. If any of these occurs, the provider should consider discontinuation of the drug. Gastrointestinal upset may be reduced by using enteric-coated aspirin.

## Selected References

American Academy of Family Physicians, Commission on Public Health and Scientific Affairs. *Age Charts for Periodic Health Examination*. Kansas City, Mo: American Academy of Family Physicians; 1993.

American College of Obstetricians and Gynecologists. *The Obstetrician-Gynecologist and Primary-Preventive Health Care*. Washington, DC: American College of Obstetricians and Gynecologists; 1993.

American Heart Association. Physicians' Health Study report on aspirin. *Circulation*. 1988;77:1447A.

Buring JE, Hennekens CH. The Women's Health Study: summary of the study design. *Journal of Myocardial Ischemia*. 1992;4:27-29.

Canadian Task Force on the Periodic Health Examination. Periodic health examination: 6. 1991 update. Acetyl-salicylic acid and the primary prevention of cardiovascular disease. *Can Med Assoc J*. 1991;145:45-49.

Fuster V, Dyken ML, Vohonas PS, Hennekens C. AHA medical/scientific statement: Aspirin as a therapeutic agent in cardiovascular disease. *Circulation*. 1993;87:659-675.

Fuster V, Cohen M, Halperin J. Aspirin in the prevention of coronary disease. *N Engl J Med*. 1989;321:183-186.

Manson JE, Stampfer MJ, Colditz GA, et al. A prospective study of aspirin use and primary prevention of cardiovascular disease in women. *JAMA*. 1991;266:521-527.

Physicians' Health Study Research Group, Steering Committee. Final report from the aspirin component of the ongoing Physicians' Health Study. *N Eng J Med*. 1989;321:129-135.

Peto R, Gray R, Collins R, et al. A randomized trial of the effects of prophylactic daily aspirin among male British doctors. *Br Med J.* 1988;296:320-331.

Thun MJ, Namboodiri MM, Heath CW. Aspirin use and reduced risk of fatal colon cancer. *N Engl J Med.* 1991;325:1593-1596.

US Preventive Services Task Force. Aspirin prophylaxis. In: *Guide to Clinical Preventive Services.* Baltimore, Md: Williams & Wilkins; 1989:chap 60.

Willard JE, Lange RA, Hillis LD. The use of aspirin in ischemic heart disease. *N Eng J Med.* 1992;327:175-181.

Adults/Older Adults — IMMUNIZATION/PROPHYLAXIS

# 46. Estrogen and Progestin

Estrogen supplementation after menopause can reduce the risk of coronary heart disease and osteoporosis in women. Coronary heart disease causes approximately 30% of deaths of women over 50 years of age. Estrogen supplementation has been shown in observational studies to be associated with a 35% reduction in relative risk of death from coronary heart disease. Osteoporosis leads to approximately 1.2 million fractures in the United States annually. About two thirds of these occur in women. Women who are older, white, slender, or have had a bilateral oophorectomy or an early menopause are at increased risk for developing osteoporosis-related fractures. Approximately 15% of white women over 50 years of age suffer hip fractures, and approximately 1.5% die as a result of hip fractures. A recent meta-analysis found a 25% decrease in the relative risk of suffering a hip fracture for women over the age of 50 years who have ever used estrogen (see Table 46-1). Estrogen supplementation also provides several benefits that improve the quality of life—such as a decrease of vasomotor symptoms (hot flushes or flashes) and an improvement of genitourinary symptoms (dryness, urgency, incontinence, frequency).

Estrogen supplementation may, however, also lead to significant negative health outcomes. Women with intact uteri who use estrogen for 10 to 20 years have an eight-fold increase in the incidence of endometrial cancer. The concomitant use of progestin decreases the risk of endometrial cancer to a level comparable to that of women not taking estrogen. Progestin use, however, also seems to decrease the cardiovascular benefits of estrogen, although the risk of coronary heart disease is probably still reduced by combination therapy. Controversy surrounds the question of whether women taking estrogen supplementation are at increased risk for breast cancer. This risk, if real, does not seem to be affected by short-term estrogen use (less than 5 years), but it may be increased by approximately 25% with usage over 10 years. Adding progestin is not protective and may increase breast cancer risk.

**Recommendations of Major Authorities**

- **American Academy of Family Physicians, American College of Obstetricians and Gynecologists (ACOG), American College of Physicians (ACP),** and **U.S. Preventive Services Task Force (USPSTF)**—All women should understand the probable risks and benefits of hormone replacement therapy, decide how valuable they consider each of the potential effects of therapy, and participate with their physician in deciding whether to take preventive hormone therapy. **ACP** also states: "All women, regardless of race, should consider preventive hormone therapy. Women who have had a hysterectomy are likely to benefit from estrogen therapy. There is no reason to add a progestin to the hormone regimen in such women. Women who have coronary heart disease or who are at increased risk for coronary heart disease are likely to benefit from hormone therapy. If such women have a uterus, a progestin should be added to the estrogen therapy unless careful endometrial monitoring is performed. The risks of hormone therapy may outweigh its benefits in women who are at increased risk for breast cancer. For other women, the best course of action is not clear." In a recent review (in preparation), **USPSTF** emphasizes the importance of counseling all women about the use of these agents.

## Ch. 46. Estrogen and Progestin — Adults/Older Adults — IMMUNIZATION/PROPHYLAXIS

- **Canadian Task Force on the Periodic Health Examination**—Because neither the absolute benefit nor the absolute risk of estrogen therapy is quantified, a recommendation advocating the widespread use of estrogen to prevent osteoporosis appears to be premature. This policy is currently under review. A policy regarding the use of estrogen/progestin in prevention of coronary heart disease has not been formulated.

### Basics of Estrogen/Progestin Prophylaxis

1. *Indications:* There is considerable controversy about the indications for estrogen/progestin use in primary prevention (see Recommendations of Major Authorities). Clinicians should consider the following factors in assessing whether a woman should receive estrogen replacement:

   - Coronary heart disease risk factors, such as family history, blood pressure, weight, smoking status, cholesterol.

   - Osteoporosis risk factors, such as race, body build, physical activity level, bone mineral density.

   - Breast cancer risk factors, such as personal and family history, late parity (after 30), early menarche (before 12), and late menopause (after 50).

   - Patient desire for quality-of-life benefits, such as decreased vasomotor and genitourinary tract symptoms.

   - Patient tolerance for side effects, such as endometrial bleeding and breast tenderness.

   - Patient willingness to participate in follow-up, such as endometrial sampling and mammography.

**Table 46-1. Relative Risk of Selected Conditions for a 50-Year-Old White Woman Treated With Long-Term Hormone Replacement**

| Condition | Estrogen Therapy | Estrogen Plus Progestin |
|---|---|---|
| Coronary Heart Disease | 0.65 | 0.65-0.80 |
| Stroke | 0.96 | 0.96 |
| Hip Fracture | 0.75 | 0.75 |
| Breast Cancer | 1.25 | 1.25-2.00 |
| Endometrial Cancer | 8.22 | 1.00 |

*Best estimate of the relative risk for developing each condition in long-term hormone users compared with nonusers.

From: Grady D, Rubin SM, Petitti DB, et al. Hormone therapy to prevent disease and prolong life in postmenopausal women. *Ann Intern Med.* 1992;117:1016-0137. Reproduced by permission of the American College of Physicians; copyright © 1992.

In order to prevent irreversible bone loss, it may be desirable to begin estrogen replacement soon after the onset of menopause. An absolute upper age limit for estrogen replacement has not been established. The use of progestin or careful endometrial monitoring is recommended for women with intact uteri.

2. *Dosage and Administration:* Several different regimens for hormone replacement have been developed. Oral preparations have been better evaluated for primary prevention than transdermal or other routes of administration. The most common initial oral dosage in the United States is 0.625 mg of conjugated estrogen taken every day. For women who cannot tolerate this dosage, 0.3 mg of conjugated estrogen daily with 1500 mg of calcium daily may provide protection against bone loss. Cyclic regimens of estrogen have been widely used, but they provide no physiologic advantages while causing patient confusion. Progestin may be given cyclically or continuously. The usual dosage for cyclic administration is 5 mg to 10 mg of progesterone acetate (or equivalent) daily for the first 10 to 14 days of the month. The usual dosage for continuous administration of progesterone acetate is 2.5 mg daily.

3. *Contraindications:* Contraindications for estrogen replacement include:

- Unexplained vaginal bleeding.
- Active liver disease.
- Chronic impaired liver function.
- Recent vascular thrombosis (with or without emboli).
- Carcinoma of the breast.
- Endometrial carcinoma, except in certain circumstances.

Conditions that may constitute relative contraindications include:

- Seizure disorders.
- Hypertension.
- Uterine leiomyomas.
- Familial hyperlipidemia.
- Migraine headaches.
- Thrombophlebitis.

- Endometriosis.

- Gallbladder disease.

From: American College of Obstetricians and Gynecologists. *Hormone Replacement Therapy.* Washington, DC: American College of Obstetricians and Gynecologists; 1992. ACOG Technical Bulletin 166. Reproduced with permission of the publisher; copyright © 1992.

4. *Adverse Reactions:* The most common side effects of estrogen include endometrial bleeding, breast tenderness, nausea, bloating, and headaches. The increase in endometrial cancer risk and potential increase in breast cancer risk are discussed above. The most common side effects when a progestin is added to estrogen therapy are bloating, weight gain, nausea, irritability, breast tenderness, and depression. These can generally be alleviated by decreasing the dose of progestin. Thromboembolic phenomena, such as pulmonary embolism and thrombophlebitis, have also been occasionally reported. If used in a continuous regimen, progestin causes unpredictable endometrial bleeding in 30% to 50% of women. This abates after 6 to 8 months of use due to uterine atrophy.

5. *Surveillance*: ACP (1992) has issued the following recommendations for surveillance of endometrial cancer in women taking estrogen:

*For Women Taking Estrogen Without Progestin*

At onset of treatment:

- Pelvic examination.

- Endometrial evaluation* to rule out hyperplasia or cancer.

Evaluation of vaginal bleeding*:

- For any episode of vaginal bleeding unless the woman has had a normal evaluation in the previous 6 months.

Frequency of screening while on treatment:

- Probably yearly.

*For Women Taking Estrogen and Progestin*

At onset of treatment:

- Pelvic examination.

- No endometrial evaluation required.

* Office-based biopsy, transvaginal ultrasound, or dilation and curettage.

Evaluation of vaginal bleeding*:

- For women on cyclic estrogen plus progestin therapy: If bleeding occurs other than at the time of expected withdrawal bleeding (days 10 to 15 of the month if the progestin is given on days 1 to 10 of the month).

- For women on continuous estrogen plus progestin therapy: If bleeding is heavy (heavier than normal menstrual period), prolonged (longer than 10 days at a time), or frequent (more often than monthly), and if bleeding persists longer than 10 months after beginning therapy.

Frequency of screening while on treatment:

- No routine screening required.

* Office-based biopsy, transvaginal ultrasound, or dilation and curettage.

6. *Breast Cancer Surveillance*: Both ACOG and ACP recommend that breast cancer screening be performed at the same frequency and with the same methods as for women not taking estrogen/progestin replacement.

## Patient Resources

*Age Page—Osteoporosis: The Bone Thinner*; *Age Page—Should You Take Estrogen?* National Institute on Aging, Bldg 31, Rm 5C27, Bethesda, MD 20892; (301) 496-1752.

*Hormone Replacement Therapy*; *Preventing Osteoporosis*. American College of Obstetricians and Gynecologists, 409 12th Street SW., Washington, DC 20024; 1-800 762-2664.

*Hormone Replacement Therapy: Facts To Help You Decide*; *Action for a Healthier Life: A Guide for Mid-Life and Older Women*. American Association of Retired Persons, Fulfillment Services, 601 E Street NW., Washington, DC 20049; (202) 434-2277.

*Osteoporosis in Women: Keeping Your Bones Healthy and Strong*. American Academy of Family Physicians, 8880 Ward Parkway, Kansas City, MO 64114-2797; 1-800 944-0000.

## Selected References

American Academy of Family Physicians, Commission on Public Health and Scientific Affairs. *Age Charts for Periodic Health Examination*. Kansas City, Mo: American Academy of Family Physicians; 1993.
American College of Obstetricians and Gynecologists, Committee on Technical Bulletins. *Hormone Replacement Therapy*. Washington, DC: American College of Obstetricians and Gynecologists; 1992. ACOG Technical Bulletin 166.
American College of Obstetricians and Gynecologists. *Standards for Obstetric and Gynecologic Services*. Washington, DC: American College of Obstetricians and Gynecologists; 1992.

## Ch. 46. Estrogen and Progestin    Adults/Older Adults — IMMUNIZATION/PROPHYLAXIS

American College of Obstetricians and Gynecologists. *The Role of the Obstetrician-Gynecologist and Primary-Preventive Health Care.* Washington, DC: American College of Obstetricians and Gynecologists; 1993.

American College of Physicians. Guidelines for counseling postmenopausal women about preventive hormone therapy. *Ann Intern Med.* 1992;117:1038-1041.

Barrett-Connor E, Bush TL. Estrogen and coronary heart disease in women. *JAMA.* 1992;265:1861-1867.

Canadian Task Force on the Periodic Health Examination. The periodic health examination: 2. 1987 update. *Can Med Assoc J.* 1988;138:618-626.

Grady D, Rubin SM, Petitti DB, et al. Hormone therapy to prevent disease and prolong life in postmenopausal women. *Ann Intern Med.* 1992;117:1016-1037.

Henrich JB. The postmenopausal estrogen/breast cancer controversy. *JAMA.* 1992;268:1900-1902.

Mann KV, Wiese WH, Stachenko S. Postmenopausal osteoporosis and fractures. In: Goldbloom RB, Lawrence RS. *Preventing Disease: Beyond the Rhetoric.* New York, NY: Springer-Verlag; 1990:chap 24.

US Preventive Services Task Force. Estrogen prophylaxis. In: *Guide to Clinical Preventive Services.* Baltimore, Md: Williams & Wilkins; 1989:chap 59.

## Adults/Older Adults — IMMUNIZATION/PROPHYLAXIS

# 47. Hepatitis B

Between 200,000 and 300,000 new cases of hepatitis B (HBV) infection occur yearly in the United States. Most of these occur in young adults, primarily as a result of blood or sexual contact (see Table 47-1 for a list of groups at high risk for HBV infection). HBV infection causes significant morbidity and mortality. Approximately 25% of patients become ill with jaundice. Approximately 15,000 hospitalizations and 250 deaths yearly are due to acute HBV infection. Between 5% and 10% of individuals with acute HBV infection become chronic carriers of the virus. Approximately 25% of carriers develop chronic active HBV, with many (3000 to 4000 annually) ultimately developing cirrhosis and liver failure. HBV carriers are also at significantly increased risk for developing liver cancer. HBV-related liver cancer leads to 1000 to 1500 deaths annually in the United States.

HBV vaccine is up to 95% effective in preventing HBV infection. Among the 90% of recipients who develop adequate antibody levels, effectiveness is virtually 100%. Patients with HIV infection, on hemodialysis, and 50 years of age and older have decreased antibody responses to the vaccine. Antibody levels decrease with time. After 7 years, up to 50% of recipients have low or undetectable antibody levels. Nonetheless, patients with normal immune systems continue to be protected from infection.

For prophylaxis after percutaneous or sexual contact with HBV infection, HBV immune globulin (HBIG) has an effectiveness of approximately 75% in preventing infection.

See chapter 14 for information on HBV immunization and prophylaxis for children and adolescents.

### Recommendations of Major Authorities

*Immunization*

- All major authorities, including **Advisory Committee on Immunization Practices (ACIP), American Academy of Family Physicians (AAFP), American College of Obstetricians and Gynecologists, American College of Physicians (ACP), Canadian Task Force on the Periodic Health Examination,** and **U.S. Preventive Services Task Force**—Individuals in groups at increased risk for HBV infection (see Table 47-1) should be immunized.

**ACIP, AAFP,** and **ACP** make the following recommendations regarding pre- and postvaccination antibody testing: Prevaccination antibody testing (either anti-HBc or anti-HBs) of adults may be cost-effective in groups at high risk for HBV infection. The decision to do prevaccination testing should take into account the cost of vaccination, the cost of testing for susceptibility, and the expected prevalence of immune individuals. Consideration should also be given to the likelihood of patient follow-up and vaccine delivery after prevaccination testing. Postvaccination testing is recommended only for those patients whose subsequent clinical management depends on knowledge of their immune status, such as dialysis patients and patients with HIV infection. Postvaccination testing also should be considered for individuals at occupational risk due to

Ch. 47. Hepatitis B                    Adults/Older Adults — IMMUNIZATION/PROPHYLAXIS

exposure to sharp instruments. Postvaccination testing should occur 1 to 6 months after vaccination. Revaccination with one or more additional doses should be considered for individuals who do not adequately respond to vaccination initially. Despite the decline of antibody levels with time, routine booster doses and serologic monitoring are not recommended for patients with normal immune status. Routine testing and administration of a booster vaccination (if the antibody level falls below 10 mIU/mL) are recommended for hemodialysis patients. According to **ACIP**, this testing should occur annually; **ACP** recommends hemodialysis patients receive testing semiannually.

## *Prophylaxis*

- All major authorities, including **Advisory Committee on Immunization Practices (ACIP)**, **American Academy of Family Physicians**, **American College of Physicians**, **Canadian Task Force on the Periodic Health Examination**, and **U.S. Preventive Services Task Force**—HBIG should be used for prophylaxis of unimmunized or inadequately immunized individuals exposed to active HBV infection. In adults, exposures warranting prophylaxis include percutaneous or mucosal contact with HBsAg-positive blood or body fluids and sexual contact with an HBsAg-positive person.

## Basics of Hepatitis B Immunization and Prophylaxis

### *Immunization*

1. *Vaccine Types:* There are currently two types of recombinant-derived HBV vaccines licensed for use in the United States—Recombivax HB® and Engerix-B®. These vaccines may be used interchangeably at any point in the vaccination schedule. Plasma-derived vaccine is no longer distributed in the United States.

2. *Schedule:* Both types of vaccine are given as a three-dose series, with the second and third doses administered 1 and 6 months after the first dose. If a three-dose series is interrupted after the first dose, the second dose should be administered as soon as possible. The second and third doses should be separated by an interval of at least 2 months. A four-dose series (0, 1, 2, and 12 months), which may induce immunity faster than a three-dose series, has been approved for Engerix-B® vaccine but has not been shown to be advantageous in clinical trials. Upon completion, both the three- and four-dose regimens confer essentially the same level of immunity. For hemodialysis patients, the fourth dose of Engerix-B® vaccine should be given 6 months (rather than 12 months) after the first dose. Patients in whom postvaccination testing shows inadequate antibody response after their initial vaccination series may receive one or more additional doses of vaccine (see Recommendations of Major Authorities).

3. *Dosage and Administration:* For adults over 19 years of age, the recommended dosage of both types of vaccine is 1 mL given intramuscularly. See Table 14-2 for recommended dosages of HBV vaccine for individuals 19 years of age and younger. The proper injection site is the deltoid muscle, as injection into the buttock results in decreased antibody response because of deposition of vaccine into fat. HBV vaccine may be given at the same time as, but at a different site than, HBIG and other vaccines. For hemodialysis patients and other patients who are immunocompromised, the dose should be increased. ACIP recommends using either 1 mL of a special formulation of Recombivax HB® containing 40 µg or two 1-mL doses of Engerix-B® given at the same site.

## Table 47-1. Groups at High Risk for Hepatitis B Infections

| |
|---|
| Health care workers and others at occupational risk |
| Clients and staff of institutions for the developmentally disabled—including nonresidential day-care programs if attended by known HBV carriers |
| Hemophiliacs and other recipients of certain blood products |
| Hemodialysis patients |
| Household contacts and sex partners of HBsAg-positive persons |
| Household contacts of adoptees from HBV-endemic, high-risk countries who are HBsAg-positive |
| International travelers who spend more than 6 months in areas with high HBV infection rates and have close contact with the local population; also short-term travelers who have contact with blood, or sexual contact with residents in high- or intermediate-risk areas |
| Injection drug users |
| Sexually active homosexual or bisexual males |
| Heterosexual individuals who have had more than one sex partner in the previous 6 months and/or those with a recent episode of a sexually transmitted disease |
| Inmates of long-term correctional institutions |

Note: This table duplicates Table 14-1.

Adapted from: Advisory Committee on Immunization Practices (ACIP). Hepatitis B virus: a comprehensive strategy for eliminating transmission in the United States through universal childhood vaccination. *MMWR.* 1991;40:(RR-13)1-25.

4. *Precautions:* The only contraindication to HBV vaccination is known serious adverse reaction to the vaccine. Pregnancy and lactation are not contraindications to vaccination.

5. *Adverse Reactions:* The side effects of HBV vaccination are relatively minor, such as pain at the injection site (3% to 29%) and temperature greater than 37.7°C (100°F) (1% to 6%). The occurrence of Guillain-Barré syndrome was reported at a very low rate (0.5 per 100,000) for adults receiving plasma-derived HBV vaccine. No such association has been found with the use of recombinant hepatitis vaccines, although data are insufficient to draw firm conclusions on this issue. Possible serious side effects should be reported to the Vaccine Adverse Event Reporting System (VAERS) with a Vaccine Adverse Reaction Report form. VAERS forms and instructions are available in *FDA Drug Bulletin* (Food and Drug Administration) and the *Physician's Drug Reference*, or by calling the 24-hour VAERS information recording at 1-800 822-7967.

6. *Vaccine Storage and Handling:* Vaccine should be stored at 2° to 8°C (36° to 46°F) but not frozen, which would destroy the potency of the vaccine. Vaccine that has been frozen should not be used. Handle all vaccine preparations according to manufacturers' instructions.

## Prophylaxis

1. *Indications:* The recommendations of ACIP for HBV prophylaxis following percutaneous and mucosal exposure are given in Table 47-2. In the case of sexual exposure to an HBsAg-positive person, it is desirable to test the patient's anti-HBc level before administering HBIG, if this can be accomplished without delaying treatment beyond 14 days after the last exposure. In addition to HBIG, HBV vaccine should also be given to susceptible patients. An alternate treatment for exposed individuals who would not routinely be considered at high risk and in need of vaccination is to administer one dose of HBIG (without vaccine) and retest the sex partner's HBsAg status 3 months later. If the sex partner has become HBsAg-negative, no further treatment is needed. If the sex partner is still HBsAg-positive, a second dose of HBIG should be given and vaccination begun. Adult household contacts of individuals with acute HBV infection do not need prophylaxis with HBIG unless they have had identifiable blood exposure, such as by sharing a toothbrush or razor with the infected individual. Patients with such exposures should be treated in the same manner as patients with sexual exposure. If the index patient becomes an HBV carrier, all household contacts should receive HBV vaccine.

Table 47-2. Recommendations for Hepatitis B Prophylaxis Following Percutaneous and Mucosal Exposure

| Exposed Person | HBsAg-Positive | HBsAg-Negative | Unknown or Not Tested |
|---|---|---|---|
| Unvaccinated | Administer HBIG x 1 and initiate vaccine | Initiate vaccine | Initiate vaccine |
| Previously vaccinated, known responder | Test exposed person for anti-HBs* 1. If adequate, no treatment 2. If inadequate, vaccine booster dose | No treatment | No treatment |
| Previously vaccinated, known non-responder | HBIG x 2 or HBIG x 1, plus 1 dose of vaccine | No treatment | If known high-risk source, may treat as if source were HBsAg-positive |
| Previously vaccinated, response unknown | Test exposed person for anti-HBs* 1. If inadequate, HBIG x 1, plus vaccine booster dose 2. If adequate, no treatment | No treatment | Test exposed person for anti-HBs* 1. If inadequate, vaccine booster dose 2. If adequate, no treatment |

\* Adequate anti-HBs level is ≥10 mIU/mL.

Adapted from: Advisory Committee on Immunization Practices (ACIP). Hepatitis B virus: a comprehensive strategy for eliminating transmission in the United States through universal childhood vaccination. *MMWR.* 1991;40:(RR-13)1-25.

2. *Schedule:* HBIG should be given as soon after exposure to infection as possible. It may be given as late as 14 days after exposure but is of uncertain effectiveness 7 days or more after exposure. If the patient is known not to have responded to a primary HBV vaccination series (by anti-HBs level), a second injection of HBIG may be given 1 month later in lieu of a vaccine booster dose.

3. *Dosage and Administration:* The recommended dosage of HBIG is 0.06 mL/kg given intramuscularly. The preferred site for administration in adults is the deltoid muscle. If the gluteal region is used, care should be taken to use only the upper, outer quadrant. Before injection, the plunger should be drawn back to verify that injection into a vein or artery will not occur. HBIG may be given at the same time as, but at a different site from, HBV vaccine.

4. *Precautions:* HBIG should be used with caution in patients with a history of hypersensitivity to human IG preparations or thimerosal.

5. *Adverse Reactions:* The main side effects of HBIG injection are pain and swelling at the injection site. Urticaria, angioedema, and very rarely, anaphylaxis can occur. HIV is not known to be transmitted by HBIG injection.

## Patient Resources

*Immunization of Adults: A Call to Action.* Technical Information Services, Centers for Disease Control and Prevention, Division of Immunization, Atlanta, GA 30333; (404) 639-3747.

## Selected References

Advisory Committee on Immunization Practices (ACIP). Hepatitis B virus: a comprehensive strategy for eliminating transmission in the United States through universal childhood vaccination. *MMWR.* 1991;40(RR-13):1-25.

Advisory Committee on Immunization Practices (ACIP). Protection against viral hepatitis. *MMWR.* 1990;39(RR-2):1-26.

American Academy of Family Physicians. *Recommendations for Hepatitis B Preexposure Vaccination and Postexposure Prophylaxis.* Kansas City, Mo: American Academy of Family Physicians; 1992.

American College of Obstetricians and Gynecologists. *The Obstetrician-Gynecologist and Primary-Preventive Health Care.* Washington, DC: American College of Obstetricians and Gynecologists; 1993.

American College of Physicians Task Force on Adult Immunization and Infectious Diseases Society of America. *Guide for Adult Immunization.* 2nd ed. Philadelphia, Pa: American College of Physicians; 1990:66-73.

Canadian Task Force on the Periodic Health Examination. The periodic health examination: 2. 1984 update. *Can Med Assoc J.* 1984;130:1278-1285.

US Preventive Services Task Force. Adult immunizations. In: *Guide to Clinical Preventive Services.* Baltimore, Md: Williams & Wilkins; 1989:chap 57.

US Preventive Services Task Force. Postexposure prophylaxis. In: *Guide to Clinical Preventive Services.* Baltimore, Md: Williams & Wilkins; 1989:chap 58.

## Adults/Older Adults — IMMUNIZATION/PROPHYLAXIS

# 48. Influenza
## (Including Childhood Immunization)

Influenza is a significant cause of mortality and morbidity in the United States. Between 1977 and 1988, at least 10,000 deaths occurred in each of seven separate influenza epidemics in the United States. More than 40,000 deaths occurred in three of these epidemics. Approximately 80% to 90% of deaths occur in individuals 65 years of age or older. Older adults with underlying health problems, such as pulmonary or cardiovascular disorders, are particularly at risk of death and serious illness from influenza. Nonelderly adults and children with certain chronic medical problems are also at increased risk for influenza-related complications (see Table 48-1).

Influenza vaccine is approximately 30% to 40% effective in preventing clinical illness and 80% effective in preventing death in older adults. Approximately 40% of noninstitutionalized older adults receive immunization annually. Amantadine prophylaxis is 70% to 90% effective for preventing influenza type A illness in adults, but it does not prevent influenza type B illness.

### Recommendations of Major Authorities

*Immunization*

- **Advisory Committee on Immunization Practices, American Academy of Family Physicians, American College of Physicians, Canadian Task Force on the Periodic Health Examination**, and **U.S. Preventive Services Task Force**—Influenza immunization should be provided annually to all individuals 65 years of age or older. Immunization should also be provided to adults and children at least 6 months of age who are at increased risk for influenza-related complications due to certain medical conditions, such as chronic pulmonary and cardiovascular disorders (see Table 48-1), or who may transmit influenza to individuals at increased risk, such as health-care workers and household members (see Table 48-2).

- **American College of Obstetricians and Gynecologists**—All women 60 years of age and older should receive immunization against influenza yearly.

*Prophylaxis*

- **Advisory Committee on Immunization Practices, American College of Physicians, American Geriatrics Society, Canadian Task Force on the Periodic Health Examination**, and **U.S. Preventive Services Task Force**—Amantadine should be given prophylactically to the following individuals: residents of institutions housing high-risk patients in which an influenza A outbreak occurs; older adults and others at high risk for whom immunization is contraindicated; older adults and other high-risk patients who have been recently exposed to influenza A, but are unimmunized or only recently immunized; immunocompromised patients and others expected to have a suboptimal response to immunization.

## Basics of Influenza Immunization and Prophylaxis

*Immunization*

1. *Vaccine Types:* There are two basic types of influenza vaccine available—one prepared from whole virus particles and the other from split virus particles. Either type of vaccine is equally appropriate for use with adults and children over the age of 12 years. Only the split virus preparation should be used with children 12 years of age or younger. The vaccines are trivalent—containing viruses or virus particles from three strains: two type A and one type B. The mixture of viruses used is updated annually according to antigenic change in the viruses causing infection.

2. *Schedule:* Influenza vaccine should be administered annually, preferably shortly before the onset of the influenza season. Because antibody levels decline with time, the immunization should not be given too early. Since the influenza season in the United States usually begins in December, the period between mid-October and mid-November is usually the optimal time for immunization campaigns. Clinicians should, however, take advantage of the opportunity to begin immunizing all high-risk patients, including older adults, who are seen for health care beginning in September. Immunization programs may be undertaken as soon as current vaccine is available if regional influenza activity is expected to begin earlier than December. Immunization may be offered up to and even after influenza virus activity is documented in a community. This may be as late as April in some years.

3. *Dosage and Administration*: The recommended dosage in adults and children 3 years of age and over is 0.5 mL, administered intramuscularly. The recommended dosage for children 6 to 35 months of age is 0.25 mL. Children 12 years of age and younger should receive split vaccine only. Children less than 9 years of age who have not previously been

### Table 48-1. Groups at Increased Risk for Influenza-Related Complications

| |
|---|
| Persons ≥65 years of age |
| Residents of nursing homes and other chronic-care facilities housing persons of any age with chronic medical conditions |
| Adults and children with chronic disorders of the pulmonary or cardiovascular systems, including children with asthma |
| Adults and children who have required regular medical follow-up or hospitalization during the preceding year because of chronic metabolic diseases (including diabetes mellitus), renal dysfunction, hemoglobinopathies, or immunosuppression (including immunosuppression caused by medications) |
| Children and teenagers (6 months-18 years of age) who are receiving long-term aspirin therapy and therefore may be at risk of developing Reye's syndrome after influenza |

From: Advisory Committee on Immunization Practices (ACIP). Prevention and control of influenza: part 1, vaccines. *MMWR.* 1993;42:(RR-6)1-14.

vaccinated should receive two doses of vaccine at least a month apart to maximize the chance of a satisfactory antibody response. The second dose should be administered before December, if possible. The vaccine may be given at the same time as pneumococcal vaccine and all childhood vaccines except pertussis. Influenza vaccine should not be given within 3 days of pertussis vaccination (including DTP and DTaP).

4. *Precautions:* Individuals who have developed hives, had swelling of the lips or tongue, or experienced acute respiratory distress or collapse after eating eggs should not be given influenza vaccine. Individuals with documented immunoglobulin E (IgE)-mediated hypersensitivity to eggs—including those who have had occupational asthma or other allergic responses to egg protein—may also be at increased risk for reactions from influenza vaccine. Patients at particularly high risk for complications from influenza who are allergic to vaccine components may receive the vaccine after appropriate allergy evaluation and desensitization (Murphy and Strunk, 1985). Patients with acute febrile illnesses should not be vaccinated until their symptoms have abated.

5. *Adverse Reactions:* Because it contains only noninfectious viruses, influenza vaccine cannot cause influenza. Respiratory disease after vaccination represents coincidental illness unrelated to influenza vaccination. Adverse reactions are generally mild. Soreness at the site of injection persisting up to 2 days is the most common side effect, affecting less than one third of patients. Fever, malaise, myalgia, and other systemic symptoms are infrequent; they may occur as early as 6 hours after immunization and persist up to 48 hours. Rarely, an immediate allergic reaction can occur. Guillain-Barré syndrome was associated with swine flu immunization in 1976, but subsequently it has not been clearly associated with influenza immunization. Providers are encouraged to report adverse reactions of all kinds, particularly if serious or unusual, to the Vaccine Adverse Event Reporting System (VAERS). VAERS forms and instructions are available in the *FDA Drug Bulletin* (Food and Drug Administration) and the *Physician's Drug Reference*, or by calling the 24-hour VAERS information recording at 1-800 822-7967.

6. *Patient Education:* Educational efforts and outreach to older adults are necessary to attain better influenza immunization rates. The distribution of informational brochures, use of waiting room posters, and mailing of reminder postcards are useful interventions to improve immunization rates.

**Table 48-2. Groups That Can Transmit Influenza to Persons at High Risk**

| |
|---|
| Physicians, nurses, and other personnel in both hospital and outpatient-care settings |
| Employees of nursing homes and chronic-care facilities who have contact with patients or residents |
| Providers of home care to persons at high risk (e.g., visiting nurses, volunteer workers) |
| Household members (including children) of persons in high-risk groups |

From: Advisory Committee on Immunization Practices (ACIP). Prevention and control of influenza: part 1, vaccines. *MMWR*. 1993;42:(RR-6)1-14.

7. *Vaccine Storage and Handling:* Unused vaccine from the previous year should be discarded and never used. Vaccine should be stored at 2° to 8°C (36° to 46°F) and not frozen. Handle all vaccine preparations according to manufacturers' instructions.

## Prophylaxis

1. *Indications:* See Recommendations of Major Authorities.

2. *Schedule:* When given as an adjunct to immunization in the case of a community outbreak of influenza, amantadine should be taken daily for 2 weeks. When used for prophylaxis of patients in institutions (regardless of immunization status), immunodeficient patients, and patients for whom influenza vaccine is contraindicated, amantadine should be taken daily for the duration of influenza activity.

3. *Dosage and Administration*: The recommended dosage of amantadine for adults 65 years of age or older is 100 mg daily. For adults and children aged 9 to 64 years, the recommended dosage is 100 mg twice daily. If unacceptable side effects develop, a reduced dosage of 100 mg daily should be considered. For children less than 9 years old, the recommended dosage is 4.4 mg/kg/day, not to exceed 150 mg daily. For adults and children with reduced renal function, appropriately reduced dosages should be used. Licensing of rimantadine, an analog of amantadine, is currently pending.

4. *Precautions:* Amantadine should be used with caution in patients who have reduced renal function, a history of seizures or neuropsychiatric disorders, or who take psychotropic medication.

5. *Adverse Reactions:* Side effects occur among 5% to 10% of patients receiving amantadine. These mainly affect the central nervous system (nervousness, anxiety, insomnia, difficulty concentrating, lightheadedness) and gastrointestinal tract (anorexia or nausea). Congestive heart failure and urinary retention may be exacerbated by amantadine use. More serious but less frequent central nervous system side effects (seizures, confusion) associated with amantadine use have affected older people, those with renal failure, and those with seizure, mental, or behavioral disorders. Side effects tend to decrease or resolve after 1 week of continuous use and cease after discontinuation of the drug.

## Patient Resources

*Immunization of Adults: A Call to Action.* Technical Information Services, Centers for Disease Control and Prevention, Division of Immunization, Atlanta, GA 30333; (404) 639-1819.

*Age Page—What to Do About Flu*; *Age Page—"Shots" for Safety.* National Institute on Aging, Bldg 31, Rm 5C27, Bethesda, MD 20892; (301) 496-1752.

*Flu.* National Institute of Allergy and Infectious Diseases, 9000 Rockville Pike, Bethesda, MD 20892; (301) 496-5717.

**Selected References**

Advisory Committee on Immunization Practices (ACIP). Prevention and control of influenza: part 1, vaccines. *MMWR*. 1993;42(RR-6):1-14.

Advisory Committee on Immunization Practices (ACIP). Prevention and control of influenza. *MMWR*. 1992;41 (RR-9):1-17.

Advisory Committee on Immunization Practices (ACIP). Update on adult immunization. *MMWR*. 1991;40 (RR-12):1-94.

American Academy of Family Physicians, Commission on Public Health and Scientific Affairs. *Age Charts for Periodic Health Examination*. Kansas City, Mo: American Academy of Family Physicians; 1993.

American Academy of Pediatrics, Committee on Infectious Diseases. *Report of the Committee on Infectious Diseases*. 22nd ed. Elk Grove Village, Ill: American Academy of Pediatrics; 1991:274-281.

American College of Obstetricians and Gynecologists. *The Obstetrician-Gynecologist and Primary-Preventive Health Care*. Washington, DC: American College of Obstetricians and Gynecologists; 1993.

American College of Physicians Task Force on Adult Immunization and Infectious Diseases Society of America. *Guide for Adult Immunization*. 2nd ed. Philadelphia, Pa: American College of Physicians; 1990:78-83.

American Geriatrics Society, Clinical Practices Committee. Prevention and Treatment of Influenza in the Elderly. New York, NY: American Geriatrics Society; 1988. Policy statement.

Canadian Task Force on the Periodic Health Examination. The periodic health examination 1979. *Can Med Assoc J*. 1979;121:1193-1254.

Murphy KR, Strunk RC. Safe administration of influenza vaccine in asthmatic children hypersensitive to egg proteins. *J Pediatr* 1985;106:931-933.

US Preventive Services Task Force. Adult immunizations. In: *Guide to Clinical Preventive Services*. Baltimore, Md: Williams & Wilkins; 1989:chap 57.

## Adults/Older Adults — IMMUNIZATION/PROPHYLAXIS

# 49. Pneumococcus
## (Including Childhood Immunization)

*Streptococcus pneumoniae* infections are a major cause of morbidity and mortality in the United States, causing 15% to 20% of all cases of pneumonia. Pneumococcal infection causes approximately 40,000 deaths annually in the United States. As many as 20% of patients with pneumococcal pneumonia develop bacteremia. Older adults are particularly at risk of mortality from pneumococcal infection. In older adults, mortality from pneumococcal bacteremia may be as high as 60%. Other groups at increased risk include the very young and individuals with chronic cardiovascular and pulmonary conditions, organ transplants, diabetes mellitus, alcoholism, cirrhosis, functional or anatomic asplenia (e.g. sickle cell disease or splenectomy), Hodgkin's and non-Hodgkin's lymphomas, multiple myeloma, renal failure, nephrotic syndrome, and HIV infection (see Table 49-1).

The current 23-valent pneumococcal vaccine, which replaced a 14-valent vaccine in 1983, contains antigens for 88% of the serotypes of *S. pneumoniae* causing bacteremia in the United States. Human antibody studies demonstrate cross-reactivity with an additional 8% of serotypes causing bacteremia. The vaccine has a protective efficacy of approximately 60% (for included serotypes) for all patients. Efficacy of the vaccine may decrease with increasing age and time since vaccination. Among older adults, antibody levels may decrease after 6 years to levels that are not protective. In immunocompromised patients and patients with certain chronic illnesses, the initial antibody response to pneumococcal vaccine is lower and declines more rapidly.

Implementation of immunization recommendations has been poor, with only about 20% of patients at risk for pneumococcal disease, including older adults, receiving the vaccine. Many opportunities for vaccination are missed, such as during hospitalization or on discharge. Two thirds of patients with serious pneumococcal disease have been hospitalized at least once within the preceding 5 years. Recent research indicates that predischarge vaccination of patients hospitalized for pneumonia of any etiology decreases their rates of subsequent hospitalization for pneumococcal disease.

**Recommendations of Major Authorities**

- **Advisory Committee on Immunization Practices (ACIP), American Academy of Family Physicians, American College of Physicians (ACP), American College of Obstetricians and Gynecologists**, and **U.S. Preventive Services Task Force (USPSTF)**—All people 65 years of age or older should be immunized at least once with pneumococcal vaccine. Patients with medical and living conditions putting them at high risk for pneumococcal disease (including immune compromise) should also be immunized (see Table 49-1). **ACIP** and **USPSTF** recommend that revaccination be strongly considered for patients who received the 14-valent vaccine and who are at highest risk of serious or fatal pneumococcal infections (such as patients with surgical or functional asplenia). **ACP** recommends revaccination for such patients. **ACIP**, **ACP**, and **USPSTF** recommend that adults who received the 23-valent vaccine 6 or more years ago and who are at the highest risk for pneumococcal infection should be considered for revaccination. According to **ACIP**, revaccination should be considered for children with nephrotic syndrome, asplenia, or sickle cell disease who would be 10 years old or younger at revaccination.

- **Canadian Task Force on the Periodic Health Examination**—There is insufficient evidence to include vaccination in or exclude it from the periodic health examination of immunocompetent elderly people living independently. There is good evidence to include vaccination in the periodic health examination of immunocompetent elderly people living in institutions and patients with sickle cell disease or a history of splenectomy. There is fair evidence to exclude vaccination from the periodic health examination of immunosuppressed patients.

## Basics of Pneumococcal Immunization

1. *Vaccine Types:* Only 23-valent vaccine is currently available in the United States. A protein-polysaccharide conjugate vaccine is currently under development.

2. *Schedule:* There is some disagreement among authorities regarding the indications for vaccination and revaccination (see Recommendations of Major Authorities). Clinicians should use health-care contacts of all types, including hospitalizations, to provide immunization to appropriate patients. If possible, patients should receive vaccination before undergoing splenectomy.

3. *Dosage and Administration*: The recommended dosage for adults and children is 0.5 mL given intramuscularly or subcutaneously. Pneumococcal vaccine may be given at the same time as, but in a different site from, influenza vaccine.

4. *Precautions:* Known hypersensitivity to any of the vaccine components is a contraindication to vaccination. Revaccination may lead to increased incidence of adverse reactions, particularly if at intervals of 3 years or less.

**Table 49-1. Groups at Increased Risk for Pneumococcal Disease**

| |
|---|
| Persons ≥65 years of age |
| Adults and children with chronic illness—cardiovascular disease, pulmonary disease, diabetes mellitus, alcoholism, cirrhosis, cerebrospinal fluid leaks. This does not include recurrent upper respiratory tract infections, including otitis media and sinusitis, in children. |
| Immunocompromised individuals—splenic dysfunction (e.g. sickle cell anemia) or anatomic asplenia, Hodgkin's or non-Hodgkin's lymphoma, multiple myeloma, chronic renal failure, nephrotic syndrome, organ transplantation or other conditions associated with immunosuppression |
| Those with HIV infection (asymptomatic or symptomatic) who are ≥2 years of age |
| Residents of special environments or social settings with an identified increased risk of pneumococcal disease or its complications (e.g., certain Native American populations) |

Adapted from: Advisory Committee on Immunization Practices (ACIP). Update on adult immunization. *MMWR*. 1991;40:(RR-12)1-94.

5. *Adverse Reactions:* Approximately 50% of patients develop mild, local side effects, such as erythema and pain at the injection site. Fever, myalgia, and severe local reactions have been reported in less than 1% of vaccinations. Anaphylactic reactions are rare (approximately 5 per 1 million doses). Providers are encouraged to report adverse reactions of all kinds, particularly if serious or unusual, to the Vaccine Adverse Event Reporting System (VAERS). VAERS forms and instructions are available in the *FDA Drug Bulletin* (Food and Drug Administration) and the *Physician's Drug Reference*, or by calling the 24-hour VAERS information recording at 1-800 822-7967.

6. *Vaccine Storage and Handling.* Vaccine should be stored at 2° to 8°C (36° to 46°F). Handle all vaccine preparations according to manufacturers' instructions.

**Patient Resources**

*Immunization of Adults: A Call to Action.* Technical Information Services, Centers for Disease Control and Prevention, Division of Immunization, Atlanta, GA 30333; (404) 639-3747.

*Age Page—"Shots" for Safety.* National Institute on Aging, Bldg 31, Rm 5C27, Bethesda, MD 20892; (301) 496-1752.

**Selected References**

Advisory Committee on Immunization Practices (ACIP). Update on adult immunization. *MMWR.* 1991;40 (RR-12):1-94.

American Academy of Family Physicians, Commission on Public Health and Scientific Affairs. *Age Charts for Periodic Health Examination.* Kansas City, Mo: American Academy of Family Physicians; 1993.

American Academy of Pediatrics, Committee on Infectious Diseases. *Report of the Committee on Infectious Diseases.* 22nd ed. Elk Grove Village, Ill: American Academy of Pediatrics; 1991:373-378.

American College of Obstetricians and Gynecologists. *The Obstetrician-Gynecologist and Primary-Preventive Health Care.* Washington, DC: American College of Obstetricians and Gynecologists; 1993.

American College of Physicians Task Force on Adult Immunization and Infectious Diseases Society of America. *Guide for Adult Immunization.* 2nd ed. Philadelphia, Pa: American College of Physicians; 1990:91-96.

Broome CV, Breiman RF. Pneumococcal vaccine—past, present, and future. *N Eng J Med.* 1991;325:1506-1508.

Canadian Task Force on the Periodic Health Examination. Periodic health examination: 2. 1991 update: administration of pneumococcal vaccine. *Can Med Assoc J.* 1991;144:665-671.

Fedson DS, Harward MP, Reid RA, Kaiser DL. Hospital-based pneumococcal immunization: epidemiologic rationale from the Shenandoah study. *JAMA.* 1990;264:1117-1122.

Gable CB, Holzer SS, Engelhart L, et al. Pneumococcal vaccine: efficacy and associated cost savings. *JAMA.* 1990;264:2910-2915.

Shapiro ED, Berg AT, Austrian R, et al. The protective efficacy of polyvalent pneumococcal polysaccharide vaccine. *N Eng J Med.* 1991;325:1453-1460.

US Preventive Services Task Force. Adult immunizations. In: *Guide to Clinical Preventive Services.* Baltimore, Md: Williams & Wilkins; 1989:chap 57.

## Adults/Older Adults — IMMUNIZATION/PROPHYLAXIS

# 50. Rubella

Rubella is a generally mild illness that when contracted by pregnant women, particularly in the first trimester, can lead to miscarriage, stillbirth, and congenital rubella syndrome (CRS)—the common features of which are hearing loss, developmental delay, growth retardation, and cardiac and ocular defects. The incidence of rubella and CRS decreased markedly after introduction of rubella vaccine in 1969. In 1988, there were only 225 cases of rubella and 6 cases of CRS reported in the United States. Between 1988 and 1991, however, the number of reported cases of rubella increased 6-fold and the incidence of CRS increased 15-fold. The majority of new cases of rubella occur in young adults who are unvaccinated, particularly in settings of mass congregation, such as colleges, prisons, and religious communities.

Rubella vaccine is approximately 95% effective at conferring immunity. This immunity is probably lifelong. Screening and subsequent immunization of susceptible women of childbearing age has been shown to decrease the incidence of CRS. Evidence that screening and immunization of susceptible men and older women decreases incidence of CRS is weak. For this reason, most authorities recommend concentrating screening and immunization efforts on women of childbearing age.

See chapter 15 for information on immunization of children and adolescents against measles, mumps, and rubella.

### Recommendations of Major Authorities

- All major authorities, including **Advisory Committee on Immunization Practices (ACIP), American Academy of Family Physicians, American Academy of Pediatrics (AAP), American College of Obstetricians and Gynecologists, American College of Physicians (ACP), Canadian Task Force on the Periodic Health Examination**, and **U.S. Preventive Services Task Force**—Women of childbearing age who lack documented evidence of immunity or prior immunization should be immunized. All of these authorities emphasize the importance of immunizing women, and some (**ACIP, AAP, ACP**) recommend immunization of susceptible males as well.

### Basics of Rubella Immunization

1. *Indications:* All women of childbearing age should be screened for immunity to rubella. Those who have neither documentation of prior immunization after 12 months of age nor documented immunity by antibody testing should be immunized. Reported history of infection should not be taken as evidence of immunity. Antibody testing may be offered to those suspected of lacking immunity, but authorities agree that immunization may be provided without this testing. Screening and vaccination of other adults may be considered, especially in high-risk settings (e.g., colleges, military bases).

Ch. 50. Rubella                    Adults/Older Adults — IMMUNIZATION/PROPHYLAXIS

2. *Vaccine Types*: Rubella vaccine is made from a live virus. The currently available vaccine is designated RA 27/3 and is available in either a monovalent form (rubella only) or in combinations: measles-rubella (MR), rubella-mumps, and measles-mumps-rubella (MMR). Any of these vaccines may be used in adults, but authorities recommend using MMR, unless contraindicated.

3. *Dosage and Administration*: A dose of 0.5 mL of reconstituted vaccine (of any type) should be administered subcutaneously, using a ⁵/₈- to ³/₄-inch 23-25 gauge needle.

4. *Precautions*: Although limited studies have shown no evidence of vaccine-induced CRS, pregnant women should not be given rubella vaccine, and all women receiving vaccine should be advised not to become pregnant for 3 months after vaccination. Women who do become pregnant within 3 months of vaccination should be counseled about concern for the fetus, but they generally should not be advised that interruption of the pregnancy is necessary. Patients who are immunocompromised (except for HIV-positive patients) should not be immunized.

   Immune globulin-containing preparations, such as IG, HBIG, VZIG, packed red blood cell, whole blood, or plasma, may interfere with immune response to MMR vaccination. MMR should not be given from 2 weeks before to 3-11 months (depending on the immune globulin content of the preparation) after such preparations are given. Vaccination should be repeated after the window of immune globulin interference has expired, or antibody testing should be performed to determine immunity status. See Advisory Committee on Immunization Practices (*MMWR*, in press) for more detailed information regarding this issue.

   The postpartum vaccination of rubella-susceptible women with rubella or MMR vaccine should not be delayed because of the receipt of anti-$Rh_o$(D)Ig (human) or any other blood product containing IG. Women given a postpartum rubella immunization who have received anti-$Rh_o$(D)Ig (human) during the last trimester or at delivery should have immunity confirmed by antibody level testing 3 months after the immunization.

   Immunization should be delayed for adults with febrile illnesses. Caution should be taken in administering rubella vaccine in the form of MMR to adults with a history of allergy to eggs. Adults who have experienced anaphylactic reactions to topically or systemically administered neomycin should not be given rubella vaccine.

5. *Adverse Reactions:* Approximately 25% of adults immunized with rubella vaccine develop arthralgia, and 13% to 15% report arthritis-like symptoms. These symptoms generally develop 1 to 3 weeks after vaccination, persist for 1 day to 3 weeks, and rarely recur. Rarely, recurrent arthralgia and sometimes arthritis persist for an extended length of time. Paresthesias and pain in the arms and legs may also rarely develop and follow the same course as arthralgias. These adverse reactions seem to occur more often in non-immune patients after vaccination. Other adverse reactions include low-grade fever, rash, and lymphadenopathy. Providers are encouraged to report adverse reactions of all kinds, particularly if serious or unusual, to the Vaccine Adverse Event Reporting System

(VAERS). VAERS forms and instructions are available in the *FDA Drug Bulletin* (Food and Drug Administration) and the *Physician's Drug Reference*, or by calling the 24-hour VAERS information recording at 1-800 822-7967.

6. *Vaccine Storage and Handling:* Reconstituted vaccine should be discarded if not used within 8 hours. Unreconstituted vaccine should be stored at 2° to 8°C (36° to 46°F) or colder and should be protected from light. Handle all vaccine preparations according to manufacturers' instructions.

**Selected References**

Advisory Committee on Immunization Practices (ACIP). General recommendations on immunization. *MMWR*. In press.

Advisory Committee on Immunization Practices (ACIP). Rubella prevention. *MMWR*. 1990;39(RR-15):1-18.

American Academy of Family Physicians, Commission on Public Health and Scientific Affairs. *Age Charts for Periodic Health Examination*. Kansas City, Mo: American Academy of Family Physicians; 1993.

American Academy of Pediatrics, Committee on Infectious Diseases. *Report of the Committee on Infectious Diseases*. Elk Grove Village, Ill: American Academy of Pediatrics; 1991:410-417.

American College of Obstetricians and Gynecologists. *The Obstetrician-Gynecologist and Primary-Preventive Health Care*. Washington, DC: American College of Obstetricians and Gynecologists; 1993.

American College of Physicians. *Guide for Adult Immunization*. 2nd ed. Philadelphia, Pa: American College of Physicians; 1990:105-109.

Canadian Task Force on the Periodic Health Examination. The periodic health examination 1979. *Can Med Assoc J*. 1979; 121:1193-1254.

US Preventive Services Task Force. Screening for rubella. In: *Guide to Clinical Preventive Services*. Baltimore, Md: Williams & Wilkins; 1989:chap 36.

## Adults/Older Adults — IMMUNIZATION/PROPHYLAXIS

# 51. Tetanus and Diphtheria

Tetanus occurs almost entirely in unimmunized or incompletely immunized persons. Approximately 50 to 100 cases occur each year in the United States. Adults over 60 years of age account for 60% of the cases. The overall case fatality rate is approximately 30%, but it is considerably higher for older adults. Serologic studies have demonstrated that approximately 40% of adults over 60 years of age lack protective levels of antitoxin antibodies. Immunization with tetanus toxoid is almost 100% effective at preventing illness. Tetanus immune globulin (TIG) is highly protective when given prophylactically for wound management.

Diphtheria immunization of children has reduced its incidence in the United States to less than 10 cases yearly, primarily among adults. As with tetanus, most cases occur in nonimmunized or incompletely immunized individuals. The case fatality rate is 5% to 10%. Immunization has resulted in serologic evidence of immunity in most children, but 22% to 62% of adults aged 18 to 39 years and 41% to 84% of adults 60 years of age or older lack protective levels of antitoxin antibodies. A complete vaccination series substantially reduces the risk of developing diphtheria, and vaccinated individuals who develop disease have milder illnesses. Carriage of *Corynebacterium diphtheriae* is not prevented by vaccination.

See chapter 12 for information on diphtheria, tetanus, and pertussis immunization and tetanus prophylaxis in children and adolescents.

**Recommendations of Major Authorities**

- All major U.S. authorities, including **Advisory Committee on Immunization Practices, American Academy of Family Physicians, American College of Obstetricians and Gynecologists, American College of Physicians**, and **U.S. Preventive Services Task Force**—Adults should receive a tetanus-diphtheria (Td) booster vaccination every 10 years.

- **Canadian Task Force on the Periodic Health Examination**—Adults in good health should receive a tetanus booster vaccination every 10 years. Concomitant booster vaccination against diphtheria is optional.

**Basics of Tetanus and Diphtheria Immunization and Tetanus Prophylaxis**

*Immunization*

1. *Vaccine Types:* There are three basic types of toxoid available for immunization of adults: tetanus and diphtheria toxoids adsorbed for adult use (Td), tetanus toxoid (T), and tetanus toxoid (fluid). Td should be used unless immunization against diphtheria is not desired. U.S. authorities recommend combined tetanus-diphtheria booster immunizations for adults because of the prevalence of low diphtheria antitoxin antibody levels in adults. Of the two single-antigen preparations available for tetanus immunization, T is preferable for

use because it induces more persistent antitoxin antibody titers than the fluid preparation. Diphtheria and tetanus toxoids and pertussis vaccine adsorbed (DTP) and diphtheria and tetanus toxoids adsorbed (DT) are for use in children under 7 years of age and should not be used in adults.

2. *Schedule:* Booster vaccinations should be given every 10 years. If childhood immunizations have been received according to the usual schedule, with a booster dose at 14 to 16 years of age, the first adult vaccination will be needed at about 25 years of age. Adults who have not received a primary series should receive 3 vaccinations (the second 4 to 8 weeks after the first, and the third 6 to 12 months after the second) followed by booster vaccinations every 10 years. A primary series may be completed without restarting, regardless of excess elapsed time between vaccinations. Since immunosuppressive therapies may reduce the immune response, vaccination should be deferred for 1 month after the discontinuation of immunosuppressive therapy. For management of certain wounds, administration of a tetanus booster may be indicated if 5 years have elapsed since the last vaccination (see Table 51-1).

3. *Dosage and Administration:* The recommended dosage for all adult tetanus and diphtheria vaccines is 0.5 mL given intramuscularly, preferably in the deltoid muscle using a 1- to 1$^{1}$/$_{2}$-inch 20-25 gauge needle. Tetanus toxoid (fluid) may be given subcutaneously. If administered at the same time as TIG, separate sites and separate syringes should be used.

4. *Precautions:* A history of a neurologic reaction or a severe hypersensitivity reaction (e.g., generalized urticaria or anaphylaxis) after a previous dose is a contraindication to diphtheria and tetanus toxoids. If a prior systemic reaction suggests allergic hypersensitivity,

Table 51-1. Summary Guide to Tetanus Prophylaxis in Routine Wound Management

| Number of previous tetanus vaccinations | Clean, minor wounds | | All other wounds[a] | |
|---|---|---|---|---|
| | Give Td[b] | Give TIG | Give Td[b] | Give TIG |
| Uncertain or less than 3 | Yes | No | Yes | Yes |
| 3 or more[c] | No[d] | No | No[e] | No |

[a]Such as, but not limited to: wounds contaminated with dirt, feces, and saliva; puncture wounds; avulsions; and wounds resulting from missiles, crushing, burns, and frostbite.

[b]For adults and children 7 years of age or older, Td is preferred to tetanus toxoid alone. For children less than 7 years of age, DTP (DT, if pertussis vaccine is contraindicated) is preferred to tetanus toxoid alone.

[c]If only 3 doses of fluid toxoid have been received, a fourth dose of toxoid, preferably an adsorbed toxoid, should be given.

[d]A booster should be given if more than 10 years since last dose.

[e]A booster should be given if more than 5 years since last dose.

Adapted from: Advisory Committee on Immunization Practices (ACIP). Diptheria, tetanus, and pertussis: guidelines for vaccine prophylaxis and other preventive measures. *MMWR.* 1985;34:1-17 and Diptheria, tetanus, and pertussis: recommendations for vaccine use and other preventive measures. *MMWR.* 1991;40:1-28.

appropriate skin testing to document immediate hypersensitivity may be useful before discontinuing tetanus toxoid vaccinations. Mild, nonspecific skin-test reactivity is common. The administration of vaccinations more frequently than every 10 years (except for management of certain wounds) should be avoided because induction of high serum tetanus antitoxin antibody levels may lead to Arthus hypersensitivity reactions (severe local reactions starting 2 to 8 hours after a vaccination and often associated with fever and malaise). Patients who have experienced an Arthus reaction should not receive booster vaccinations more frequently than every 10 years, even for wound treatment. Vaccinations should not been given to women during the first trimester of pregnancy.

5. *Adverse Reactions:* Local reactions (usually erythema and induration, with or without tenderness) can occur after vaccination with Td or other preparations. Fever and other systemic reactions can occur, but are less common. Arthus reactions can occur (as discussed above), particularly among patients who have received multiple tetanus boosters using the adsorbed preparations. Severe reactions, such as generalized urticaria, anaphylaxis, or neurologic complications, have been reported rarely.

6. *Storage and Handling:* Toxoids should be stored at 2° to 8°C (36° to 46°F) and not frozen. Vaccine that has been frozen should not be used. Handle all vaccine preparations according to manufacturers' instructions.

## *Tetanus Prophylaxis*

1. *Indications:* The use of tetanus immune globulin (TIG) is indicated in the management of other than minor, clean wounds in individuals who have had fewer than 3 previous tetanus toxoid vaccinations or whose vaccination status is unknown or uncertain (see Table 51-1).

2. *Dosage and Administration:* The recommended dosage of TIG is 250 units, injected intramuscularly, preferably in the deltoid muscle of adults. It can be given at the same time as tetanus toxoid, but should be given at a different site and with a different syringe.

3. *Precautions:* Care should be taken to avoid intravenous injection, which can cause an anaphylactic reaction.

4. *Adverse Reactions:* Adverse reactions are primarily limited to soreness at the site and slight temperature elevation. More serious reactions, such as anaphylaxis and angioneurotic edema, are rare. Providers are encouraged to report adverse reactions of all kinds, particularly if serious or unusual, to the Vaccine Adverse Event Reporting System (VAERS). VAERS forms and instructions are available in the *FDA Drug Bulletin* (Food and Drug Administration) and the *Physician's Drug Reference*, or by calling the 24-hour VAERS information recording at 1-800 822-7967.

## Patient Resources

*Immunization of Adults: A Call to Action.* Technical Information Services, Centers for Disease Control and Prevention, Division of Immunization, Atlanta, GA 30333; (404) 639-3747.

## Ch. 51. Tetanus and Diphtheria    Adults/Older Adults — IMMUNIZATION/PROPHYLAXIS

*Age Page—"Shots" for Safety*. National Institute on Aging, Bldg 31, Rm 5C27, Bethesda, MD 20892; (301) 496-1752.

**Selected References**

Advisory Committee on Immunization Practices (ACIP). General recommendations on immunization. *MMWR*. In press.

Advisory Committee on Immunization Practices (ACIP). Diphtheria, tetanus, and pertussis: guidelines for vaccine prophylaxis and other preventive measures. *MMWR*. 1985;34:1-17.

Advisory Committee on Immunization Practices (ACIP). Diphtheria, tetanus and pertussis: recommendations for vaccine use and other preventive measures. *MMWR*. 1991;40:1-28.

Advisory Committee on Immunization Practices (ACIP). Update on adult immunization. *MMWR*. 1991;40(RR-12):1-94.

American Academy of Family Physicians, Commission on Public Health and Scientific Affairs. *Age Charts for Periodic Health Examination*. Kansas City, Mo: American Academy of Family Physicians; 1993.

American College of Obstetricians and Gynecologists. *The Obstetrician-Gynecologist and Primary-Preventive Health Care*. Washington, DC: American College of Obstetricians and Gynecologists; 1993.

American College of Physicians Task Force on Adult Immunization and Infectious Diseases Society of America. *Guide for Adult Immunization*. 2nd ed. Philadelphia, Pa: American College of Physicians; 1990:110-113.

Canadian Task Force on the Periodic Health Examination. The periodic health examination 1979. *Can Med Assoc J*. 1979;121:1193-1254.

US Preventive Services Task Force. Adult immunizations. In: *Guide to Clinical Preventive Services*. Baltimore, Md: Williams & Wilkins; 1989:chap 57.

## Adults/Older Adults — COUNSELING

# 52. Alcohol and Other Drug Abuse

Substance abuse is the harmful or hazardous use of alcohol, tobacco, or other (legal and illegal) drugs. It is a leading cause of premature and preventable illness, disability, and death in the United States. Alcohol abuse is related to more than half of all traffic fatalities, 67% of drownings and murders, 70% to 80% of deaths in fires, and 35% of suicides. The abuse of alcohol costs society nearly twice as much as all other drugs combined—approximately $85.8 billion annually. This figure includes medical treatment and indirect economic losses, such as reduced worker productivity, early death, and property damage. The emotional costs to alcohol abusers, victims of alcohol-related crimes, and family members are also very high.

The abuse of other drugs costs society approximately $47 billion per year. In 1991, 12.7% of individuals reported currently using illicit drugs, and 37% reported use in the past. Marijuana is used more than once per week by an estimated 4.6 million adults, and nearly 580,000 adults use cocaine one or more times per week. Drug abuse is an increasingly important risk factor for HIV infection. Approximately 27% of HIV-infected patients have injection drug use as a risk factor, either alone or in combination with homosexual activity. In addition to providing a route of entry into the body for the HIV virus, some types of drug use may lower resistance to the HIV virus by impairing cell-mediated immunity.

Primary care providers often fail to recognize alcohol and drug abuse problems in their patients. Some studies report detection rates as low as 30%. Minimal interventions by primary care clinicians, such as advice to modify current use patterns and warnings about adverse health consequences, can have beneficial effects, especially for patients in the early stages of addiction. More intensive interventions, such as referral to outpatient or inpatient treatment facilities, can be life-saving for patients in more advanced stages of alcohol and other drug dependence problems.

For information on counseling children and adolescents on alcohol and other drug abuse, refer to chapter 17. Counseling children and adolescents on tobacco use prevention is discussed in chapter 23, and counseling adults on smoking cessation is covered in chapter 59.

**Recommendations of Major Authorities**

- **American Academy of Family Physicians** and **U.S. Preventive Services Task Force**—All adults should be asked to describe their use of alcohol and other drugs. Routine measurement of biochemical markers and drug testing is not recommended as the primary method of detecting alcohol and other drug abuse in asymptomatic individuals. Individuals in whom alcohol or drug abuse or dependence is confirmed should receive appropriate counseling, treatment, and referrals. All people who use intoxicating drugs should be counseled about the hazards of operating a motor vehicle or performing other potentially dangerous activities while intoxicated. Injection drug users should be counseled to avoid sharing or using unsterilized needles and syringes.

- **American College of Obstetricians and Gynecologists**—Women should be asked about their use of alcohol and other drugs.

- **American College of Physicians**—The physician's role in recognizing and treating chemical dependence requires knowledge of the symptoms of chronic and excessive drug use and increased sensitivity to and awareness of behavior associated with such problem use. The physician's role in preventing chemical dependency includes patient education and counseling about the appropriate use of substances upon which dependence is likely. Thoughtful and knowledgeable prescribing practices that minimize the likelihood of producing or maintaining iatrogenic chemical dependence are essential.

- **American Medical Association**—All physicians with clinical responsibility for diagnosis of and referral for alcoholism and drug abuse problems should be able to recognize alcohol- or drug-caused dysfunction and should be aware of the medical complications, symptoms, and syndromes with which alcoholism or drug abuse commonly presents. All complete health examinations should include an in-depth history of alcohol and other drug use. The physician should evaluate patient requirements and community resources so that an adequate level of care may be prescribed, with patients' needs matched to appropriate resources and with referrals made to a resource that provides appropriate medical care.

- **Canadian Task Force on the Periodic Health Examination**—Although no single screening instrument has shown optimal accuracy in detecting problem drinking, there is good evidence that case-finding, counseling, and follow-up are effective in managing the problem. Research has indicated that specific questions and approaches may be incorporated into the periodic health examination to raise clinical suspicion and prompt further inquiry; approaches may be combined sequentially to increase either sensitivity or specificity.

## Basics of Counseling for Abuse of Alcohol and Other Drugs

### *Identification*

1. *Conducting an alcohol/drug history:* Identifying the patient with substance abuse problems is the necessary first step toward providing help. History-taking should begin with questions about relatively nonthreatening subjects—such as the number of cups of caffeinated beverages the patient drinks per day—before moving on to questions about the types, amounts, duration, and patterns of use of legal and illegal substances. Questions about frequency and quantity are of limited utility in detecting substance abuse because of the tendency of patients to underreport use. However, such questions may be helpful in identifying individuals who drink large quantities (e.g. binge drinkers, who consume 9 or more drinks per occasion). Corroboration of information by family and others who know the patient well may be helpful. Questions about the negative consequences of abuse can also be helpful in assessing the magnitude of the problem. Areas that may be addressed include: driving history, employment history, educational progress, legal problems, family life, social activities, and enrollment in treatment programs. Asking about family history of substance abuse will help the clinician assess the patient's genetic vulnerability. If the patient has made previous attempts to stop or moderate alcohol or drug use, he or she should be asked about the methods, barriers encountered, and degree of success.

2. *Use of brief screening questionnaires:* The use of brief, self-administered screening questionnaires can help identify patients in need of more detailed evaluation. The CAGE questionnaire (see Table 52-1) for alcohol abuse screening is the shortest of such

**Table 52-1. CAGE Questionnaire**

| |
|---|
| "Have you ever felt you ought to **C**ut down on drinking?" |
| "Have people **A**nnoyed you by criticizing your drinking?" |
| "Have you ever felt bad or **G**uilty about your drinking?" |
| "Have you ever had a drink first thing in the morning to steady your nerves or get rid of a hangover (**E**ye-opener)?" |

One "yes" response should raise suspicions of alcohol abuse. More than one "yes" response should be considered a strong indication that alcohol abuse exists.

From: Ewing JA. Detecting alcoholism: the CAGE questionnaire. *JAMA*. 1984;252:1905-1907. Reproduced by permission of the American Medical Association; copyright © 1984.

---

instruments and has relatively good sensitivity (approximately 85%) and specificity (approximately 89%). The CAGE questions have been recently adapted to include other drugs and evaluated as the CAGEAID questionnaire (Brown, 1992). A World Health Organization 6-country collaborative project recently developed the 10-item Alcohol Use Disorders Identification Test (AUDIT—see Table 52-2). In initial testing, this questionnaire has been found to have sensitivity and specificity values of greater than 90%. Some authorities recommend the use of a brief trauma questionnaire, such as that in Table 52-3, to screen for the frequent injuries that alcoholics sustain.

Also available are several excellent but more lengthy screening questionnaires, some self-administered, that may be more appropriate for research and special applications than for routine use in primary care (Magruder-Habib et al, 1991). Examples include the Michigan Alcoholism Screening Test (MAST) and the Drug Abuse Screening Test (DAST).

3. *Asking about physical symptoms*: The clinician should ask the patient about physical symptoms of substance abuse. Examples include frequent headaches or other chronic tension states, absence from work based on vague physical complaints, insomnia, unexplained mood changes, gastrointestinal disorders, uncontrolled hypertension, impotence and other sexual disorders, and neuropathies.

4. *Physical examination:* The physical examination is a relatively insensitive and non-specific method of detecting alcohol or drug abuse. Some signs of alcohol abuse include weight gain or loss, labile or refractory hypertension, abnormal skin vascularization, conjunctival injection, tongue or hand tremor, epigastric tenderness, and hepatomegaly. Damaged nasal mucosa and weight loss may be present with cocaine use. Hypodermic marks may be present with injection drug use. Signs of previous or current trauma are other clues to substance abuse problems.

5. *Laboratory tests:* The use of laboratory tests, such as liver enzymes and erythrocyte mean corpuscular volume, are helpful in evaluating physiological damage, but are not good screening tools for detecting alcohol abuse. Gamma-glutamyl transferase level is the most

## Table 52-2. Alcohol Use Disorders Identification Test (AUDIT)

1. How often do you have a drink containing alcohol?

| Never | Monthly or less | 2 to 4 times a month | 2 to 3 times a week | 4 or more times a week |

2. How many drinks containing alcohol do you have on a typical day when you are drinking?

| 1 or 2 | 3 or 4 | 5 or 6 | 7 to 9 | 10 or more |

3. How often do you have six or more drinks on one occasion?

| Never | Less than monthly | Monthly | Weekly | Daily or almost daily |

4. How often during the last year have you found that you were not able to stop drinking once you had started?

| Never | Less than monthly | Monthly | Weekly | Daily or almost daily |

5. How often during the last year have you failed to do what was normally expected from you because of drinking?

| Never | Less than monthly | Monthly | Weekly | Daily or almost daily |

6. How often during the last year have you needed a first drink in the morning to get yourself going after a heavy drinking session?

| Never | Less than monthly | Monthly | Weekly | Daily or almost daily |

7. How often during the last year have you had a feeling of guilt or remorse after drinking?

| Never | Less than monthly | Monthly | Weekly | Daily or almost daily |

8. How often during the last year have you been unable to remember what happened the night before because you had been drinking?

| Never | Less than monthly | Monthly | Weekly | Daily or almost daily |

9. Have you or has someone else been injured as a result of your drinking?

| No | Yes, but not in the last year | Yes, during the last year |

10. Has a relative or friend, or a doctor or other health worker been concerned about your drinking or suggested you cut down?

| No | Yes, but not in the last year | Yes, during the last year |

Scoring

| 0 | 1 | 2 | 3 | 4 |

Questions 1-8 are scored 0, 1, 2, 3, 4. Questions 9 and 10 are scored 0, 2 or 4 only. A total score of 8 or more indicates a strong likelihood of hazardous or harmful alcohol consumption.

From: Saunders JB, Aasland OG, Babor TF, De La Fuente JR, Grant M. Development of the Alcohol Use Disorders Identification Test (AUDIT): WHO Collaborative Project on Early Detection of Persons with Harmful Alcohol Consumption—II. *Addiction.* 1993;88:791-804.

### Table 52-3. Trauma Questionnaire*

| |
|---|
| "Have you had any fractures or dislocations since you were 18?" |
| "Have you been injured in a traffic accident?" |
| "Have you had your head injured?" |
| "Have you been injured in an assault or a fight?" |
| "Have you been injured after drinking?" |

*2 or more "yes" answers indicates a history of significant trauma.

From: National Institute on Alcohol Abuse and Alcoholism. *Seventh Special Report to the U.S. Congress on Alcohol and Health*. Rockville, MD: U.S. Department of Health and Human Services; 1990. USDHHS Publication ADM 90-1656.

sensitive biochemical test for alcohol abuse, but even this has a sensitivity of only 25% to 36%. Urine drug screens can help confirm drug use but give no information about the quantity or frequency of the use. An estimated 5% to 30% of positive drug screens are false positives, depending on the drug, the method of analysis, and the population being tested. In general, these tests should not be used as screening tools in the primary care setting, and certainly they should not be used without patient consent.

6. *Screening protocols:* Some authorities recommend combining a variety of different screening approaches into a protocol. An example of such a protocol, adapted from one developed by the National Institute on Alcohol Abuse and Alcoholism, is in Fig 52-1.

## *Counseling*

1. *Establishing a therapeutic relationship:* The provider should express genuine concern and maintain an honest, nonjudgmental approach with substance abuse patients. Arguing with, confronting, or labeling the patient should be avoided. An attempt should be made to maintain a partnership with the patient, in which the clinician functions as an expert consultant. Trust is essential; the patient should be assured that information disclosed will be kept confidential to the maximum extent possible.

2. *Making the medical office or clinic off-limits for substance abuse:* This should be true for tobacco, alcohol, and other drugs. Counseling a patient who is under the influence of alcohol or other drugs is not productive and may be counterproductive because of the indirect encouragement it gives to the patient for abuse. Such patients should be scheduled for return appointments to occur when they are not under the influence.

3. *Presenting information about negative health consequences:* This should be done in a straightforward, nonjudgmental manner. For example, "Your trouble sleeping, the difficulty in controlling your blood pressure, and the recent problems at home with your family make me concerned that alcohol may be the main problem. I would like to discuss this possibility with you more."

**Figure 52-1. Alcoholism Screening Protocol**

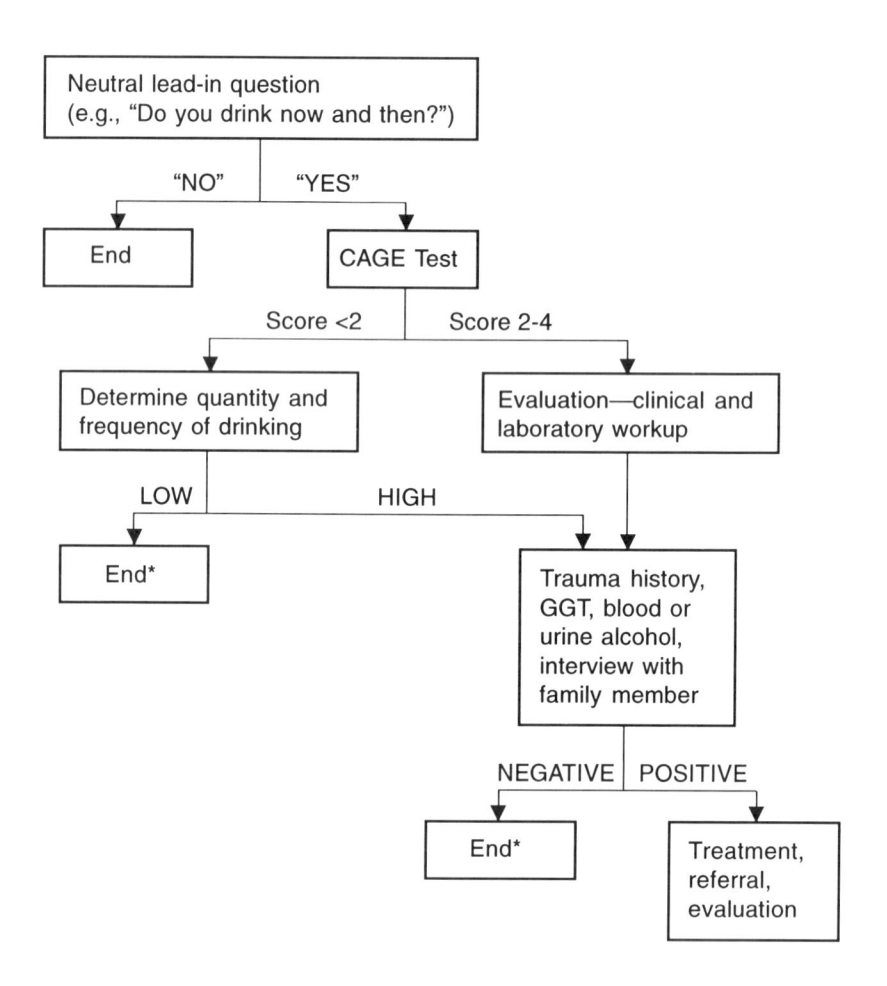

```
        Neutral lead-in question
        (e.g., "Do you drink now and then?")
              /              \
           "NO"            "YES"
            ↓                ↓
           End           CAGE Test
                        /         \
                  Score <2      Score 2-4
                     ↓              ↓
        Determine quantity and   Evaluation—clinical and
        frequency of drinking    laboratory workup
            /        \                    ↓
          LOW       HIGH                  ↓
           ↓          ↓                   ↓
          End*       Trauma history, GGT, blood or
                     urine alcohol, interview with
                     family member
                        /          \
                   NEGATIVE      POSITIVE
                      ↓              ↓
                     End*         Treatment,
                                  referral,
                                  evaluation
```

*However, follow-up visits may be appropriate.

Adapted from: National Institute on Alcohol Abuse and Alcoholism. *Seventh Special Report to the U.S. Congress on Alcohol and Health.* Rockville, MD: U.S. Department of Health and Human Services; 1990. USDHHS Publication ADM 90-1656.

Injection drug users should be warned about the risk of HIV, hepatitis B, and other disorders from using contaminated or shared needles. Information about cleaning needles with bleach should be provided (see chapter 58.)

4. *Emphasizing personal responsibility and self-efficacy:* The clinician should convey to the patient a sense of optimism and confidence that he or she can control his or her substance use.

5. *Conveying a clear message and setting goals:* The clinician should communicate clearly and firmly to the patient a recommendation to stop substance abuse. It may be helpful to assist the patient in setting a date for abstinence or goals for step-wise moderation of substance use. The patient should be helped to anticipate physiologic and psychologic withdrawal symptoms and plan for potential relapses or "slips."

6. *Involving family and other supports:* The assistance and patience of family members can be critical for the success of the patient's efforts at abstinence or moderation. Involving others must be done only with patient consent.

7. *Establish a working relationship with community treatment resources:* Many patients may benefit from the structure provided by peer counseling, support groups, inpatient treatment, and other modalities. The clinician should become familiar with the support and treatment resources available in the community so that appropriate referrals, if needed, can be made.

8. *Providing follow-up:* Monitoring and supporting patient success is essential and desirable, even for patients referred for treatment. Return appointments should be scheduled at regular intervals, particularly during the first weeks of each patient's efforts to stop or moderate use.

**Patient Resources**

*Alcohol: What to Do If It's a Problem for You.* American Academy of Family Physicians, 8880 Ward Parkway, Kansas City, MO 64114-2797; 1-800 944-0000.

*Alcohol and Women.* American College of Obstetricians and Gynecologists, 409 12th Street SW, Washington, DC 20024; 1-800 762-2264.

*Let's Talk Facts about Substance Abuse.* American Psychiatric Association, 1400 K Street NW, Washington, DC 20005; 1-800 368-5777.

Numerous publications are available from National Clearinghouse for Alcohol and Drug Information; 1-800 729-6686.

## Selected References

American Academy of Family Physicians, Commission on Public Health and Scientific Affairs. *Age Charts for Periodic Health Examination*. Kansas City, Mo: American Academy of Family Physicians; 1993.

American College of Obstetricians and Gynecologists. *The Obstetrician-Gynecologist and Primary-Preventive Health Care*. Washington, DC: American College of Obstetricians and Gynecologists; 1993.

American College of Physicians. *Chemical Dependence*. Philadelphia, Pa: American College of Physicians; 1984. Position paper.

American Medical Association, Council on Scientific Affairs. *Guidelines for Alcoholism Diagnosis, Treatment and Referral*. Chicago, Ill: American Medical Association; 1979.

Babor TF. Alcohol and substance abuse in primary care settings. In: Mayfield J, Grady M, eds. *Primary Care Research: An Agenda for the 90s*. Washington, DC: US Dept of Health and Human Services; 1990:113-124.

Babor TF, Ritson EB, Hodgson RJ. Alcohol-related problems in the primary health care setting: a review of early intervention strategies. *Br J of Addict*. 1986;81:23-46.

Baird MA. Early detection of alcoholism. *Drug Therapy*. October 1990:29-39.

Barnes HN. Presenting the diagnosis: working with denial. In: Barnes HN, Aronson MD, Delbanco TL, eds. *Alcoholism: A Guide for the Primary Care Physician*. New York, NY: Springer-Verlag; 1987: chap 6.

Batki SL. Drug abuse, psychiatric disorders, and AIDS: dual and triple diagnosis. *West J Med*. 1990;152:547-552.

Bien TH, Miller WR, Tonigan JS. Brief interventions for alcohol problems. *Addiction*. 1993;88:315-336.

Bigby JA. Negotiating treatment and monitoring recovery. In: Barnes HN, Aronson MD, Delbanco TL, eds. *Alcoholism: A Guide for the Primary Care Physician*. New York, NY: Springer-Verlag; 1987: chap 7.

Brown RL. Identification and office management of alcohol and drug disorders. In: Fleming MF, Barry KL, eds. *Addictive Disorders*. St Louis, Mo: Mosby Year Book; 1992.

Bush B, Shaw S, Cleary P, Delbanco TL, Aronson MD. Screening for alcohol abuse using the CAGE questionnaire. *Am J Med*. 1987;82:231-235.

Canadian Task Force on the Periodic Health Examination. The periodic health examination: 2. 1989 update. *Can Med Assoc J*. 1989;141:4-24.

Cyr MG, Wartman SA. The effectiveness of routine screening questions in the detection of alcoholism. *JAMA*. 1988;259:51-54.

Delbanco TL. Patients who drink too much: where are their doctors? *JAMA*. 1992;267:702-703.

Ewing JA. Detecting alcoholism: the CAGE questionnaire. *JAMA*. 1984;252:1905-1907.

Gerstein DR, Lewin LS. Treating drug problems. *N Engl J Med*. 1990;323:844-848.

Kamerow DB, Pincus HA, Macdonald DI. Alcohol abuse, other drug abuse, and mental disorders in medical practice. *JAMA*. 1986;255:2054-2057.

Magruder-Habib K, Durand M, Frey K. Alcohol abuse and alcoholism in primary health care setting. *J Fam Pract*. 1991;32:406-413.

Moore RD, Bone LR, Geller G, Marmon JA, Stokes EJ, Levine DM. Prevalence, detection, and treatment of alcoholism in hospitalized patients. *JAMA*. 1989;261:403-407.

National Institute on Alcohol Abuse and Alcoholism. *Motivational Enhancement Therapy Manual: A Clinical Research Guide for Therapists Treating Individuals With Alcohol Abuse and Dependence*. vol 2. Rockville, Md: US Dept of Health and Human Services; 1992. DHHS Publication ADM 92-894.

National Institute on Alcohol Abuse and Alcoholism. *Seventh Special Report to the U.S. Congress on Alcohol and Health*. Rockville, Md: US Dept of Health and Human Services; 1990. DHHS Publication ADM 90-1656.

Rush BR. The use of family medical practices by patients with drinking problems. *Can Med Assoc J.* 1989;140:35-39.

Saunders JB, Aasland OG, Babor TF, De La Fuente JR, Grant M. Development of the Alcohol Use Disorders Identification Test (AUDIT): WHO Collaborative Project on Early Detection of Persons with Harmful Alcohol Consumption—II. *Addiction.* 1993;88:791-804.

Selzer ML. The Michigan Alcoholism Screening Test: the quest for a new diagnostic instrument. *Am J Psych.* 1971;127:89-94.

Skinner HA. The Drug Abuse Screening Test. *Addict Behav.* 1982;7:363-371.

US Preventive Services Task Force. Screening for alcohol and other drug abuse. In: *Guide to Clinical Preventive Services.* Baltimore, Md: Williams & Wilkins; 1989:chap 47.

Walsh DC, Hingson RW, Merrigan DM, et al. The impact of a physician's warning on recovery after alcoholism treatment. *JAMA.* 1992;267:663-667

Adults/Older Adults — COUNSELING

# 53. Dental and Oral Health

Most Americans are affected by dental and oral health problems at some point in their lives. The most common diseases are dental caries (tooth decay) and periodontal disease, both of which are largely preventable. Although dental caries is more commonly thought of as a childhood disease, adults continue to be at risk for dental decay throughout their lives. Root-surface decay associated with gingival recession is a particular concern in older adults. The National Survey of Adult Oral Health recently found that 77% of employed adults aged 18 to 65 years and 95% of adults over age 65 had experienced some loss of periodontal tissue. Periodontal diseases and recurrent caries are the predominant causes of tooth loss. Oral mucosal lesions of all types are also prevalent (10% to 30%) in adult and elderly populations.

Numerous clinical trials have demonstrated that personal oral hygiene measures can control plaque and gingivitis in most individuals. The progression of periodontal diseases can be retarded by the combination of excellent personal oral hygiene practices and regular professional care. The routine use of dentifrices with fluoride has been shown to prevent both coronal and root-surface caries in adult populations.

Oral-pharyngeal cancers also are a major concern among adults. They represent 3% to 4% of all cancers and, excluding skin cancer, are the seventh most common form of cancer. The use of tobacco in all forms and heavy alcohol use are major causal factors.

For information on counseling children and adolescents on dental and oral health, refer to chapter 18. For a discussion of the oral cavity examination, see chapter 29.

**Recommendations of Major Authorities**

- **American Cancer Society**—Patients should be counseled about oral health during cancer-related checkups, which should occur every 3 years for those aged 20 to 40 years, and then yearly for those over 40.

- **American Dental Association**—Adults should be seen for routine dental care and oral hygiene counseling at least once a year.

- **Canadian Task Force on the Periodic Health Examination**—Counseling for prevention of periodontal disease should occur yearly, generally at the time of the oral examination, which by custom is done at intervals of 6 months or 1 year.

- **U.S. Preventive Services Task Force**—All patients should be encouraged to visit a dental care provider on a regular basis. Primary care providers should counsel patients regarding daily tooth brushing and flossing, using fluoride appropriately for caries prevention, and avoiding sugary foods. All adult patients should be counseled regarding the dangers of tobacco and alcohol use. Patients with increased exposure to sunlight should be advised to protect their lips and skin from the harmful effects of ultraviolet rays from the sun.

## Basics of Dental and Oral Health Counseling

1. Patients should be encouraged to see an oral health professional regularly (in general, at least yearly) for preventive care. Older adults often do not seek regular oral health care. Patients needing dental care more frequently include diabetics, tobacco and alcohol users, the immunocompromised, and those with decreased salivary flow (xerostomia) due to many commonly prescribed medications (see Table 53-1), Sjögren's syndrome, or head and neck irradiation.

2. All patients should be encouraged to brush their teeth daily with a fluoride-containing toothpaste or other dentifrice and to use dental floss each day.

3. Individuals with a history of frequent caries should be encouraged to reduce their intake of foods containing refined sugars and to avoid sugary between-meal snacks. These patients may also benefit from the use of a fluoride-containing mouth rinse.

4. Patients should be counseled to avoid or cease the use of tobacco in any form (see chapter 59) and to limit alcohol consumption (see chapter 52).

5. Individuals with increased exposure to sunlight should be encouraged to protect their lips and skin from the harmful effects of ultraviolet rays by using sunscreens and lip balms with SPFs of 15 or more, wearing protective clothing such as hats, and avoiding direct sun exposure between the hours of 10:00 am and 3:00 pm.

6. Individuals engaged in sports with the potential for oral and dental trauma should be encouraged to use appropriate protective equipment, including mouth guards. All patients should be urged to wear safety belts while in motor vehicles and helmets while riding bicycles and motorcycles.

Table 53-1. Oral Effects of Selected Drugs

| Effect | Medication |
| --- | --- |
| Xerostomia | Anticholinergics, antidepressants, antihypertensives, antipsychotics, diuretics, gastrointestinals, systemic antihistamines/decongestants, systemic bronchodilators |
| Soft tissue reactions | Methyldopa, barbiturates, sulfonamides, penicillamine, gold salts, chloroquine, isoniazid |
| Altered host resistance | Antibiotics, insulin, oral hypoglycemics, systemic corticosteroids |
| Gingival overgrowth | Phenytoin, nifedipine, cyclosporine, diltiazem |
| Interactions with dental drugs | Barbiturates, benzodiazepines, muscle relaxants, sedative-hypnotics, nonsteroidal anti-inflammatory agents, opiate analgesics |
| Need to minimize vasoconstrictor use | Antiarrhythmics, cardiac glycosides, tricyclic antidepressants, calcium channel blockers |

Adapted from: Park BZ, Kinney MB, Steffensen JEM. Putting your teeth into your physical exam. 2: adults. *J Fam Pract.* 1992;35:585-587. Used with permission of the authors and Appleton & Lange; copyright © 1992.

# Ch. 53. Dental and Oral Health — Adults/Older Adults — COUNSELING

7. Patients, particularly those who use tobacco or alcohol, should be encouraged to see a dentist or physician if they notice any irregularities in the oral cavity—such as color changes, cracks, ulcers, bleeding, swelling or thickening in the lips, cheeks, gums, tongue, or roof of the mouth—that last longer than 2 weeks.

8. Clinicians should counsel patients on the oral effects and complications of medications (see Table 53-1).

9. Transient bacteremia is common during dental procedures, including cleaning. Patients with certain cardiac conditions should be given antibiotic prophylaxis prior to any dental cleaning or other procedure known to induce gingival or mucosal bleeding (see Tables 53-2 and 53-3).

**Table 53-2. Cardiac Conditions\* for Which Endocarditis Prophylaxis Is and Is Not Recommended**

| Prophylaxis recommended | Prophylaxis NOT recommended |
|---|---|
| Prosthetic cardiac valves, including bioprosthetic and homograft valves | Isolated secundum atrial septal defect |
| Previous bacterial endocarditis, even in the absence of heart disease | Surgical repair, without residua, beyond 6 months in: secundum atrial septal defect, ventricular septal defect, patent ductus arteriosus |
| Surgically constructed systemic-pulmonary shunts | Previous coronary artery bypass surgery |
| Most congenital cardiac malformations | Mitral valve prolapse without valvular regurgitation\*\* |
| Rheumatic and other acquired valvular dysfunction, even after valve surgery | Physiologic, functional, or innocent heart murmurs |
| Hypertrophic cardiomyopathy | Previous Kawasaki disease without valvular dysfunction |
| Mitral valve prolapse with valvular regurgitation | Previous rheumatic fever without valvular dysfunction |
| | Cardiac pacemakers and implanted defibrillators |

\*This table lists selected conditions but is not all-inclusive.

\*\*Persons who have mitral valve prolapse associated with thickening and/or redundancy of valve leaflet(s) may be at increased risk for bacterial endocarditis, particularly men 45 years of age or older.

Adapted from: Dajani AS, Bisno AL, Chung KJ, et al. Prevention of bacterial endocarditis: recommendations by the American Heart Association. *JAMA.* 1990;264:2919-2922. Used with permission from the American Medical Association; copyright © 1990.

## Ch. 53. Dental and Oral Health — Adults/Older Adults — COUNSELING

**Table 53-3. Standard Antibiotic Prophylaxis Regimens for Dental or Operative Procedures in the Oral Cavity of Patients Subject to Bacterial Endocarditis***

**For patients able to take amoxicillin/penicillin****
Amoxicillin, 3 g orally 1 hour before procedure, then 1.5 g 6 hours after initial dose

**For amoxicillin/penicillin-allergic patients****
Erythromycin ethylsuccinate, 800 mg, or erythromycin stearate, 1 g, orally 2 hours before procedure, then half the dose 6 hours after initial dose
OR
Clindamycin, 300 mg orally 1 hour before procedure and 150 mg 6 hours after initial dose

*Includes those with prosthetic heart valves and other high-risk patients.

**Initial pediatric doses are as follows: amoxicillin, 50 mg/kg; erythromycin ethylsuccinate or stearate, 20 mg/kg; clindamycin, 10 mg/kg. Follow-up dose 6 hours later should be one-half the initial dose. Total pediatric dose should not exceed total adult dose.

From: Dajani AS, Bisno AL, Chung KJ, et al. Prevention of bacterial endocarditis: recommendations by the American Heart Association. *JAMA*. 1990;264:2919-2922.

Used with permission from the American Medical Association; copyright © 1990.

## Patient Resources

*Facts on Oral Cancer*; *Self Oral Screen in Six Orderly Steps*. American Cancer Society, 1559 Clifton Rd. NE, Atlanta, GA 30329-4251; 1-800 ACS-2345.

*What You Need to Know about Oral Cancer*. Office of Cancer Communications, National Cancer Institute, Bldg 31, Rm 10A24, Bethesda, MD 20892; 1-800 4-CANCER.

*Dental Tips for Diabetics* (English and Spanish); *Dry Mouth (Xerostomia)*; *Fact Sheet: Periodontal (Gum) Disease*; *Fact Sheet: Tooth Decay*; *Fever Blisters and Canker Sores*; *Fluorides Aren't Just for Kids*; *Periodontal Disease and Diabetes: A Guide for Patients*. National Institute of Dental Research, Public Information and Reports Section, PO Box 54793, Washington, DC 20032; (301) 496-4261.

*A Beautiful Smile is Ageless*; *For a Lifetime of Smiles...*; *Know Your Oral Health IQ*; and others. American Dental Hygienists' Association, 444 N. Michigan Avenue, Suite 3400, Chicago, IL 60611; (312) 440-8900.

*Diet and Dental Health*; *Fluoride Helps Prevent Tooth Decay*; *Smoking and Oral Health*; *Smokeless Tobacco: Think Before You Chew*. These and other materials available from: American Dental Association, Dept. of Salable Materials, 211 E. Chicago Ave., Chicago, IL 60611; 1-800 947-4746.

## Provider Resources

*Detection and Prevention of Periodontal Disease: A Guide for Health Care Providers*. National Institute of Dental Research, Public Information and Reports Section, PO Box 54793, Washington, DC 20032; (301) 496-4261.

## Selected References

American Dental Association. *Statement on Diet and Dental Caries*. Chicago, Ill: American Dental Association; 1982.

American Dental Association. Current preventive concepts. In: *Accepted Dental Therapeutics*. 40th ed. Chicago, Ill: American Dental Association; 1984.

American Dental Association. *Importance of Professional Teeth Cleaning*. Chicago, Ill: American Dental Association; 1985.

Canadian Task Force on the Periodic Health Examination. *Periodic Health Examination Monograph*. Hull, Quebec: Minister of Supply and Services Canada; 1980.

Centers for Disease Control. Deaths from oral cavity and pharyngeal cancer—United States, 1987. *MMWR*. 1991; 39:457-472.

Dajani AS, Bisno AL, Chung KJ, et al. Prevention of bacterial endocarditis: recommendations by the American Heart Association. *JAMA*. 1990;264:2919-2922.

Greene JC, Louie R, Wycoff SJ. US Preventive Services Task Force: preventive dentistry: I. dental caries. *JAMA*. 1989;262:3459-3563.

Greene JC, Louie R, Wycoff SJ. US Preventive Services Task Force: preventive dentistry: II. periodontal diseases, malocclusion, trauma, and oral cancer. *JAMA*. 1990;263;421-423.

Mandel ID. Preventive dental services for the elderly. *Dental Clinics of North America*. 1989;33:81-90.

Niessen, LC, George, CW. Oral health. *MMJ*. 1989;38:126-128.

Park BZ, Kinney MB, Steffensen JEM. Putting teeth into your physical exam. 2: adults. *J Fam Pract*. 1992;35:585-587.

Thomas JE, Faecher RS. A physician's guide to early detection of oral cancer. *Geriatrics*. 1992;47:58-63.

US Preventive Services Task Force. Counseling to prevent dental disease. In: *Guide to Clinical Preventive Services*. Baltimore, Md: Williams & Wilkins; 1989:chap 55.

## Adults/Older Adults — COUNSELING

# 54. Injury and Violence Prevention

Unintentional injuries are the fourth leading cause of death in the United States and the leading cause of death for those aged 5 to 34 years. Motor vehicle crashes cause half of all unintentional injury deaths and are the leading cause of work-related injury deaths. Most motor vehicle trauma is related to alcohol use or failure to use safety belts, or both. The use of safety belts decreases the chance of injury or death in an automobile crash by 50%. Other major causes of unintentional injury deaths are falls, poisoning, drowning, and residential fires.

Unintentional injury is also a major cause of morbidity and mortality for older adults. It is the sixth leading cause of death in people 75 years and older. Falls are the most common cause of serious unintentional injury, accounting for 40% of all injury mortality in people over 75 years of age. The death rate due to falls in the 65-to-74 age group is twice that of the general population, and among those over 85 years of age it is 15 times that of the general population. Hip fracture is the most common fall-related injury leading to hospitalization in older adults. Roughly half of all people sustaining hip fractures never regain full function. Between $1 billion and $2 billion is spent annually in the United States for the acute medical treatment of hip fractures in older adults.

Injury to women as a result of violence should be of special concern to clinicians because it is one of America's most widespread health problems—and yet one of the least reported. The great majority of abused adults—over 90%—are women. It is difficult to ascertain the exact incidence of violence against women. One estimate, based on the work of several investigators, has placed the annual number of cases at 2 to 4 million; abuse has been estimated to occur in up to 25% of all familial relationships. Abuse of women knows no socioeconomic, racial, ethnic, religious, or age barriers. The consequences of this abuse are serious and alarming: over one-third of female murder victims are killed by their male partners, and about 6% of the visits made by women to emergency rooms are for injuries related to abuse.

Although primary care clinicians treat a wide range of injuries, studies indicate that they deliver little counseling to adults about injury prevention and do not detect and treat domestic violence in an optimal manner. Considering the amount of death and disability caused by preventable injuries and violence, these topics should be discussed with all patients.

For information on counseling children and adolescents on violent behavior and firearms, refer to chapter 25. Related information on counseling children and adolescents on safety can be found in chapter 21, on screening children and adolescents for depression and suicide in chapter 5, and on screening adults for depression in chapter 32.

## Recommendations of Major Authorities

*Adults*

- Most major authorities, including **American Academy of Family Physicians**, **American College of Physicians**, **Canadian Task Force on the Periodic Health Examination**, **National Transportation Safety Board**, and **U.S. Preventive Services Task Force**—Health-care professionals should counsel patients about car safety belt use and the avoidance of driving while using or after use of alcohol or other drugs.

- **American Academy of Family Physicians** and **U.S. Preventive Services Task Force**—Clinicians should provide counseling about injury prevention in the home, at work, and in the community.

- **American College of Obstetricians and Gynecologists**—Injury prevention should be part of the evaluation and counseling portions of the periodic examination of women of all ages, with particular attention to abuse, safety belts and safety helmets, firearms, recreational and occupational hazards, and sports involvement.

- **American Medical Association**—All women patients in emergency, surgical, primary care, pediatric, prenatal, and mental health settings should be screened for domestic violence.

- **Canadian Task Force on the Periodic Health Examination**—Although scientific justification is lacking to include counseling to prevent unintentional injuries (other than motor vehicle crashes), the periodic health examination provides the health professional with an opportunity to stress the need for safe practices in the home and in the community environment.

*Older Adults*

- **U.S. Preventive Services Task Force**—Regular injury prevention counseling should be provided to all older adults or their caretakers, or both.

- **Canadian Task Force on the Periodic Health Examination**—Because older adults are at particular risk for injury, counseling on safety in the home and community should be included in periodic health examinations at the discretion of the clinician.

## Basics of Injury Prevention Counseling

*Adults*

1. Safety counseling should be made an integral part of the provider's practice. Questions about safety issues should be included on intake questionnaires. Significant safety issues should be entered on the patient problem list. A record should be kept of counseling interventions delivered to patients. Interventions should be tailored to address concerns and motivations important to the patient. Care should be taken by the clinician to avoid sounding moralistic.

2. All patients should be advised to use safety belts when operating or riding in a motor vehicle. Table 54-1 provides guidelines on proper safety belt use.

**Table 54-1. Proper Safety Belt Use**

| |
|---|
| The belt should be worn over the shoulder, across the chest, and low on the lap, avoiding excess slack—not behind the back, under the arm, or over the abdomen. |
| Safety belts should be worn even for short trips. Three out of four motor vehicle crashes occur within 25 miles of home. Unbelted motorists have been killed in crashes when going as slowly as 12 miles per hour. |
| Safety belts should be worn even when the automobile has airbags. Airbags are effective primarily in frontal collisions and provide little protection in collisions from the side. |

Adapted from: National Committee for Injury Prevention and Control. Injury Prevention: meeting the challenge. *Am J Prev Med.* 1989;5(suppl.):1-303. Used with permission of Oxford University Press Journals; copyright © 1989.

3. All patients should be counseled on the importance of avoiding alcohol when driving, boating, swimming, and using motorized tools and firearms. The use of a nondrinking "designated driver" should be encouraged for return trips from parties and other events at which alcohol will be available.

4. All patients should be counseled to wear safety helmets while operating or riding motorcycles or bicycles and to wear mouth guards when playing contact sports.

5. All patients should be counseled to install and maintain smoke detectors in their residences. The batteries should be changed yearly (or, if needed, every 6 months). A good way to remember this is to do it when resetting clocks in the spring and fall. It is also advisable to test smoke detectors monthly to make sure they are operating correctly.

6. Patients should be advised about the dangers of keeping guns in the home. Many more children, friends, and family members than intruders are killed every year by guns in the home. If guns are kept in the home, they should be locked up unloaded and stored in a location separate from ammunition.

7. Patients should be counseled to be aware of the hazards and safety rules at the work site. Patients at increased risk of back injuries because of occupation or personal history should be counseled to learn safe lifting techniques and to perform appropriate back strengthening exercises.

## *Older Adults*

1. Older adults or their caretakers should be periodically counseled to:

    - Inspect the home for adequate lighting.

    - Remove or repair floor structures that predispose to tripping, such as loose rugs, electrical cords, and toys.

- Install handrails and traction strips in stairways and bathtubs.
- Keep hot water set at 49°C (120°F) or lower.

Counseling for safety can be facilitated with patient or caretaker use of a home-safety checklist (see Table 54-2). Home visits are also an excellent opportunity to assess home safety for older adults.

2. Patient visual acuity should be checked periodically (see chapter 44), and physical mobility assessed.

3. The prescribing of drugs associated with falls (ie. long-acting benzodiazapines, tricyclic antidepressants, major tranquilizers, and other sedatives) should be avoided or closely monitored. Many falls in older adults are due to side effects from polypharmacy (see chapter 57).

4. Older adults without medical contraindications should be encouraged to engage in an exercise program to maintain muscle and bone strength, mobility, and flexibility.

5. The need for estrogen replacement therapy to help prevent fractures from osteoporosis in postmenopausal women should be assessed (see chapter 46). The need for counseling about weight-bearing exercises, calcium supplementation, and other nutritional issues should also be assessed in these women.

**Basics of Detecting and Counseling Women Who are Victims of Violence**

1. Common characteristics of abused women include a history of having been beaten as a child; raised in a single-parent home; married as a teenager; and pregnant before marriage. Frequent somatic complaints among these individuals include: headaches, insomnia, choking sensation, hyperventilation, gastrointestinal symptoms, pain in the chest, back and pelvis. They are more likely than other women to abuse alcohol and drugs, attempt suicide, and transfer their aggression to children. Pregnant women are three times as likely as nonpregnant women to be victims of abuse.

2. Violence toward women can sometimes be detected on the physical examination. The areas most commonly injured in women are the head, neck, chest, abdomen, breasts and upper extremities. Burns, bruises in patterns resembling hands, belts, cords, or other weapons, and multiple traumatic injuries may be seen.

3. Women should be asked directly whether they have ever been physically abused, particularly if there is evidence of injury. Questions such as "Has anyone at home hit you or tried to injure you?" and "Have you ever been physically abused, either recently or in the past?" are appropriate ways in which to introduce the subject.

4. It is important for the clinician to acknowledge the problem and to affirm that battering is unacceptable. The first step is to listen nonjudgmentally and to attempt to assess the

## Ch. 54. Injury and Violence Prevention — Adults/Older Adults — COUNSELING

**Table 54-2. Home Safety Checklist for Older Adults**

Place a check mark next to each question if the answer is yes. Use this checklist to correct all hazards in the home.

### Housekeeping
- _____ Do you clean up spills as soon as they occur?
- _____ Do you keep floors and stairways clean and free of clutter?
- _____ Do you put away books, magazines, sewing supplies, and other objects as soon as you are through with them and never leave them on floors or stairways?
- _____ Do you store frequently used items on shelves that are within easy reach?

### Floors
- _____ Do you keep everyone from walking on freshly washed floors before they are dry?
- _____ If you wax floors, do you apply 2 thin coats and buff each thoroughly or use self-polishing wax?
- _____ Do all area rugs have nonslip backings?
- _____ Have you eliminated small rugs at the tops and bottoms of stairways?
- _____ Are all carpet edges tacked down?
- _____ Are rugs and carpets free of curled edges, worn sports, and rips?
- _____ Have you chosen rugs and carpets with short, dense pile?
- _____ Are rugs and carpets installed over good-quality, medium-thick pads?

### Lighting
- _____ Do you have light switches near every doorway?
- _____ Do you have enough good lighting to eliminate shadowy areas?
- _____ Do you have a lamp or light switch within easy reach of every bed?
- _____ Do you have night lights in your bathrooms and in hallways leading from bedrooms to bathrooms?
- _____ Are all stairways well lit with light switches at both top and bottom?

### Bathrooms
- _____ Do you use a rubber mat or nonslip decals in tubs and showers?
- _____ Do you have a grab bar securely anchored over each tub and shower?
- _____ Do you have a nonslip rug on all bathroom floors?
- _____ Do you keep soap in easy-to-reach receptacles?

### Traffic Lanes
- _____ Can you walk across every room in your home, and from one room to another, without detouring around furniture?
- _____ Is the traffic lane from your bedroom to the bathroom free of obstacles?
- _____ Are telephone and appliance cords kept away from areas where people walk?

### Stairways
- _____ Do securely fastened handrails extend the full length of the stairs on each side of the stairways?
- _____ Do the handrails stand out from the walls so you can get a good grip?
- _____ Are handrails distinctly shaped so you are alerted when you reach the end of a stairway?
- _____ Are all stairways in good condition, with no broken, sagging, or sloping steps?
- _____ Are all stairway carpeting and metal edges securely fastened and in good condition?
- _____ Have you replaced any single-level steps with gradually rising ramps or made sure such steps are well lighted?

*(Continued)*

**Table 54-2. Home Safety Checklist for Older Adults—Continued**

Place a check mark next to each question if the answer is yes. Use this checklist to correct all hazards in the home.

**Ladders and Step Stools**
_____ Do you always use a step stool or ladder that is tall enough for the job?
_____ Do you always set up your ladder or step stool on a firm, level base that is free of clutter?
_____ Before you climb a ladder or step stool, do you always make sure it is fully open and that the stepladder spreaders are locked?
_____ When you use a ladder or step stool, do you face the steps and keep your body between the side rails?
_____ Do you avoid standing on the top step of a step stool or climbing beyond the second step from the top on a stepladder?

**Outdoor Areas**
_____ Are walks and driveways in your yard and other areas free of breaks?
_____ Are lawns and gardens free of holes?
_____ Do you put away garden tools and hoses when they are not in use?
_____ Are outdoor areas kept free of rocks, loose boards, and other tripping hazards?
_____ Do you keep outdoor walkways, steps, and porches free of wet leaves and snow?
_____ Do you sprinkle icy outdoor areas with deicers as soon as possible after a snowfall or freeze?
_____ Do you have mats at doorways for people to wipe their feet on?
_____ Do you know the safest way of walking when you can't avoid walking on a slippery surface?

**Footwear**
_____ Do your shoes have soles and heels that provide good traction?
_____ Do you avoid walking in stocking feet and wear house slippers that fit well and don't fall off?
_____ Do you wear low-heeled oxfords, loafers, or good-quality sneakers when you work in your house or yard?
_____ Do you replace boots or galoshes when their soles or heels are worn too smooth to keep you from slipping on wet or icy surfaces?

*(Continued)*

seriousness of the victim's circumstances. Trust is essential; the patient should be assured that information disclosed will be kept confidential to the maximum extent possible.

5. Clinicians should help abused women understand the dynamics of their relationships and the dangers faced by themselves and their children.

6. Information about available community, social, and legal resources, legal rights, and a plan for dealing with the abusive partner should be made available to these women. Local referral numbers for assistance and further information on detection and treatment of domestic violence are available from the National Council on Child Abuse and Family Violence, 1-800 222-2000.

Ch. 54. Injury and Violence Prevention          Adults/Older Adults — COUNSELING

**Table 54-2. Home Safety Checklist for Older Adults—Continued**

Place a check mark next to each question if the answer is yes. Use this checklist to correct all hazards in the home.

**Personal Precautions**

_____ Are you always alert for unexpected hazards, such as out-of-place furniture?
_____ If young children visit or live in your home, are you alert for children playing on the floor and toys left in your path?
_____ If you have pets, are you alert for sudden movements across your path and pets getting underfoot?
_____ When you carry packages, do you divide them into smaller loads and make sure they do not obstruct your vision?
_____ When you reach or bend, do you hold onto a firm support and avoid throwing your head back or turning it too far?
_____ Do you always move deliberately and avoid rushing to answer phone or doorbell?
_____ Do you take time to get your balance when you change position from lying down to sitting and from sitting to standing?
_____ Do you keep yourself in good condition with moderate exercise, good diet, adequate rest, and regular medical checkups?
_____ If you wear glasses, is your prescription up to date?
_____ Do you know how to reduce injury in a fall?
_____ If you live alone, do you have daily contact with a friend or neighbor?

Adapted from: National Safety Council. *Falling—The Unexpected Trip: A Safety Program for Older Adults* (Program Leader's Guide). Chicago, IL: National Safety Council; 1982. Used with permission of the National Safety Council; copyright © 1982.


**Patient Resources**

*Age Page—Accidents and the Elderly*; *Age Page—Safety Belt Sense*; *Age Page—Preventing Falls and Fractures*; *Age Page—Heat, Cold, and Being Old*. National Institute on Aging, Bldg 31, Rm 5C27, Bethesda, MD 20892; (310) 496-1752.

*Auto Safety Hot Line*. National Highway Traffic Safety Administration: 1-800 424-9393.

*The Abused Woman*. American College of Obstetricians and Gynecologists, 409 12th St. SW, Washington, DC 20024-2188; (202) 638-5577.

*Your Home Safety Checklist; Preventing Falls: A Safety Program for Older Adults*; *Facts About Backs*; *Playing it Safe: A Pocket Guide to Fitness*, and other materials. National Safety Council, 444 N. Michigan Ave., Chicago, IL 60601; 1-800 621-7619, ext 1300.

**Provider Resources**

*Diagnostic and Treatment Guidelines on Domestic Violence*. American Medical Association, Department of Mental Health, 515 North State Street, Chicago, IL 60610; (312) 464-5066.

*Is 40 Years of a Patient's Life Worth 3 Seconds of Your Time?*; *HELP: Motor Vehicle Trauma.* American Academy of Family Physicians, 8880 Ward Parkway, Kansas City, MO 64114-2797; 1-800 274-2237.

*How to Plan a Comprehensive Community Occupant Protection Program.* National Highway Traffic Safety Administration, Office of Occupant Protection, NTS-13, 400 7th St. SW, Washington, DC 20590; (202) 366-2696.

*Injury Control News.* Association for the Advancement of Injury Control, 900 17th St. NW, Washington, DC 20006; (202) 659-8844.

*The Battered Woman.* The American College of Obstetricians and Gynecologists, 409 12th St. SW, Washington, DC 20024-2188; (202) 638-5577.

**Selected References**

American College of Physicians. *Health Promotion/Disease Prevention: Seat Belt Use.* Philadelphia, Pa: American College of Physicians; 1984.

American Academy of Family Physicians, Commission on Public Health and Scientific Affairs. *Age Charts for Periodic Health Examination.* Kansas City, Mo: American Academy of Family Physicians; 1993.

American College of Obstetricians and Gynecologists. *The Obstetrician-Gynecologist and Primary-Preventive Health Care.* Washington, DC: American College of Obstetricians and Gynecologists; 1993.

American Medical Association, Council on Scientific Affairs. Violence against women. Relevance for medical practitioners. *JAMA.* 1992;267:3184-3189.

Baker SP, O'Neill B, Ginsberg MJ, Li G. *The Injury Fact Book.* New York, NY: Oxford University Press; 1991.

Canadian Task Force on the Periodic Health Examination. *Periodic Health Examination Monograph.* Hull, Quebec: Ministry of Supply and Services Canada; 1980.

Carnaveli D, Patrick M. *Nursing Management of the Elderly.* Philadelphia, Pa: JB Lippincott; 1986.

Hindmarsh JJ, Estes EH. Falls and older persons: causes and interventions. *Arch Intern Med.* 1989;149:2217-2222.

Johnson K, Ford D, Smith G. The current practices of internists in prevention of residential fire injury. *Am J Prev Med.* 1993;9:39-44.

McFarlane J, Parker B, Soeken K, Bullock L. Assessing for abuse during pregnancy. Severity and frequency of injuries and associated entry into prenatal care. *JAMA.* 1992;267:3176-3178.

National Committee for Injury Prevention and Control. Injury prevention: meeting the challenge. *Am J Prev Med.* 1989;5(suppl.):1-303.

National Safety Council. *Falling—The Unexpected Trip: A Safety Program for Older Adults* (Program Leader's Guide). Chicago, Ill: National Safety Council; 1982.

Polen MR, Friedman GD. Automobile injury: selected risk factors and prevention in the health care setting. *JAMA.* 1988;259:76-80.

U.S. Department of Health and Human Services. *Surgeon General's Workshop on Violence and Public Health: Report.* DHHS Publ. No. HRS-D-MC 86-1. Washington, DC: U.S. Public Health Service, 1986.

US Preventive Services Task Force. Counseling to prevent motor vehicle injuries.In: *Guide to Clinical Preventive Services.* Baltimore, Md: Williams & Wilkins; 1989:chap 51.

US Preventive Services Task Force. Counseling to prevent household and environmental injuries. In: *Guide to Clinical Preventive Services.* Baltimore, Md: Williams & Wilkins; 1989:chap 52.

## Adults/Older Adults — COUNSELING

# 55. Nutrition

Good nutrition is important for good health throughout life. Dietary intervention is an important component of both prevention and treatment of many chronic conditions, including coronary heart disease, diabetes, certain cancers, and hypertension. Nutritional deficiencies, which were endemic at the beginning of the century, now occur infrequently in otherwise healthy individuals. Overconsumption of calories (particularly as fat) and declining levels of physical activity, however, have made obesity a major public health problem in the United States. Approximately 25% of adult Americans are overweight. Overconsumption of other dietary components, such as sodium and alcohol, have contributed to serious health problems for many individuals. Underconsumption of certain nutrients, such as calcium, iron, and folate, cause health problems for some individuals—particularly women.

Patients express a desire for nutritional guidance from primary care clinicians. Fewer than half of all clinicians, however, report regularly providing even basic nutrition assessment and counseling to patients. As with other types of life-style counseling, simple, focused interventions can be beneficial to patients.

See chapter 19 for information on nutrition counseling for children.

### Recommendations of Major Authorities

- Most major authorities, including **American Academy of Family Physicians, American College of Obstetricians and Gynecologists, American College of Physicians, American Dietetic Association, American Heart Association**, and **U.S. Preventive Services Task Force**—Clinicians should routinely provide nutritional assessment and counseling to their patients.

### Basics of Nutrition Counseling

1. Every patient should be weighed and measured regularly. Chapter 28 contains information on performing and assessing body measurement. Patients should be advised of their healthy weight range based on such factors as age, gender, and distribution of body fat.

2. Clinicians should talk with all patients about their dietary habits. Short patient questionnaires can be useful in identifying patients in need of more in-depth evaluation. Table 55-1 gives a brief questionnaire developed for use with older adults. Questionnaires for more general use have also been developed (Block, et al., 1989).

## Ch. 55. Nutrition
### Adults/Older Adults — COUNSELING

**Table 55-1. Determining Your Nutritional Health: Checklist for Older Adults***

|  | YES |
|---|---|
| I have an illness or condition that made me change the kind and/or amount of food I eat. | 2 |
| I eat fewer than 2 meals per day. | 3 |
| I eat few fruits and vegetables, or milk products. | 2 |
| I have 3 or more drinks of beer, liquor or wine almost every day. | 2 |
| I have tooth or mouth problems that make it hard for me to eat. | 2 |
| I don't always have enough money to buy the food I need. | 4 |
| I eat alone most of the time. | 1 |
| I take 3 or more different prescribed or over-the-counter drugs a day. | 1 |
| Without wanting to, I have lost or gained 10 pounds in the last 6 months. | 2 |
| I am not always physically able to shop, cook, or feed myself. | 2 |
|  | **TOTAL** |

*Instructions: Read the statements above. Circle the number in the yes column for those that apply. For each "yes" answer, score the number in the box. Total your nutrition score. If it is:

- 0-2 Good! Recheck your nutritional score in 6 months.

- 3-5 You are at moderate risk. See what can be done to improve your eating habits and lifestyle. Your office on aging, senior nutrition program, senior citizens center or health department can help. Recheck your nutritional score in 3 months.

- ≥6 You are at high nutritional risk. Talk with your doctor, dietitian or other qualified health or social service professional about this checklist. Talk with them about any problems you may have. Ask for help to improve your nutritional health.

Adapted from: The Nutrition Screening Initiative. (Educational material and office aids for screening elderly patients for nutritional deficiencies). Washington, DC: Nutrition Screening Initiative. Reprinted with permission of the Nutrition Screening Initiative; copyright © 1993.

3. Patients should be given basic information about managing a healthy diet. The U.S. Department of Agriculture and the U.S. Department of Health and Human Services recommend the following in *Dietary Guidelines for Americans*:

- Eat a variety of foods.

- Maintain a healthy weight.

- Choose a diet low in total fat (less than 30% of calories), saturated fat (less than 10% of calories), and cholesterol.

- Choose a diet with plenty of vegetables, fruits, and grain products (5 or more servings daily).

- Use sugars only in moderation.

- Use salt and sodium only in moderation.

- If you drink alcoholic beverages, do so only in moderation (no more than 1 drink daily for women or 2 drinks daily for men). Women who are pregnant or planning to become pregnant should not drink alcohol at all.

4. Use of a pictorial guide, such as the Food Guide Pyramid (Fig 55-1), can be a useful tool for helping patients plan a healthful diet.

5. Fig 55-2 explains the new food label mandated by the U.S. Food and Drug Administration for use on all packaged foods. Clinicians should be familiar with the label and encourage and, as needed, instruct patients in its use.

6. Women have special dietary needs. Chief among these are needs for calcium and folic acid. Women of all ages should be counseled to consume adequate calcium, which during the teen years and early adulthood helps build optimal bone mass and after menopause helps control bone loss and delays the development of osteoporosis. Dairy products are major sources of calcium. Other dietary sources are fish, vegetables, such as broccoli and spinach, and fortified cereals and grains.

   The U.S. Public Health Service recommends that all women of childbearing age in the United States consume 0.4 mg of folic acid per day to reduce their risk of having a pregnancy affected with spina bifida or other neural tube defect (NTD). Women should be advised of their options for complying with this recommendation. Consumption of a diet consistent with the *Dietary Guidelines* and Food Guide Pyramid is likely to provide the proper amount of folic acid. Fortified foods, such as breakfast cereals, may help patients consume enough folic acid. Folic acid supplement pills and multivitamin preparations containing 0.4 mg folic acid are also available. Patients should be cautioned against consuming more than 1 mg daily, because the effects of excess folic acid are not well known; they may include delaying the detection of vitamin $B_{12}$ deficiency, allowing neurologic damage to progress. However, women who have had a previous NTD-affected pregnancy should talk with their doctor several months before planning to become pregnant about using a higher dose of folic acid. Public health measures to supplement the U.S. food supply with folic acid currently are being studied.

7. For patients who are overweight, a diet with fewer total calories from fat and a modest increase in physical activity should be recommended. (See chapter 56 for information on physical activity counseling.) In general, the goal should be a weight loss of from $1/2$ to 1 pound per week. Although more rapid weight loss may be achieved with a very low-calorie (800 kcal/day or less) diet, weight loss from these diets usually is not well maintained and may lead to health problems. Selected patients who have failed at conservative methods of weight loss and who are severely obese or have obesity-related medical problems may benefit from the short-term weight loss of very low-calorie diets, under medical supervision. Behavior therapy and physical activity have been shown to help maintain weight loss.

## Ch. 55. Nutrition

Adults/Older Adults — COUNSELING

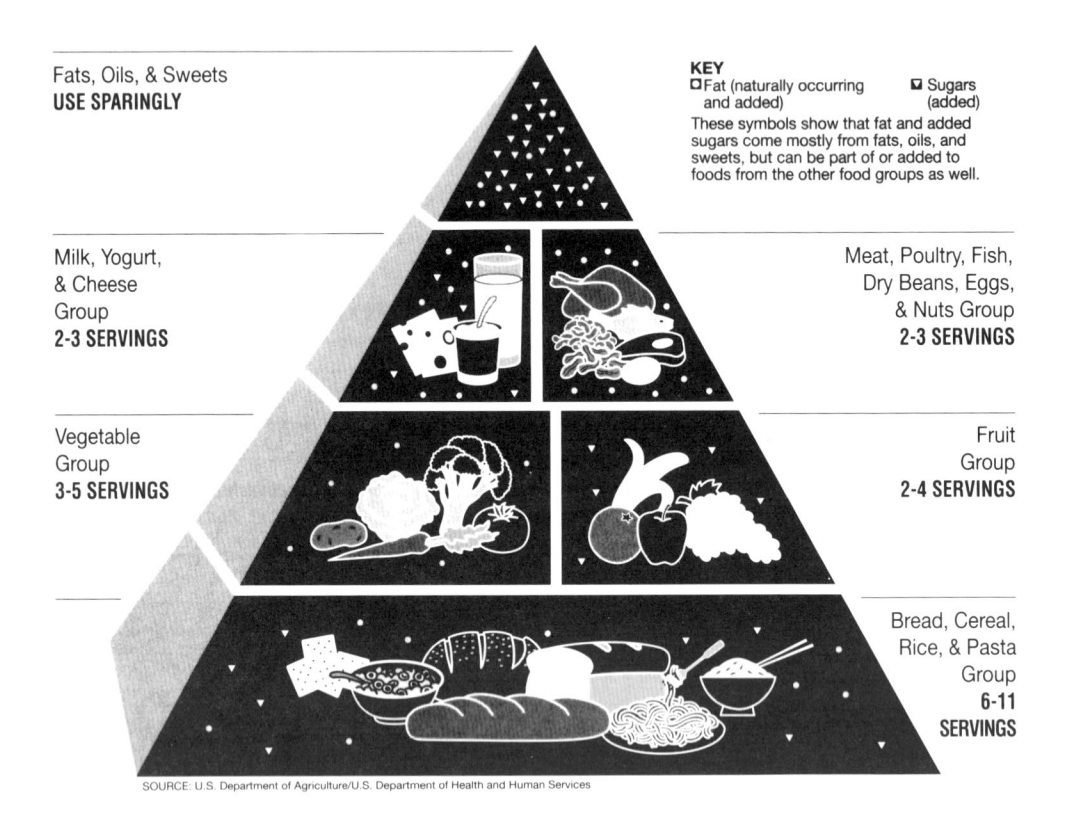

**Figure 55-1. Food Guide Pyramid: A Guide to Daily Food Choices**

Fats, Oils, & Sweets
**USE SPARINGLY**

**KEY**
☐ Fat (naturally occurring and added)    ▼ Sugars (added)

These symbols show that fat and added sugars come mostly from fats, oils, and sweets, but can be part of or added to foods from the other food groups as well.

Milk, Yogurt, & Cheese Group
**2-3 SERVINGS**

Meat, Poultry, Fish, Dry Beans, Eggs, & Nuts Group
**2-3 SERVINGS**

Vegetable Group
**3-5 SERVINGS**

Fruit Group
**2-4 SERVINGS**

Bread, Cereal, Rice, & Pasta Group
**6-11 SERVINGS**

SOURCE: U.S. Department of Agriculture/U.S. Department of Health and Human Services

**Figure 55-1. Food Guide Pyramid: A Guide to Daily Food Choices—Continued**

**What Counts as One Serving?**

**Breads, Cereals, Rice, and Pasta**
1 slice of bread
½ cup of cooked rice or pasta
½ cup of cooked cereal
1 ounce of ready-to-eat cereal

**Vegetables**
½ cup of chopped raw or cooked vegetables
1 cup of leafy raw vegetables

**Fruits**
1 piece of fruit or melon wedge
¾ cup of juice
½ cup of canned fruit

**Milk, Yogurt, and Cheese**
1 cup of milk or yogurt
1½ to 2 ounces of cheese

**Meat, Poultry, Fish, Dry Beans, Eggs, and Nuts**
2½ to 3 ounces of cooked lean meat, poultry, or fish
Count ½ cup of cooked beans, or 1 egg, or 2 tablespoons of peanut butter as 1 ounce of lean meat (about ⅓ of a serving)

**Fats, Oils, and Sweets**
Limit calories from these, especially if weight loss is needed

The amount eaten may be more than one serving. For example, a dinner portion of spaghetti would count as two or three servings of pasta.

**How Many Servings Are Needed?**

Teenage boys and active men need the highest number of servings shown. Women and some older adults need the lowest number of servings shown. Children, teenage girls, active women, and most men need a number of servings somewhere in the middle of those shown.

From: Human Nutrition Information Service. *Food Guide Pyramid: A Guide to Daily Food Choices.* Washington, DC: U.S. Department of Agriculture; 1992. (Leaflet No. 572)

---

8. For patients with borderline or elevated cholesterol levels, the National Cholesterol Education Program (NCEP) recommends that primary care providers instruct patients in the use of a cholesterol-lowering diet. The Step I diet recommended by the NCEP has less than 300 mg per day of cholesterol and 8% to 10% of total calories from saturated fatty acids. For patients who fail to adequately reduce their cholesterol levels on this diet, the Step II diet is recommended, which has less than 200 mg per day of cholesterol and less than 7% of total calories from saturated fatty acids. Referral to a dietitian is recommended for patients in need of the Step II diet. The NCEP guidelines for foods to choose or decrease for the Step I or Step II diets are given in Table 55-2.

9. It is important to provide ongoing support and reinforcement to patients undertaking significant dietary changes. This can take several forms, including follow-up visits, telephone calls, and postcards. It is important to encourage patients through the plateaus and regressions that occur as a normal part of efforts at long-term change.

**Figure 55-2. Guide To Using the New Food Label**

| | |
|---|---|
| **Serving sizes** are now more consistent across product lines, stated in both household and metric measures, and reflect the amounts people actually eat. | **New title** signals that the label contains the newly required information. |

## Nutrition Facts

Serving Size ½ cup (114g)
Servings Per Container 4

**Amount Per Serving**

**Calories** 90    Calories from Fat 30

| | **% Daily Value*** |
|---|---|
| **Total Fat** 3g | **5%** |
| Saturated Fat 0g | **0%** |
| **Cholesterol** 0mg | **0%** |
| **Sodium** 300mg | **13%** |
| **Total Carbohydrate** 13g | **4%** |
| Dietary Fiber 3g | **12%** |
| Sugars 3g | |
| **Protein** 3g | |

| | | | | |
|---|---|---|---|---|
| Vitamin A | 80% | • | Vitamin C | 60% |
| Calcium | 4% | • | Iron | 4% |

\* Percent Daily Values are based on a 2,000 calorie diet. Your daily values may be higher or lower depending on your calorie needs:

| | | Calories | 2,000 | 2,500 |
|---|---|---|---|---|
| Total Fat | Less than | | 65g | 80g |
| Sat Fat | Less than | | 20g | 25g |
| Cholesterol | Less than | | 300mg | 300mg |
| Sodium | Less than | | 2,400mg | 2,400mg |
| Total Carbohydrate | | | 300g | 375g |
| Fiber | | | 25g | 30g |

Calories per gram:
Fat 9  •  Carbohydrate 4  •  Protein 4

\* This label is only a sample. Exact specifications are in the final rules.

**Calories from fat** are now shown on the label to help consumers meet dietary guidelines that recommend people get no more than 30 percent of their calories from fat.

**% Daily Value** shows how a food fits into the overall daily diet.

**The list of nutrients** covers those most important to the health of today's consumers, most of whom need to worry about getting too much of certain items (fat, for example), rather than too few vitamins or minerals, as in the past.

**The label of larger packages** must now tell the number of calories per gram of fat, carbohydrate, and protein.

**Daily Values** are also something new. Some are maximums, as with fat (65 grams or less); others are minimums, as with carbohydrate (300 grams or more). The daily values for a 2,000- and 2,500- calorie diet must be listed on the label of larger packages. Individuals should adjust the values to fit their own calorie intake.

From: U.S. Food and Drug Administration. The new food label. *FDA Backgrounder*. Dec. 10, 1992:1-9.

10. Patients with multiple or severe nutritional problems should be referred, if possible, for counseling from a nutrition professional. Information on registered consulting nutrition professionals in the community can be obtained from the American Dietetic Association: 1-800 877-1600, ext. 4898.

11. Clinicians should monitor their own diet and make necessary adjustments. Research indicates that clinicians who follow good nutrition practices are more likely to provide good nutrition counseling to their patients.

**Patient Resources**

*CHATS: A Guide to Sensible Eating* (scripted slide show); *Osteoporosis in Women: Keeping Your Bones Healthy and Strong*. American Academy of Family Physicians, 8880 Ward Parkway, Kansas City, MO 64114-2797; 1-800 944-0000.

*Diet, Nutrition and Cancer Prevention: The Good News*. Office of Cancer Communications, National Cancer Institute, Bldg 31, Rm 10A24, Bethesda, MD 20892; 1-800 4-CANCER.

*Eating Right To Lower Your Blood Cholesterol*; *Eating Right to Lower Your High Blood Pressure*, and other materials. National Heart, Lung, and Blood Institute Information Center, PO Box 30105, Bethesda, MD 20824-0105; (301) 251-1222.

*Dietary Guidelines and Your Diet*; *The Food Guide Pyramid*; *Nutrition and Your Health: Dietary Guidelines for Americans* (3rd ed); *Nutritive Value of Foods*, and other materials. Superintendent of Documents, U.S. Government Printing Office, Washington, DC 20402; (202) 783-3238.

**Provider Resources**

*Physician's Guide to Outpatient Nutrition*. American Academy of Family Physicians, 8880 Ward Parkway, Kansas City, MO 64114-2797; 1-800 944-0000.

*Diet, Nutrition and Cancer Prevention: A Guide to Food Choices*. Office of Cancer Communications, National Cancer Institute, Bldg 31, Rm 10A24, Bethesda, Maryland 20892; 1-800 4-CANCER.

*Nutrition Screening Initiative* (Educational material and office aids for screening elderly patients for nutritional deficiencies). Nutrition Screening Initiative, 1010 Wisconsin Avenue NW., Suite 800, Washington, DC 20007; (202) 625-1662. A project of the American Academy of Family Physicians, the American Dietetic Association, and the National Council on the Aging, Inc.

Table 55-2. Examples of Foods To Choose or Decrease for the NCEP Step I* and Step II Diets

| Food Group | Choose | Decrease |
|---|---|---|
| Lean meat, poultry, and fish<br><br>≤5-6 oz. per day | Beef, pork, lamb—lean cuts well trimmed before cooking | Beef, pork, lamb—regular ground beef, fatty cuts, spare ribs, organ meats |
|  | Poultry without skin | Poultry with skin, fried chicken |
|  | Fish, shellfish | Fried fish, fried shellfish |
|  | Processed meat—prepared from lean meat, e.g., lean ham, lean frankfurters, lean meat with soy protein or carrageen | Regular luncheon meat, e.g., bologna, salami, sausage, frankfurters |
| Eggs<br><br>≤4 yolks per week, Step I<br>≤2 yolks per week, Step II | Egg whites (two whites can be substituted for one whole egg in recipes), cholesterol-free egg substitute | Egg yolks (if more than 4 per week on Step I or if more than 2 per week on Step II); includes eggs used in cooking and baking |
| Low-Fat Dairy Products<br><br>2-3 servings per day | Milk—skim, ½%, or 1% fat (fluid, powdered, evaporated), buttermilk | Whole milk (fluid, evaporated, condensed), 2% fat milk (lowfat milk), imitation milk |
|  | Yogurt—nonfat or low-fat yogurt or yogurt beverages | Whole milk yogurt, whole milk yogurt beverages |
| Dairy products | Cheese—low-fat natural or processed cheese | Regular cheeses (American, blue, Brie, cheddar, Colby, Edam, Monterey Jack, whole-milk mozzarella, Parmesan, Swiss), cream cheese, Neufchatel cheese |
|  | Low-fat or nonfat varieties, e.g., cottage cheese—low-fat, nonfat, or dry curd (0% to 2%) | Cottage cheese (4% fat) |
|  | Frozen dairy dessert—ice milk, frozen yogurt (low-fat or nonfat) | Ice cream |
|  | Low-fat coffee creamer | Cream, half & half, whipping cream |
|  | Low-fat or nonfat sour cream | Nondairy creamer, whipped topping, sour cream |

*(Continued)*

**Table 55-2. Examples of Foods To Choose or Decrease for the NCEP Step I\* and Step II Diets—Continued**

| Food Group | Choose | Decrease |
|---|---|---|
| Fats and oils<br><br>≤6-8 teaspoons per day | Unsaturated oils—safflower, sunflower, corn, soybean, cottonseed, canola, olive, peanut | Coconut oil, palm kernel oil, palm oil |
| | Margarine—made from unsaturated oils listed above, light or diet margarine, especially soft or liquid forms | Butter, lard, shortening, bacon fat, hard margarine |
| | Salad dressings—made with unsaturated oils listed above, low-fat or fat-free | Dressings—made with egg yolk, cheese, sour cream, whole milk |
| | Seeds and nuts—peanut butter, other nut butters | Coconut |
| | Cocoa powder | Milk chocolate |
| Breads and Cereals<br><br>6 or more servings per day | Breads—whole-grain bread, English muffins, bagels, buns, corn or flour tortilla | Bread in which eggs, fat, and/or butter are a major ingredient; croissants |
| | Cereals—oat, wheat, corn, multigrain | Most granolas |
| | Pasta | |
| | Rice | |
| | Dry beans and peas | |
| | Crackers, low-fat—animal-type, graham, soda crackers, breadsticks, melba toast | High-fat crackers |
| | Homemade baked goods using unsaturated oil, skim or 1% milk, and egg substitute—quick breads, biscuits, cornbread muffins, bran muffins, pancakes, waffles | Commercial baked pastries, muffins, biscuits |

*(Continued)*

\*Careful selection of processed foods is necessary to stay within the sodium guideline (<2400 mg).

Table 55-2. Examples of Foods To Choose or Decrease for the NCEP Step I* and Step II Diets—Continued

| Food Group | Choose | Decrease |
|---|---|---|
| Soups | Reduced- or low-fat and reduced-sodium varieties, e.g., chicken or beef noodle, minestrone, tomato, vegetable, potato, reduced-fat soups made with skim milk | Soup containing whole milk, cream, meat fat, poultry fat, or poultry skin |
| Vegetables<br><br>3-5 servings per day | Fresh, frozen, or canned, without added fat or sauce | Vegetables fried or prepared with butter, cheese, or cream sauce |
| Fruits<br><br>2-4 servings per day | Fruit—fresh, frozen, canned, or dried<br><br>Fruit juice—fresh, frozen, or canned | Fried fruit or fruit served with butter or cream sauce |
| Sweets and modified-fat desserts | Beverages—fruit-flavored drinks, lemonade, fruit punch | |
| | Sweets—sugar, syrup, honey, jam, preserves, candy made without fat (candy corn, gumdrops, hard candy), fruit-flavored gelatin | Candy made with milk chocolate, coconut oil, palm kernel oil, palm oil |
| | Frozen dessert—low-fat and nonfat yogurt, ice milk, sherbet, sorbet, fruit ice, popsicles | Ice cream and frozen treats made with ice cream |
| | Cookies, cake, pie, pudding—prepared with egg whites, egg substitutes, skim milk or 1% milk, and unsaturated oil or margarine; ginger snaps, fig and other fruit bar cookies, fat-free cookies, angel food cake | Commercial baked pies, cakes, doughnuts, high-fat cookies, cream pies |

*Careful selection of processed foods is necessary to stay within the sodium guideline (<2400 mg).

From: National Cholesterol Education Program. *Second Report of the National Cholesterol Education Program Expert Panel on Detection, Evaluation, and Treatment of High Blood Cholesterol in Adults (Adult Treatment Panel II)*. Bethesda, MD: National Institutes of Health, National Heart, Lung, and Blood Institute. NIH Pub. No. 93-3095, 1993.

## Selected References

American Academy of Family Physicians, Commission on Public Health and Scientific Affairs. *Age Charts for Periodic Health Examinations*. Kansas City, Mo: American Academy of Family Physicians; 1993.

American College of Obstetricians and Gynecologists. *The Obstetrician-Gynecologist and Primary-Preventive Health Care*. Washington, DC: American College of Obstetricians and Gynecologists; 1993.

American College of Physicians. *Nutrition*. Washington, DC: American College of Physicians; 1985. Position paper.

American Heart Association. Dietary guidelines for healthy American adults: a statement for physicians and health professionals by the Nutrition Committee. *Circulation*. 1988;77:721A-724A.

American Medical Association, Counsel on Scientific Affairs. *Medical Evaluation of Healthy Persons*. Chicago, Ill: American Medical Association; 1983.

Ammerman AS, DeVellis RF, Carey TS, et al. Physician-based diet counseling for cholesterol reduction: current practices, determinants, and strategies for improvement. *Prev Med*. 1993;22:96-109.

Block G, Clifford C, Naughton MD, Henderson M, McAdams M. A brief dietary screen for high fat intake. *J. Nutrit Educ*. 1989;21:199-207.

Expert Panel on Detection, Evaluation, and Treatment of High Blood Cholesterol in Adults. Summary of the second report of the National Cholesterol Education Program (NCEP) Expert Panel on Detection, Evaluation, and Treatment of High Blood Cholesterol in Adults (Adult Treatment Panel II). *JAMA*. 1993;269:3015-3023.

Lin-Fu JS, Anthony MA. *Folic Acid and Neural Tube Defects: A Fact Sheet for Health Care Providers*. Rockville, Md: Maternal and Child Health Bureau, Health Resources and Services Administration, Public Health Service; May 1993.

National Cholesterol Education Program. *Report of the Expert Panel on Population Strategies for Blood Cholesterol Reduction*. Bethesda, Md: National Institutes of Health, National Heart, Lung, and Blood Institute; 1990. US Dept of Health and Human Services, Public Health Service, publication NIH 90-3046.

National Cholesterol Education Program. *Second Report of the National Cholesterol Education Program Expert Panel on Detection, Evaluation, and Treatment of High Blood Cholesterol in Adults (Adult Treatment Panel II)*. Bethesda, MD: National Institutes of Health, National Heart, Lung, and Blood Institute. NIH Pub. No. 93-3095, 1993.

National Task Force on the Prevention and Treatment of Obesity. Very low-calorie diets. *JAMA*. 1993;270:967-974.

US Department of Health and Human Services. *Surgeon General's Report on Nutrition and Health*. Washington, DC: Dept. of Health and Human Services, 1988. DHHS Publication PHS 88-50210.

US Food and Drug Administration. The new food label. *FDA Backgrounder*. Dec 10, 1992:1-9.

US Preventive Services Task Force. Nutrition counseling. In: *Guide to Clinical Preventive Services*. Baltimore, Md: Williams & Wilkins; 1989:chap 50.

## Adults/Older Adults — COUNSELING

# 56. Physical Activity

Physical inactivity is associated with many of the leading causes of death and disability in the United States, including coronary heart disease, hypertension, noninsulin-dependent diabetes mellitus, obesity, osteoporosis, and falls. Regular exercise reduces cardiovascular disease risk, promotes weight loss and control, improves musculoskeletal functioning, helps prevent diabetes, and may help prevent bone loss with aging. Even light exercise is beneficial for health. Less than half of the adult population exercises 3 or more days per week for at least 20 minutes. Less than 20% of adults exercise vigorously and frequently enough to produce cardiopulmonary conditioning benefits. Most older adults also do not exercise sufficiently to improve muscle strength and flexibility, aspects of fitness particularly important for their health.

Surveys of primary care clinicians indicate that only about 30% routinely provide counseling on physical activity to their sedentary patients. Some studies suggest that physical exercise counseling can be provided by primary care clinicians with limited time and effort. If needed, there are an increasing number of well-trained exercise physiologists and rehabilitation specialists to whom patients can be referred for evaluation and in-depth counseling.

**Recommendations of Major Authorities**

- **American Academy of Family Physicians, American College of Obstetricians and Gynecologists, U.S. Department of Health and Human Services**, and **U.S. Preventive Services Task Force (USPSTF)**—Providers should routinely assess patients' physical activity practices and counsel them in engaging in a program of regular physical activity that is tailored to their health status and life-style. **USPSTF** recommends that women receive counseling regarding the use of weight-bearing exercise to help prevent postmenopausal osteoporosis. **Canadian Task Force on the Periodic Health Examination** states that, although evidence is preliminary, exercise may help prevent osteoporosis.

**Basics of Physical Activity Counseling**

1. All patients should be asked about their physical activity habits, including both organized (i.e., sports and exercise) and general activities (i.e., house and yard work, walking).

2. An assessment should be made as to whether the patient's activities are sufficient to confer health benefits. The American College of Sports Medicine (ACSM) has issued guidelines for different types of activity.

    - *General Activity:* Every patient should accumulate 30 minutes or more of moderate-intensity physical activity on most days of the week (5 days per week is a suggested goal). Activities that can contribute to the 30-minute total include walking up stairs (instead of taking the elevator), gardening, raking leaves, dancing, and walking part or all of the way to work. The recommended 30 minutes of physical activity may also come from planned exercise or recreation. This recommendation has also been endorsed by the Centers for Disease Control and Prevention.

- *Organized Activity:* In order to confer health benefits, sports and exercise should involve use of large muscle groups in a prolonged, rhythmic manner for at least 15 minutes, at least 3 days per week, at moderate or greater intensity. Additional fitness benefits are expected to accrue to those who exercise at least 20 minutes, at least 4 days per week at moderate or greater intensity. There are several methods for assessing intensity of exercise; the simplest involves measurement of heart rate. According to ACSM, moderate intensity for health benefits should be defined as maintaining a heart rate that is at least 55% of maximum for age; for building fitness, moderate intensity should be defined as maintaining a heart rate of at least 60% of maximum for age. ACSM has recommended that for routine exercise and sports that heart rate not exceed 90% of maximum for age. See Table 56-1 for heart rate values according to age.

3. Patients lacking sufficient activity for health benefits and those wishing to improve physical activity habits should be assisted in planning a program of physical activity. Such a program should be:

- *Medically Safe:* Heart disease is the biggest risk. ACSM has issued guidelines for assessing coronary risk factors, symptoms, and age with regard to participation in exercise programs and the need for exercise tolerance testing for those significantly increasing their level of exercise (see Tables 56-2, 56-3, 56-4). Some authorities, including the American College of Cardiology and American Heart Association, have questioned the utility of exercise tolerance testing for asymptomatic individuals. Patients who have been sedentary, however, should increase their level of exercise gradually, rather than abruptly. The potential for musculoskeletal injury must also be assessed in planning an exercise program. Alternate-day exercise and the use of stretching exercises in the warm-up and cool-down phases of exercise sessions will decrease the risk of musculoskeletal injuries. This is particularly important for older adults and those who have not been physically active recently.

- *Enjoyable:* Patients will not continue activities that they do not enjoy. Patients should be counseled to choose activities they find inherently pleasurable, to vary activities, and to share activities with friends or family. They should be encouraged to identify barriers to enjoyment and ways to overcome these barriers. See Table 56-5 for examples of methods to overcome barriers.

- *Convenient:* Expensive or specialized equipment and facilities, long commutes, and inflexible hours can be significant barriers. Activities that can be enjoyed with a minimum of special preparation, ideally those that fit into daily activities, should be encouraged. The effort should go into the exercise, not the preparation.

- *Realistic:* A program that is too difficult in terms of goals and integration with other daily activities will lead to disappointment. The importance of gradual increases in intensity, frequency, and duration that can be accomplished without too much difficulty should be stressed. Use of an exercise log may help patients keep track of gradual progress toward attainable goals.

- *Structured:* Having defined activities, goals for performance, and a set schedule and location may help improve some patients' compliance. Signing a physical activity "contract" may be helpful for some patients. Too much structure may cause some patients to lose interest, however. This should be individualized for each patient.

4. Even patients who are unwilling or unable to participate in a regular exercise program should be encouraged to increase the amount of physical activity in their daily lives. Examples include: taking the stairs rather than the elevator when possible; leaving the subway or bus one or two stops early and walking the rest of the way; doing household chores and yard work on a regular basis; and substituting walking or bicycling for driving whenever convenient.

5. Nursing and office staff should be involved in monitoring patient progress and providing information and support to patients. Some form of routine follow-up with patients about their progress is very helpful in physical activity counseling.

6. Posters, displays, videotapes, and other resources should be used to create an office or clinic environment that conveys positive messages about exercise and physical activity.

7. Providers should get adequate physical activity themselves. Studies show that providers who exercise regularly themselves are significantly better at providing exercise counseling to their patients.

**Patient Resources**

*Pep Up Your Life: A Fitness Book for Seniors.* American Association of Retired Persons, Fulfillment Services, 601 E Street NW, Washington, DC 20049; (202) 434-2277.

*Exercise and Fitness: A Guide for Women.* American College of Obstetricians and Gynecologists, 409 12th St. SW, Washington, DC 20024; 1-800 762-2264.

*ACSM Fitness Book.* American College of Sports Medicine. Leisure Press, PO Box 5076, Champaign, IL 61825-5076; 1-800 747-4475.

*Fitness Fundamentals and the Presidential Sports Award*, and other materials. President's Council on Physical Fitness and Sports, 701 Pennsylvania Ave. NW, Suite 250, Washington, DC 20004; (202) 272-3430.

## Ch. 56. Physical Activity — Adults/Older Adults — COUNSELING

**Table 56-1. Heart Rates (Beats/Minute) According to Age***

| Age (Years) | 55% of Maximum[a] | 60% of Maximum[b] | 90% of Maximum[c] | Maximum[d] |
|---|---|---|---|---|
| 20 | 110 | 120 | 180 | 200 |
| 25 | 107 | 117 | 177 | 195 |
| 30 | 104 | 114 | 173 | 190 |
| 35 | 102 | 111 | 168 | 185 |
| 40 | 99 | 108 | 163 | 180 |
| 45 | 96 | 105 | 159 | 175 |
| 50 | 93 | 102 | 153 | 170 |
| 55 | 91 | 99 | 149 | 165 |
| 60 | 88 | 96 | 143 | 160 |
| 65 | 85 | 93 | 140 | 155 |
| 70 | 82 | 90 | 135 | 150 |
| 75 | 80 | 87 | 132 | 145 |
| 80 | 77 | 84 | 129 | 140 |

*This formula is only an approximation of any individual's response and will not apply when certain rate-altering medications are being taken, such as beta-blockers and some calcium antagonists.

[a] Minimum exercise heart rate for health benefit designated by ACSM

[b] Minimum exercise heart rate for fitness designated by ACSM

[c] Maximum exercise heart rate designated by ACSM

[d] Maximum average heart rate adjusted for age (according to formula: maximum=220−age)

Adapted from: American College of Sports Medicine, Preventive and Rehabilitative Exercise Committee. *Guidelines for Exercise Testing and Prescription.* 4th ed. Philadelphia, PA: Lea & Febiger; 1991. Used with permission of Lea & Febiger; copyright © 1991.

---

**Table 56-2. Major Coronary Risk Factors**

Diagnosed hypertension or systolic blood pressure ≥160 mm Hg or diastolic blood pressure ≥90 mm Hg on at least two separate occasions, or on antihypertensive medications

Serum cholesterol ≥240 mg/dL (≥6.2 mmol/L), HDL ≤35 mg/dL

Cigarette smoking

Diabetes mellitus*

Family history of coronary or atherosclerotic disease in parents or siblings prior to age 55

*Persons with insulin-dependent diabetes mellitus (IDDM) who are over 30 years of age or have had IDDM for more than 15 years, and persons with noninsulin-dependent diabetes mellitus (NIDDM) who are over 35 years of age should be classified as patients with disease and treated according to the guidelines in Table 56-4.

Adapted from: American College of Sports Medicine, Preventive and Rehabilitative Exercise Committee. *Guidelines for Exercise Testing and Prescription.* 4th ed. Philadelphia, PA: Lea & Febiger; 1991. Used with permission of Lea & Febiger; copyright © 1991.

## Ch. 56. Physical Activity — Adults/Older Adults — COUNSELING

**Table 56-3. Major Symptoms and Signs Suggestive of Cardiopulmonary or Metabolic Disease***

| |
|---|
| Pain or discomfort in the chest or surrounding areas that appears to be ischemic in nature |
| Unaccustomed shortness of breath or shortness of breath with mild exertion |
| Dizziness or syncope |
| Orthopnea/paroxysmal nocturnal dyspnea |
| Ankle edema |
| Palpitations or tachycardia |
| Claudication |
| Known heart murmur** |

*These symptoms must be interpreted in the clinical context in which they appear, since they are not all specific for cardiopulmonary or metabolic disease.

**Of organic type

Adapted from: American College of Sports Medicine, Preventive and Rehabilitative Exercise Committee. *Guidelines for Exercise Testing and Prescription.* 4th ed. Philadelphia, PA: Lea & Febiger; 1991. Used with permission of Lea & Febiger; copyright © 1991.

**Table 56-4. ACSM Guidelines for Medical Examination and Diagnostic Exercise Testing Prior to Beginning an Exercise Program**

| Medical examination and diagnostic exercise test recommended prior to: | Apparently Healthy — Age ≤40 years (men) ≤50 years (women) | Apparently Healthy — Age >40 years (men) >50 years (women) | Higher Risk[a] — No Symptoms | Higher Risk[a] — Symptoms | With Disease[b] |
|---|---|---|---|---|---|
| Moderate exercise[c] | No | No | No | Yes | Yes |
| Vigorous exercise[d] | No | Yes | Yes | Yes | Yes |

[a] Individuals with 2 or more coronary risk factors (Table 56-2) or symptoms (Table 56-3)

[b] Individuals with known cardiac, pulmonary, or metabolic disease

[c] Moderate exercise—exercise intensity well within the individual's current capacity and that can be comfortably sustained for a prolonged period of time (i.e. 60 minutes), slow progression, and generally noncompetitive

[d] Vigorous exercise—exercise intense enough to represent a substantial challenge and that would ordinarily result in fatigue within 20 minutes

Adapted from: American College of Sports Medicine, Preventive and Rehabilitative Exercise Committee. *Guidelines for Exercise Testing and Prescription.* 4th ed. Philadelphia, PA: Lea & Febiger; 1991. Used with permission of Lea & Febiger; copyright © 1991.

**Table 56-5. Overcoming Barriers to Exercise**

| Barrier | Suggested Response |
|---|---|
| Exercise is hard work. | Pick an activity that you enjoy and that is easy for you. |
| I do not have the time. | We are only talking about three 20-minute sessions per week. Could you do without three TV shows each week? |
| I am usually too tired for exercise. | Tell yourself, "This activity will give me more energy." See if it doesn't happen. |
| I hate to fail, so I will not start. | Physical activity is not a test. You will not fail if you choose an activity you like and start off slowly. |
| I do not have anyone to work out with. | Maybe you have not asked. A neighbor or a coworker may be a willing partner. Or you can choose an activity that you enjoy doing by yourself. |
| There is not a convenient place. | Pick an activity you can do at a convenient place. Walk around your neighborhood or do exercises with a TV show or a videotape at home. |
| I am afraid of being injured. | Walking is very safe and is excellent exercise. Choose a safe, well-lit area. |
| The weather is too bad. | There are many activities that you can do in your own home, in any weather. |
| Exercise is boring. | Listening to music during your activity keeps your mind occupied. Walking, biking, or running can take you past lots of interesting things. |
| I am too overweight. | You can benefit regardless of your weight. Pick an activity that you are comfortable with, like walking. |
| I am too old. | It is never too late to start. People of any age, including older people, can benefit from physical exercise. |

Adapted from: Project PACE, *Physician-based Assessment and Counseling for Exercise*. San Diego, CA: San Diego State University; 1991. Used with permission of the publisher; copyright © 1991.

## Provider Resources

*The Physician's Rx: Exercise.* President's Council on Physical Fitness and Sports, 701 Pennsylvania Ave. NW, Suite 250, Washington, DC 20004; (202) 272-3430.

*Physician-based Assessment and Counseling for Exercise.* Project PACE, San Diego State University, San Diego, CA 92182-0567; (619) 594-5949.

## Selected References

American Academy of Family Physicians, Commission on Public Health and Scientific Affairs. *Age Charts for Periodic Health Examination*. Kansas City, Mo: American Academy of Family Physicians; 1993.

American College of Cardiology and American Heart Association. Guidelines for exercise testing. *Circulation*. 1986;74:653A-667A.

American College of Obstetricians and Gynecologists. *The Obstetrician-Gynecologist and Primary-Preventive Health Care*. Washington, DC: American College of Obstetricians and Gynecologists; 1993.

American College of Obstetricians and Gynecologists. *Women and Exercise*. Washington, DC: American College of Obstetricians and Gynecologists; 1985. Technical bulletin 173.

American College of Sports Medicine, Preventive and Rehabilitative Exercise Committee. *Guidelines for Exercise Testing and Prescription*. 4th ed. Philadelphia, Pa: Lea & Febiger; 1991.

American College of Sports Medicine. The recommended quantity and quality of exercise for developing and maintaining cardiorespiratory and muscular fitness in health adults. *Med Sci Sports Exerc*. 1990;22:265-274.

Canadian Task Force on the Periodic Health Examination. The periodic health examination: 2. 1987 update. *Can Med Assoc J*. 1988;138:618-626

Centers for Disease Control and Prevention. Prevalence of sedentary lifestyle—Behavioral Risk Factor Surveillance System, United States, 1991. *MMWR*. 1993:42:576-579.

Harris SS, Caspersen CJ, DeFriese GH, Estes EH. Physical activity counseling for healthy adults as a primary preventive intervention in the clinical setting. *JAMA*. 1989;261:3590-3598.

King AC, Blair SN, Bild DE, et al. Determinants of physical activity and interventions in adults. *Med Sci Sports Exerc*. 1992;24(suppl):S221-S236.

Haskell WL, Leon AS, Caspersen CJ, et al. Cardiovascular benefits and assessment of physical activity and physical fitness in adults. *Med Sci Sports Exerc*. 1992;24(suppl):S201-S215.

Lewis BS, Lynch WD. The effect of physician advice on exercise behavior. *Prev Med*. 1993;22:110-121.

US Dept of Health and Human Services. Physical activity and fitness. In: *Healthy People 2000: National Health Promotion and Disease Prevention Objectives*. Washington DC: US Dept of Health and Human Services, Public Health Service; 1991:part II, chap 1. USDHHS publication PHS 91-50212.

US Preventive Services Task Force. Exercise counseling. In: *Guide to Clinical Preventive Services*. Baltimore, Md: Williams & Wilkins; 1989:chap 49.

# Adults/Older Adults — COUNSELING

## 57. Polypharmacy

Polypharmacy, the prescribing of multiple drugs for a patient, is most common in older adults because they tend to have more illnesses for which medications are prescribed. Adults aged 65 years and older comprise 12% of the population but consume 30% of all prescription medications. Nonprescription drug use among patients over age 65 years is seven times that of the general population. The incidence of adverse drug reactions increases with age and the number of drugs taken. Older adults make many mistakes in taking medications due to deteriorating vision and cognitive function, often with serious consequences. Up to 10% of all hospital admissions for patients over 65 years of age involve medication toxicity. Clinicians contribute significantly to the problem by not taking into account changes in drug metabolism that occur with aging. Renal and hepatic function decrease with age, slowing the clearance of medications. Increases in the proportion of body fat and decreases in the proportion of body water that occur with aging lead to an accumulation of fat-soluble medications in adipose tissue and increases in the concentration of hydrophilic medications in the blood.

Polypharmacy can occur in younger patients as well. As the number of symptoms and diseases increases in an individual, so does the risk of polypharmacy and the attendant risk of overmedication and adverse effects.

### Recommendations of Major Authorities

- **American Academy of Family Physicians**—Providers should assess the use of prescription and nonprescription medication by older adults during periodic health examinations.

- **American College of Obstetricians and Gynecologists**—Clinicians should assess the use of prescription and nonprescription medications by women 65 years of age and older at each periodic health evaluation (annually or as appropriate).

- **American Nurses Association**—Clinicians should maintain a drug profile on older adults to evaluate/monitor for unnecessary and excessive drug use.

- **Public Health Service, U.S. Department of Health and Human Services**—Clinicians should routinely review all prescribed and over-the-counter medications with patients aged 65 years and older each time a new medication is prescribed.

### Basics of Polypharmacy Counseling

1. Flow sheets or summary lists should be used in patient charts to document prescription and nonprescription medication dosages, frequencies, dates of use, and adverse reactions. A computerized medication list, if available, is helpful for this purpose.

2. Patients should be encouraged to keep an up-to-date list of medications with dosage and usage schedules. Older adults, particularly if visually or cognitively impaired, should be asked to bring all medications for inspection at each health-care visit.

3. Patients should be asked about alcohol and other "recreational" substance use that may interact with medications.

4. All patients and caretakers should be informed of the possible side effects and symptoms of toxicity caused by medications. Printed information sheets are helpful for this purpose.

5. Potential medication interactions should be evaluated each time a new medication is prescribed or dosages of existing medications are changed. There are several good printed references and software programs for this purpose. If available, computerized medication monitoring systems are very helpful.

6. Consideration should be given to discontinuing any medications that have not shown clear benefit in well-designed studies or for the individual patient. Prescribing medications for minor or self-limiting symptoms that may be treated safely with counseling and reassurance should be avoided. Medication regimens should be simplified whenever possible. Colley and Lucas (1993) have proposed helpful guidelines to simplify medication regimens. See Table 57-1.

7. In older adults, consideration should be given to reducing initial dosage of medication to as little as one half the usual adult dosage, unless an initial high plasma concentration is needed—as with antibiotics and certain cardiac medications. The longer time needed to reach therapeutic effect should be weighed against the risk of toxicity.

**Table 57-1. How To Simplify the Medication Regimen**

**Eliminate pharmacologic duplication**
Avoid combinations that augment side effects
Avoid combinations that duplicate therapy
Use monotherapy to manage multiple diseases when possible
Avoid drugs that can exacerbate the patient's other medical conditions

**Decrease dosing frequency**
Choose the best medication for the patient with the least frequent dosing interval
Consider sustained-release formulations (beware of cost)

**Review drug regimens regularly**
Include *all* medications, over-the-counter as well as from *all* health care providers
Ask the following questions:
- Is the patient taking the medication as prescribed?
- Are all agents still needed?
- Can the regimen be simplified?

Adapted from: Colley CA, Lucas LM. Polypharmacy: the cure becomes the disease. *J Gen Intern Med.* 1993;8:278-283. Used with permission from Hanley & Belfus, Inc.; copyright ©1993.

8. Particular caution should be used with older adults in prescribing medications with the following characteristics:

- Central nervous system effects.
- Anticholinergic side effects.
- Long half-lives.

## Patient Resources

*Food and Drug Interactions.* American Pharmaceutical Association, 2215 Constitution Ave. NW, Washington, DC 20037; (202) 628-4410.

*Age Page—Safe Use of Medicines by Older People*; *Age Page—Safe Use of Tranquilizers by Older People.* National Institute on Aging, Bldg 31, Rm 5C27, Bethesda, MD 20892; (301) 496-1752.

## Provider Resources

*Medicine Counseling Kit.* National Council on Patient Information and Education, 666 11th St. NW, Suite 810, Washington, DC 20001; (202) 347-6711.

## Selected References

American Academy of Family Physicians, Commission on Public Health and Scientific Affairs. *Age Charts for Periodic Health Examination.* Kansas City, Mo: American Academy of Family Physicians; 1993.

American College of Obstetricians and Gynecologists. *The Obstetrician-Gynecologist and Primary-Preventive Health Care.* Washington, DC: American College of Obstetricians and Gynecologists; 1993.

Beers MH, Ouslander JG. Risk factors in geriatric drug prescribing: a practical guide to avoiding problems. *Drugs.* 1989;37:105.

Colley CA, Lucas LM. Polypharmacy: the cure becomes the disease. *J Gen Intern Med.* 1993;8:278-283.

Everitt DE, Avorn J. Drug prescribing for the elderly. *Arch Intern Med.* 1986;146:2393-2396.

Porter J, Jick H. Drug-related deaths among inpatients. *JAMA.* 1977;237:879-881.

Royal College of General Physicians. Medication for the elderly. *J Roy Coll Physicians London.* 1984;18:7-17.

Williamson J, Chopin JM. Adverse reactions to prescribed drugs in the elderly: a multicenter investigation. *Age Aging.* 1980;9:73.

World Health Organization. Health care in the elderly: report of the technical group on use of medicaments by the elderly. *Drugs.* 1981;22:279.

US Dept of Health and Human Services. Food and drug safety. In: *Healthy People 2000: National Health Promotion and Disease Prevention Objectives.* Washington DC: US Dept of Health and Human Services, Public Health Service; 1991:part II, chap 12. USDHHS publication PHS 91-50212.

Adults/Older Adults — COUNSELING

# 58. Sexually Transmitted Diseases and HIV Infection

Almost 12 million cases of sexually transmitted diseases (STDs) occur annually in the United States, 86% of them in people aged 15 through 29 years. In addition to syphilis and gonorrhea, the list of STDs now includes human immunodeficiency virus (HIV), *Chlamydia trachomatis* infections, genital herpes, human papillomavirus, chancroid, genital mycoplasmas, cytomegalovirus, hepatitis B, vaginitis, enteric infections, and ectoparasitic diseases. Chlamydia is the most common STD, causing an estimated 4 million acute infections annually. Although the incidence of gonorrhea and syphilis has been decreasing in the early 1990s, they remain a persistent public health problem.

Acquired immunodeficiency syndrome (AIDS) is the ninth leading cause of death in the United States and the third leading cause of death among those aged 25 to 44 years. It is the sixth leading cause of years of potential life lost in the United States. Over 1 million people in the United States are infected with HIV. There is currently no available cure for AIDS, although treatment can delay symptom onset.

Women and children suffer a heavy burden from STDs. Apart from AIDS and subsequent death, the most serious complications for women are pelvic inflammatory disease (PID), an increased risk of cervical cancer, ectopic pregnancy, congenital infections and malformations, the delivery of premature and low birth weight infants, and fetal death. The poor, medically underserved, and racial and ethnic minorities also incur a disproportionate share of STDs and subsequent disabilities.

Individuals at increased risk for STDs and HIV infection are: 1) those who are contacts of, or have a previous history of, documented STD/HIV infection; 2) pregnant women; 3) individuals who are or were recently sexually active, especially those with multiple sexual partners; 4) individuals living in areas with a high prevalence of HIV/STDs; 5) homosexual or bisexual men; 6) drug and alcohol abusers; and 7) those involved in the exchange of sex for drugs or money.

Refer to chapters with related information on screening for STDs and HIV infection (chapter 39), counseling of children and adolescents on STDs and HIV infection (chapter 22), and counseling to prevent unintended pregnancy among adolescents (chapter 24) and adults (chapter 60).

### Recommendations of Major Authorities

- **American Academy of Family Physicians**—The periodic health examination for all individuals between the ages of 19 and 64 years of age should include counseling regarding STDs, partner selection, condoms, anal intercourse, unintended pregnancy, and contraceptive options.

- **American College of Obstetricians and Gynecologists (ACOG)**—HIV testing and counseling should be offered to all pregnant women, and should be strongly recommended for high-risk women (where seroprevalence is known to be 1 per 1000, or who engage in high-risk behavior), whether pregnant or not, and repeat testing should be offered for women seronegative less than six months after the last potential exposure.

- **ACOG** and **American College of Physicians**—Patients should be counseled on measures to prevent STDs.

- **Centers for Disease Control and Prevention**—Latex condoms should be made more widely available by health care providers in STD, family planning, and drug treatment clinics. HIV seronegative pregnant women and women of childbearing age who are at increased risk of becoming infected with HIV should receive additional counseling regarding the maternal and fetal risks associated with pregnancy should they become infected; they also should be advised to delay pregnancy. STD and HIV screening should be offered to high-risk individuals; counselors should take advantage of all available opportunities to provide clients with HIV-prevention messages. HIV pretest counseling must include a personalized client-risk assessment and should result in a personalized plan for the client to reduce the risk of HIV infection.

- **U.S. Preventive Services Task Force (USPSTF)**—Clinicians should take a complete sexual and drug history from all adolescent and adult patients. Patients should be advised that the most effective methods for preventing STD or HIV infection are sexual abstinence and maintaining a mutually monogamous sexual relationship with a partner known to be uninfected. Patients should be counseled about the proper use and limitations of condoms, and the health risks of anal intercourse. Injection drug users should be counseled to enroll in a treatment program and warned about the risks of needle sharing and the need to use sterile needles and syringes. Patients should be advised that a negative HIV test does not conclusively preclude HIV infection, especially if the patient or his/her partner has not been monogamous during the previous 6 months. All patients should be offered testing consistent with **USPSTF** recommendations for screening for syphilis, gonorrhea, chlamydia, genital herpes, hepatitis B, and HIV infection (see chapter 39).

## Basics of STD and HIV Counseling

1. Every patient's risk for STDs, including HIV infection, should be determined with a thorough sexual and drug history. Table 58-1 presents examples of questions for taking clinical histories about sexual behavior, contraceptive use, and drug use. The exact wording of questions should be tailored to individual patients.

2. Patients should be informed that HIV is transmitted by sexual intercourse, sharing needles, and infected blood. It can also be transmitted by an infected mother to her baby during pregnancy, birth, or very rarely, breast-feeding.

3. All patients should be advised that any unprotected sexual behavior poses a risk for STDs and HIV infection. A person who is infected can infect others during sexual intercourse, even if no symptoms are present. Patients should be cautioned to avoid sexual intercourse with people who may be infected with HIV, such as those who have injected drugs, people with multiple or anonymous sex partners, or people who have had any STD within the past 10 years even if they have no symptoms. Decisions about sexual intercourse should not be made while under the influence of alcohol or other drugs that cloud judgment and cause people to take risks that could put them in danger of becoming infected with STDs or HIV.

## Table 58-1. Examples of Questions for Taking Clinical Histories About Sexual Behavior and Drug Use

**Sexual Behaviors**
Are you currently or were you recently in a sexual relationship?
Do you have sex with men, women, or both?
How many men or women did you have sex with in the last week, last month, last year?
How often do you have sex with each man or woman?
Is each partner new, casual, or regular?
Have any of your partners been men who have had sex with other men?
Have any of your partners injected (shot) drugs?
Have you had sex with someone that you know or suspect has HIV?

**Drug Use Behaviors**
What type of prescription drugs are you taking?
Do you drink alcohol? How much and how often do you drink alcohol?
Have you ever taken or used a drug that was not prescribed for you—narcotics, marijuana, cocaine or "crack"?
Have you ever injected (shot) drugs?
Which drugs did you inject?
How often did you inject each drug in the last week, last month, last year?
Do you ever share needles, syringes, or "works"?
How often do you share?
Do you ever clean needles, syringes, or "works"?
How do you clean?
Do you clean needles, syringes, or "works" with bleach?

Adapted from: Gerber AR, Valdiserri RO, Holtgrave DR, et al. Preventive services guidelines for primary care clinicians caring for HIV-infected adults and adolescents. *Arch Fam Med.* 1993;2:969-979.

4. All patients should be counseled that STDs and HIV infection are best prevented by:

   - Abstinence.

   - Limiting sexual relationships to those between mutually monogamous partners known to be HIV-negative.

   - Avoiding sex with high-risk partners.

   - Avoiding anal intercourse.

   - Using latex condoms if having sex with anyone other than a single mutually monogamous partner known to be HIV-negative.

5. Patients should be reminded that partners can transmit infection even if the male withdraws before ejaculating and even if they only have oral sex.

6. Patients should be cautioned that the risk of HIV infection is increased through coinfection with other STDs, such as syphilis, genital herpes, and gonorrhea.

7. All sexually active patients should be counseled about the effective use and limitations of condoms, stressing that they are not foolproof, must be used properly, and may break during intercourse. The best preventive measure against transmission of HIV and other STDs, after abstinence, is the use of latex condoms (**not** "lambskin" or natural membrane condoms). Even under optimal conditions, however, condoms are not always effective in preventing disease transmission. Condom failures occur at an estimated rate of 10% to 15%, either as a result of product failure (i.e., breakage) or incorrect or inconsistent use. Guidelines for condom use can be found in Table 22-1.

8. Providers should dispel myths about HIV virus transmission by informing patients that they **cannot** become infected from mosquito bites; toilet seats or other everyday objects, such as doorknobs, telephones, or drinking fountains; or casual contact with someone who is infected with HIV or has AIDS, such as shaking hands, hugging, or a kiss on the cheek.

9. Patient-centered interviewing and counseling techniques should be used when assessing, informing, and advising about STDs and HIV prevention:

   - A trusting, caring relationship should be established with the patient in order to enhance the efficacy of counseling on safer sex practices and risks for STD and HIV infection.

   - The clinician should listen carefully to the patient in order to identify specific prevention needs, to provide appropriate assistance, and to avoid lecturing the patient.

   - Counseling should be culturally appropriate: Information and services should be presented in a style and format that is sensitive to the culture, values, and traditions of the patient.

   - Counseling should be sensitive to issues of sexual orientation.

   - Information and services should be provided at a level of comprehension consistent with the age and learning skills of the patient, using a dialect and terminology consistent with the patient's language and communication style.

10. All patients should be counseled to avoid injection drug use. Providers should be prepared to refer patients to drug treatment centers if necessary. Patients who use injection drugs should be reminded never to share needles, syringes, or any part of their "works" with another person. Before each use, injection drug users can clean their needles and syringes with full-strength household bleach, as follows: Draw up enough bleach to completely fill the syringe; let it stay in the syringe for at least 1 full minute; empty the syringe and rinse the bleach out well using clean water.

11. Providers should contact the state or local health agency responsible for communicable disease reporting to determine local prevalence of HIV and other STD infections. This agency also can provide information regarding state and local laws regulating patient testing and confidentiality. Requirements regarding which infections to report, when, and to whom, may vary from state to state.

## Patient Resources

*9 Common Sexually Transmitted Diseases.* American Council for Healthful Living, 439 Main St., Orange, NJ 07050; (201) 674-7476.

*HIV and AIDS; Giving and Receiving Blood; Testing for HIV Infection; Women, Sex, and HIV; Teenagers and AIDS.* American Red Cross; to order, contact local Red Cross chapter or American Red Cross Office of HIV-AIDS Education; (202) 973-6000.

*HIV in America: A Profile of the Challenges Facing Americans Living With HIV.* National Association of People Living with AIDS, 1413 K St. NW, Washington, DC 20005; (202) 898-0435.

*Condoms and Sexually Transmitted Diseases...Especially AIDS*, and many other materials. National AIDS Information Hot Line: 1-800 342-AIDS (English speaking); 1-800 344-SIDA (Spanish speaking); 1-800 AIDS-TTY (hearing impaired). All phone calls are confidential.

*Surgeon General's Report to the American Public on HIV Infection and AIDS* and many other materials. CDC National AIDS Information Clearinghouse, PO Box 6003, Rockville, MD 20850; 1-800 458-5231 (English and Spanish).

*National STD Hot Line*: 1-800 227-8922.

## Provider Resources

*Genital Human Papillomavirus Infections* (technical bulletin 105); *Gonorrhea and Chlamydia Infections* (technical bulletin 89); *Gynecologic Herpes Simplex Virus Infection* (technical bulletin 119). American College of Obstetricians and Gynecologists, 409 12th St. SW, Washington, DC 20024; 1-800 762-2264.

## Selected References

American Academy of Family Physicians, Commission on Public Health and Scientific Affairs. *Age Charts for Periodic Health Examination.* Kansas City, Mo: American Academy of Family Physicians; 1993.

American College of Obstetricians and Gynecologists. *Prevention of Human Immune Deficiency Virus Infection and Acquired Immune Deficiency Syndrome: Statement of Committee on Obstetrics: Maternal and Fetal Medicine and Gynecologic Practice.* Washington, DC: American College of Obstetricians and Gynecologists; 1987.

American College of Physicians. Acquired immunodeficiency syndrome. *Ann Intern Med.* 1986; 104:575-581.

American Medical Association. Prevention and control of acquired immunodeficiency syndrome: an interim report. *JAMA.* 1987; 258:2097-2103. Board of Trustees Report.

Centers for Disease Control. Sexually transmitted diseases treatment guidelines. *MMWR.* 1989;38 (S-8):1-43.

Centers for Disease Control. CDC estimates of HIV prevalence and projected AIDS cases: summary of a workshop, October 31-November 1, 1989. *MMWR.* 1990;39:110-112, 117-119.

Gerber AR, Valdiserri RO, Holtgrave DR, et al. Preventive services guidelines for primary care clinicians caring for HIV-infected adults and adolescents. *Arch Fam Med.* 1993;2:969-979.

Higgins DL, Galavotti C, O'Reilly KR, et al. Evidence for the effects of HIV antibody counseling and testing on risk behaviors. *JAMA.* 1991; 266:2419-2429.

Janssen RS, Sattan GA, Critchley SE. HIV infection among patients in U.S. acute care hospitals: strategies for the counseling and testing of hospital patients. *N Engl J Med.* 1992;327:445-452.

US Department of Health and Human Services. Sexually transmitted diseases. In: *Healthy People 2000: National Health Promotion and Disease Prevention Objectives.* Washington, DC: US Dept of Health and Human Services, Public Health Service; 1991:chap 19. USDHHS publication PHS 91-50212.

## Adults/Older Adults — COUNSELING

# 59. Smoking Cessation

Smoking is the leading cause of preventable death in the United States. Approximately 430,000 people die of tobacco-related causes annually. Smoking cessation is the single most important patient counseling topic because of its potential for patient benefit. Fig 59-1 shows the benefits of smoking cessation for different parts of the smoker's body. There is also evidence that exposure of nonsmokers to environmental tobacco smoke leads to lung cancer and possibly coronary heart disease. The exposure of children to environmental tobacco smoke leads to increased rates of chronic middle ear effusions, pneumonia, and other respiratory tract infections.

Primary care clinicians can play a key role in helping patients quit smoking. Even very simple interventions by primary care clinicians can lead to 5% to 10% long-term quit rates. More extensive interventions, including the use of nicotine gum and patches, can lead to rates that are significantly higher. If all primary care providers made even simple interventions with smoking patients, the national smoking cessation rate could be doubled. Recent studies indicate, however, that fewer than half of smoking patients receive any assistance in quitting from their health care providers.

For information on counseling children and adolescents on prevention of tobacco use, refer to chapter 23. Other related chapters include counseling on dental and oral health for children and adolescents (chapter 18) and adults (chapter 53), and counseling on alcohol and other drug abuse for children and adolescents (chapter 17) and adults (chapter 52).

### Recommendations of Major Authorities

- All major authorities, including **American Academy of Family Physicians**, **American Cancer Society**, **American College of Obstetricians and Gynecologists**, **American College of Physicians**, **Canadian Task Force on the Periodic Health Examination**, **National Heart, Lung, and Blood Institute**, **National Cancer Institute**, **National Institute of Dental Research**, and **U.S. Preventive Services Task Force**—Clinicians should provide smoking cessation counseling, treatment, and referral to patients who smoke.

- Several major authorities, including **Joint Commission on Accreditation of Healthcare Organizations**—Smoking should be prohibited in health-care facilities.

Ch. 59. Smoking Cessation  Adults/Older Adults — COUNSELING

**Figure 59-1. Benefits of Smoking Cessation**

**Key**
"CS" refers to continuing smokers,
"NS" refers to never smokers.

**Cervical Cancer** risk reduced compared to "CS" a few years after quitting.

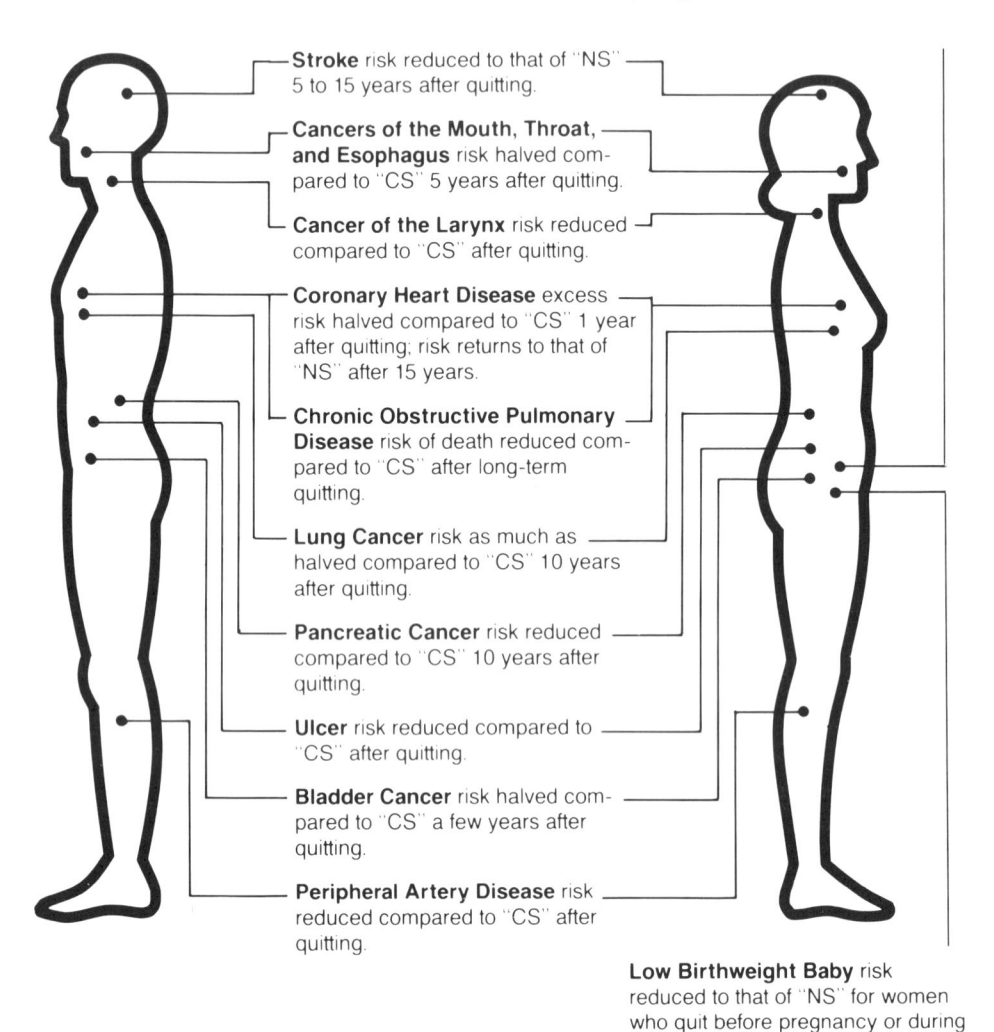

**Stroke** risk reduced to that of "NS" 5 to 15 years after quitting.

**Cancers of the Mouth, Throat, and Esophagus** risk halved compared to "CS" 5 years after quitting.

**Cancer of the Larynx** risk reduced compared to "CS" after quitting.

**Coronary Heart Disease** excess risk halved compared to "CS" 1 year after quitting; risk returns to that of "NS" after 15 years.

**Chronic Obstructive Pulmonary Disease** risk of death reduced compared to "CS" after long-term quitting.

**Lung Cancer** risk as much as halved compared to "CS" 10 years after quitting.

**Pancreatic Cancer** risk reduced compared to "CS" 10 years after quitting.

**Ulcer** risk reduced compared to "CS" after quitting.

**Bladder Cancer** risk halved compared to "CS" a few years after quitting.

**Peripheral Artery Disease** risk reduced compared to "CS" after quitting.

**Low Birthweight Baby** risk reduced to that of "NS" for women who quit before pregnancy or during first trimester.

From: Centers for Disease Control, Office on Smoking and Health. *The Health Benefits of Smoking Cessation: A Report of the Surgeon General, 1990 at a Glance*. Rockville, MD: Centers for Disease Control; 1990. USDHHS publication CDC 90-8419.

## Basics of Smoking Cessation Counseling*

1. Health-care providers should create a smoke-free office, as follows:

   - Select a date for the office to become smoke-free.
   - Advise all staff and patients of this plan.
   - Post no-smoking signs in all office areas.
   - Remove ashtrays.
   - Display nonsmoking materials and cessation information prominently.
   - Do not use waiting room magazines that contain tobacco advertising. A list of such magazines is available (Goldsmith, 1991).

2. Consideration should be given to designating an office smoking cessation coordina r who will be responsible for seeing that the smoking cessation program is carrie

3. Clinicians should ask about smoking at every opportunity:

   - "Do you smoke?"
   - "How much?"
   - "How soon after waking do you have your first cigarette?"
   - "Are you interested in stopping smoking?"
   - "Have you ever tried to stop before? If so, what happened?"

4. Assessment of patient smoking status can be facilitated by using a brief, self-administered questionnaire (see Table 59-1). Staff can help patients fill out the questionnaire or ask the questions verbally.

5. A sticker or other visual cue should be placed on the charts of patients who smoke as a reminder of the need to address the issue of smoking at every visit. Similar stickers may be placed on the charts of children of smokers to serve as cues to talk to parents about the ways their smoking endangers their children. It may also be helpful to use a flow chart in patient records to keep track of smoking cessation interventions.

*Adapted from: Glynn TJ, Manley MW. *How To Help Your Patients Stop Smoking: A National Cancer Institute Manual for Physicians*. Bethesda, Md: National Institutes of Health, 1989. USDHHS publication NIH 89-3064.

# Ch. 59. Smoking Cessation — Adults/Older Adults — COUNSELING

**Table 59-1. Smoking Assessment Form**

Name:_____  Date:_____

1. Do you now smoke cigarettes?  _____Yes  _____No

2. Does the person closest to you smoke cigarettes?  _____Yes  _____No

3. How many cigarettes do you smoke a day?  _____Cigarettes

4. How soon after you wake up do you smoke your first cigarette?
   _____Within 30 minutes  _____More than 30 minutes

5. How interested are you in stopping smoking?
   _____Not at all  _____A little  _____Some  _____A lot  _____Very

6. If you decided to quite smoking completely during the next 2 weeks, how confident are you that you would succeed?
   _____Not at all  _____A little  _____Some  _____A lot  _____Very

From: Glynn TJ, Manley MW. *How To Help Your Patients Stop Smoking: A National Cancer Institute Manual for Physicians.* Bethesda, MD: National Institutes of Health; 1989. USDHHS publication NIH 89-3064. (New edition in press)

6. All smokers should be advised to stop.

   - Clinicians should state this clearly, for example: "As your physician (or other health-care provider), I must advise you to stop smoking now."

   - The message to quit should be personalized. Reference should be made to the patient's clinical condition, smoking history, family history, personal interests, and social roles. During illnesses, especially if smoking-related, patients may be more receptive to smoking cessation interventions.

7. Providers should assist patients in stopping.

   - Setting a quit date: Patients should be helped to pick a date within the next 4 weeks, acknowledging that no time is ideal. Stopping at high-stress times is not advisable; suggesting a significant date (e.g., the patient's or a spouse's birthday or the first day of the month) may be helpful.

   - Providing self-help materials (see Patient Resources): The smoking cessation coordinator or a support staff member can review the materials with patients, if desired.

   - Consideration should be given to prescribing nicotine gum or patch, especially for highly addicted patients (those who smoke one pack a day or more or who smoke their first cigarette within 30 minutes of waking). Tables 59-2 and 59-3 present basic information about nicotine gum and patch use, respectively.

- Consideration should be given to signing a stop-smoking contract with patients.

- For patients who are not willing to quit now, motivational literature should be provided and the patients asked again at the next and subsequent visits.

- Consideration should be given to referring patients to a group clinic or intensive smoking cessation program. This option should be discussed with patients to determine if they have had experience, and are comfortable with, a group discussion format. Information on reputable programs can be obtained by calling the National Cancer Institute Information Service: 1-800 4-CANCER.

8. Follow-up is an important part of the process.

- A member of the office staff should call or write patients within 7 days after the initial visit, reinforcing the decision to stop and reminding patients of their quit date.

- A follow-up visit should be scheduled within 1-2 weeks after the patient's quit date.

- At the first follow-up visit, patients should be asked about their smoking status to provide support and help prevent relapse. Relapse is common; if it happens, patients should be encouraged to try again immediately.

- A second follow-up visit should be scheduled in 1 to 2 months. For patients who have relapsed, the circumstances of the relapse and other special concerns should be discussed.

## Patient Resources

*Clearing the Air; Guia para Dejar de Fumar; Why Do You Smoke?*; and other materials. Office of Cancer Communications, National Cancer Institute, Bldg 31, Rm 10A24, Bethesda, MD 20892; 1-800 4-CANCER.

*Check Your Smoking I.Q.: An Important Quiz for Older Smokers*; and other materials. National Heart, Lung, and Blood Institute Smoking Education Program, PO Box 30105, Bethesda, Maryland 20824-0105; (301) 251-1222.

*How To Quit Cigarettes; The Fifty Most Often Asked Questions about Smoking and Health and the Answers*; and other materials. American Cancer Society, 1559 Clifton Rd. NE, Atlanta, GA 30329-4251; 1-800 ACS-2345.

*Smoking in Women.* American College of Obstetricians and Gynecologists, 409 12th St. SW, Washington, DC 20024; 1-800 762-2264.

*Smoking: Steps To Help You Break the Habit.* American Academy of Family Physicians, 8880 Ward Parkway, Kansas City, MO 64114-2797; 1-800 944-0000.

### Table 59-2. Information About Nicotine Gum Use

| | |
|---|---|
| **Preparation** | Patients should stop smoking before beginning nicotine gum use and be involved in a smoking cessation program under the care of a physician or other health-care provider. |
| **Dosage** | Patients should use one piece of gum whenever they have the urge to smoke. Patients should be instructed not to exceed 30 pieces of 2 mg gum per day. For patients who have trouble with an as-needed approach, a fixed dosage schedule (e.g., one piece every 60-90 minutes) may be more appropriate. At least two boxes (192 pieces), of the 2 mg gum should be prescribed at the initial visit. A common problem is that patients use the gum too sparingly in the first few days after quitting and relapse because of lack of nicotine. |
| **Administration** | Each piece of nicotine gum should be chewed slowly and intermittently for about 30 minutes. Chewing quickly can release the nicotine too rapidly and reduce the effect of the gum. Each piece of gum should be chewed enough to soften it or until the taste or "tingling" from the nicotine is felt. Then it should be "parked" in contact with the oral mucosa so that the nicotine can be absorbed. The gum should be rechewed gently every few minutes to release more nicotine. |
| **Duration of therapy** | The need for refills should be assessed at follow-up visits. The dose of nicotine gum should be tapered after about 3 months. Use of the gum for more than 6 months is not recommended. |
| **Adverse reactions** | Potential side effects of nicotine gum use are sore jaw, mouth irritation, heartburn, nausea, sore throat, and palpitations. |
| **Contraindications** | Nicotine gum is contraindicated for patients who have had a recent myocardial infarction, severe or worsening angina, or life-threatening arrhythmias. It is also contraindicated for patients who are pregnant, nursing, or are unable to chew. |

Adapted from: Glynn TJ, Manley MW. *How To Help Your Patients Stop Smoking: A National Cancer Institute Manual for Physicians.* Bethesda, MD: National Institutes of Health; 1989. USDHHS publication NIH 89-3064. (New edition in press)

## Provider Resources

*Smoking and Reproductive Health.* American College of Obstetricians and Gynecologists, 409 12th St. SW, Washington, DC 20024; 1-800 762-2264. Technical Bulletin AT180.

*How To Help Your Patients Stop Smoking: A National Cancer Institute Manual for Physicians*; *How To Help Your Patients Stop Using Tobacco: A National Cancer Institute Manual for the Oral Health Team*; and other materials. Office of Cancer Communications, National Cancer Institute, Bldg 31, Rm 10A24, Bethesda, MD 20892; 1-800 4-CANCER.

## Table 59-3. Information About Nicotine Patch Use

| | |
|---|---|
| **Preparation** | Patients should stop smoking before beginning to use the nicotine patch and be involved in a smoking cessation program under the care of a physician or other health-care provider. Although the patches have proven to be beneficial even in the absence of supportive care, they are much more effective when used in conjunction with a smoking cessation program. |
| **Dosage** | All patch manufacturers recommend an initial treatment dose followed by one or two weaning doses. Most manufacturers advise starting at the highest dose patch available, except with small patients (less than 100 lb) and those with a history of cardiovascular disease. |
| **Administration** | The patch should be applied only once a day to a clean, dry and non-hairy site on the trunk or upper arm. The patch should be applied promptly on removal from its protective pouch to prevent evaporative loss of nicotine from the system. Application sites should not be reused for at least a week to prevent skin irritation. For all-day systems, the used patch should be removed after 24 hours and a new one applied to another site. For the 16-hour system, the patch should be applied on waking and removed at bedtime. |
| **Duration of therapy** | Depending on the type of patch, the recommended duration of therapy ranges from 10 to 16 weeks. |
| **Adverse reactions** | The most common side effect of the nicotine patch is a mild, transient (15 to 60 minutes) itching or burning at the site after application. Erythema, sometimes accompanied by edema, also occurs frequently at the patch site. Other common side effects include contact sensitization (rare), headache, vertigo, insomnia, somnolence, abnormal dreams, myalgia, arthralgia, abdominal pain, nausea, dyspepsia, diarrhea, and nervousness. Anxiety, irritability, and depression may also occur, but are more often symptoms of nicotine withdrawal than patch toxicity. |
| **Contraindications** | Contraindications to nicotine patch use include serious cardiac arrhythmias, severe or worsening angina, recent myocardial infarction, hypersensitivity or allergy to nicotine, and pregnancy. The patch should be used with caution in patients with psoriasis, dermatitis (atopic or eczematous), active peptic ulcers, severe renal impairment, accelerated hypertension, hyperthyroidism, pheochromocytoma, or insulin-dependent diabetes mellitus. |

Adapted from: Glynn TJ, Manley MW. *How To Help Your Patients Stop Smoking: A National Cancer Institute Manual for Physicians*. Bethesda, MD: National Institutes of Health. In press.

*Clinical Opportunities for Smoking Intervention—A Guide for the Busy Physician*; *How You Can Help Patients Stop Smoking: Opportunities for Respiratory Care Practitioners*; *Nurses: Help Your Patients Stop Smoking*. National Heart, Lung, and Blood Institute Smoking Education Program, PO Box 30105, Bethesda, Maryland 20824-0105; (301) 251-1222.

*Doctors Helping Smokers: An Office Manual*, and other materials. Doctors Helping Smokers at Blue Plus, PO Box 64179, St. Paul, MN 55164; (612) 456-1975.

*Stop Smoking Kit*. American Academy of Family Physicians, 8880 Ward Parkway, Kansas City, MO 64114-2797; 1-800 944-0000.

**Selected References**

American Academy of Family Physicians, Commission on Public Health and Scientific Affairs. *Age Charts for Periodic Health Examination*. Kansas City, Mo: American Academy of Family Physicians; 1993.

American College of Obstetricians and Gynecologists. *The Obstetrician-Gynecologist and Primary-Preventive Health Care*. Washington, DC: American College of Obstetricians and Gynecologists; 1993.

American College of Physicians, Health and Public Policy Committee. Methods for stopping cigarette smoking. *Ann Intern Med*. 1986;105:281-291.

Canadian Task Force on the Periodic Health Examination. The periodic health examination: 2. 1985 update. *Can Med Assoc J*. 1986;134:724-727.

Centers for Disease Control, Office on Smoking and Health. *The Health Benefits of Smoking Cessation: A Report of the Surgeon General, 1990 at a Glance*. Rockville, Md: Centers for Disease Control; 1990. USDHHS publication CDC 90-8419.

Fiore MC. The new vital sign: assessing and documenting smoking status. *JAMA*. 1991;266:3183-3184.

Fiore MC, Jorenby DE, Baker TB, Kenfor SL. Tobacco dependence and the nicotine patch: clinical guidelines for effective use. *JAMA*. 1992;268:2687-2694.

Frank E, Winkleby MA, Altman DG, Rockhill B, Fortmann SP. Predictors of physicians' smoking cessation advice. *JAMA*. 1991;266:3139-3144.

Glynn TJ, Manley MW. *How To Help Your Patients Stop Smoking: A National Cancer Institute Manual for Physicians*. Bethesda, Md: National Institutes of Health, 1989. USDHHS publication NIH 89-3064. (New edition in press.)

Goldsmith MS. Magazines without tobacco advertising (Medical News and Perspectives). *JAMA*. 1991;266:3099-3102.

Kottke TE, Battista RN, DeFriese GH, Brekke ML. Smoking cessation: attributes of successful interventions. *JAMA*. 1988;259:2883-2889.

Solberg LI, Maxwell PL, Kottke TE, Gepner GJ, Brekke ML. A systematic primary care office-based smoking cessation program. *J Fam Pract*. 1990;30:647-654.

Steenland K. Passive smoking and the risk of heart disease. *JAMA*. 1992;267:94-99.

Centers for Disease Control. *The Health Benefits of Smoking Cessation*. Washington, DC: US Dept of Health and Human Services; 1990. USDHHS publication CDC 90-8416.

US Preventive Services Task Force. Counseling to prevent tobacco use. In: *Guide to Clinical Preventive Services*. Baltimore, Md: Williams & Wilkins; 1989:chap 48.

## Adults/Older Adults — COUNSELING

# 60. Unintended Pregnancy

Although modern contraceptives have enabled women to increase control over their reproductive lives, in 1988 U.S. women aged 15 to 44 years reported that 39% of their births in the preceding 5 years were unintended. Most of the unintended births were mistimed—that is, they occurred sooner than wanted—but 12% were reported as unwanted at any time. Among some population groups, these figures were much higher than the general population; African-American women, for example, reported 59% of births as unintended and 29% as unwanted. Unwanted pregnancies lead to most of the 1.5 million induced abortions performed each year in the United States. Unwanted children are at increased risk of health and behavior problems in childhood and later in life.

Modern contraceptives marketed in the United States have been shown to be safe and effective (see Table 60-1 for effectiveness rates). Although most are relatively inexpensive, their costs vary. Primary care clinicians are the main source of authoritative information and advice on responsible family planning practices for patients.

For information on counseling to prevent unintended pregnancy in adolescents, see chapter 24. Also refer to related information on counseling to prevent sexually transmitted diseases (STDs) and HIV infection among adolescents (chapter 22) and adults (chapter 58).

### Recommendations of Major Authorities

- **American Academy of Family Physicians, American College of Obstetricians and Gynecologists**, and **U.S. Preventive Services Task Force**—Primary care providers should obtain a history of sexual practices and provide counseling on the prevention of unintended pregnancy and contraceptive options to all sexually active women who do not want to become pregnant and men who do not want to have a child. Counseling should also be provided regarding high-risk sexual behavior and the prevention of STDs and HIV infection.

### Basics of Counseling to Prevent Unintended Pregnancy

1. Providers should assess the sexual practices and the need for contraceptive counseling for every patient. This can be done as a part of periodic health examinations or during acute-care visits for issues of a related nature, such as STDs, postpartum care, or family stress. The main goal is to make sure family planning is a part of primary care for all sexually active patients. As with all counseling of patients regarding sensitive topics, openness and a nonjudgmental attitude is required for success.

2. Each patient's level of knowledge about contraceptive options should be determined. What methods have they tried in the past? Have these methods been acceptable and effective for the patient and partner or partners? What are the patient's medical and lifestyle factors that could influence the choice of an appropriate contraceptive?

Table 60-1. Percent of Women Experiencing an Accidental Pregnancy in First Year of Use of Contraceptives

| Method | % Pregnant in first year Typical use[1] | Perfect use[2] (estimated) |
|---|---|---|
| Male sterilization | 0.15 | 0.10 |
| Female sterilization | 0.40 | 0.40 |
| Implant (Norplant®) | 0.09 | 0.09 |
| Injectable progestogen (Depo-Provera®) | 0.30 | 0.30 |
| Intrauterine device (IUD) | | |
|     Progestasert® | 2.00 | 1.50 |
|     Copper T 380A | 0.80 | 0.60 |
|     LNg 20 | 0.10 | 0.10 |
| Pill | 3.00 | |
|     Progestin only | | 0.50 |
|     Combined | | 0.10 |
| Condom | | |
|     Male (without spermicide) | 12.00 | 3.00 |
|     Female (Reality) | 21.00 | 5.00 |
| Diaphragm with spermicide | 18.00 | 6.00 |
| Cervical cap with spermicide | 18.00 (nulliparous) 36.00 (parous) | 9.00 (nulliparous) 26.00 (parous) |
| Vaginal sponge | 18.00 (nulliparous) 36.00 (parous) | 9.00 (nulliparous) 20.00 (parous) |
| Withdrawal | 19.00 | 4.00 |
| Periodic abstinence | 20.00 | |
|     Calendar | | 9.00 |
|     Ovulation method | | 3.00 |
|     Sympto-thermal | | 2.00 |
|     Post-ovulation | | 1.00 |
| Spermicide[3] (alone) | 21.00 | 6.00 |
| None | 85.00 | 85.00 |

[1] Among typical couples who initiate use of a method (not necessarily for the first time), the percentage who experience an accidental pregnancy during the first year if they do not stop use for any other reason.

[2] Among couples who initiate use of a method (not necessarily for the first time) and who use it perfectly (both consistently and correctly), the percentage who experience an accidental pregnancy during the first year if they do not stop use for any other reason.

[3] Foams, creams, gels, vaginal suppositories, and vaginal film.

Adapted from: Hatcher RA, Trussell J, Stewart F, et al. *Contraceptive Technology 1994-1996*. New York, NY: Irvington Publishers; in press. Used with permission from the publisher; copyright © 1994.

3. Patients should be educated about the important characteristics of different contraceptive methods (Table 60-2). A range of contraceptive options, not just one method, should be presented to the patient. Patients should be assisted in carefully choosing a contraceptive method that is appropriate for their abilities, motivation, and life-style, thereby increasing the likelihood that it will be used correctly and consistently. Patients who are already using a method correctly and successfully should be encouraged to continue.

4. It is important to discuss the ability of different contraceptive methods to protect against STDs and HIV infection. Latex condoms are effective for both birth control and reducing the risk of disease. Other forms of birth control, such as IUD, diaphragm, cervical cap, and oral contraceptives, do not give the same protection. It should be stressed that even if patients use another form of birth control, those not in a mutually monogamous relationship with a person known to be free of infection also need to use condoms to reduce the risk of STDs.

5. Contraception is a responsibility of both partners. If possible, both partners should be involved in counseling and discussion of contraceptive options. Methods of male participation in family planning should also be discussed.

6. After patients choose a method, the provider should conduct an in-depth discussion of:

   - How it works.
   - Theoretical and actual effectiveness.
   - Advantages/benefits.
   - Disadvantages/risks.
   - How to use the method.
   - Nuisance side effects.
   - Warning signs.
   - Back-up methods.

   Patients should be given printed material about the contraceptive method chosen to review at home (see Patient Resources).

7. Follow-up counseling is particularly important in the first few weeks of use to deal with difficulties associated with use and side effects. The provider should ask patients how they are using the method and should correct misinformation and explore barriers to use. Counseling should continue each time patients are seen, especially until patients are very comfortable with the use of the contraceptive method. Many compliance problems can be resolved relatively simply with reassurance and changes in dose or technique of use.

Table 60-2. Complications, Side Effects, and Benefits of Major Methods of Contraception

| Methods | Complications | Side effects | Noncontraceptive benefits |
|---|---|---|---|
| Pills | Rare cardiovascular complications (stroke, heart attack, blood clots, high blood pressure, hepatic adenomas | Nausea, headaches, dizziness, spotting, weight gain, breast tenderness, chloasma, cramping, breast diseases, ovarian cysts | May offer some protection against progression to PID (but not against contracting STDs and HIV), ovarian and endometrial cancers, and benign breast masses; decreases menstrual blood loss and diminishes dysmenorrhea. |
| IUDs | PID, uterine perforation, anemia | Menstrual cramping, spotting, increased bleeding | None known except for progestin-releasing IUDs, which may decrease menstrual blood loss and pain. |
| Condoms | None known | Decreased sensation, allergy to latex, loss of spontaneity | Latex condoms protect against transmission of STDs and HIV if used properly; delay premature ejaculation. |
| Implants | Infection at implant site | Tenderness at site, menstrual changes | May offer some protection against progression to PID (but not against contracting HIV and other STDs); may decrease menstrual cramps, pain, and blood loss. |
| Injectables | None definitely proven | Menstrual changes, weight gain, headaches | May offer some protection against progression to PID (but not against contracting STDs and HIV); may be used when lactating; may have protective effects against endometrial cancer. |
| Sterilization | Infection | Pain at surgical site, psychological reactions, subsequent regret that the procedure was performed | None known; may have beneficial effects vis a vis PID. |
| Abstinence | None known | Psychological reactions | Prevents STDs and sexually transmitted HIV |

Table 60-2. Complications, Side Effects, and Benefits of Major Methods of Contraception—Continued

| Methods | Complications | Side effects | Noncontraceptive benefits |
| --- | --- | --- | --- |
| Barriers: diaphragms, caps, sponges | Mechanical irritation, vaginal infections, toxic shock syndrome | Pelvic pressure, cervical erosion, vaginal discharges if left in too long | Protects against STDs (GC and chlamydia), but data on HIV are inconclusive and conflicting. |

Adapted from: Hatcher RA, Stewart F, Trussell J, et al. *Contraceptive Technology 1990-1992*. New York, NY: Irvington Publishers; 1990. Used with permission from the publisher; copyright © 1990.

8. Oral contraceptives (OCs) can also be prescribed as a postcoital ("morning after") method to prevent pregnancy. This approach to emergency contraception has been reported to reduce the risk of pregnancy by 75% to 95% after unprotected intercourse if treatment is initiated within 72 hours. The most common method currently used in clinical practice is two doses of ethinyl estradiol in combination with either levonorgestrel or norgestrel.

The patient should be instructed to take the first dose as soon as possible (but no more than 72 hours) after unprotected intercourse. The second dose is taken 12 hours after the first dose. Postcoital contraception can be provided using the following brands of OCs: Ovral® (1 dose is 2 white pills); Nordette®, Levlen®, Lo/Ovral® (1 dose is four white pills); Triphasil®, Tri-Levlen® (1 dose is 4 yellow pills). The most common side effects of these regimens are nausea and vomiting.

Postcoital or emergency contraception has not been included in the labeling of these drugs because no company has applied to the FDA for approval to label and distribute contraceptive pills for this purpose. Physicians may prescribe an approved drug for an unlabeled indication, but no one may advertise the availability of a drug for an unlabeled use.

Adapted from: Hatcher RA, Trussell J, Stewart F, et al. *Contraceptive Technology.*. 16th Rev Ed. New York, NY: Irvington Publishers; in press. Used with permission from the publisher; copyright © 1994.

## Patient Resources

*Barrier Methods of Contraception*; *Birth Control Pills* (for low literacy audiences); *Contraception* (English and Spanish); *Family Planning by Periodic Abstinence*; *The Intrauterine Device*; *Oral Contraceptives*; *Postpartum Sterilization*; *Sterilization by Laparoscopy*; *Sterilization for Women and Men*; and other materials. American College of Obstetricians and Gynecologists, 409 12th Street SW, Washington, DC 20024; 1-800 762-2264.

*Birth Control: Choosing the Method That's Right for You*. American Academy of Family Physicians, 8880 Ward Parkway, Kansas City, MO 64114-2797; 1-800 944-0000.

*Condoms and STDs...Especially AIDS* (English version; DHHS Publication FDA 90-4239); *El Condon Proteccion Contra Las Enfermedades de Transmision, Sexual, Especialmente El SIDA* (Spanish version; DHHS Publication FDA 93-4254S). National AIDS Information Clearinghouse, PO Box 6003, Rockville, MD 20850; 1-800 458-5231; and National AIDS Information Hot Line (Spanish speaking): 1-800 344-SIDA.

*Facts About Birth Control* (English and Spanish). Planned Parenthood, 810 7th Ave., New York, NY 10019; (212) 541-7800.

*Your Contraceptive Choices For Now, For Later*. US Dept of Health and Human Services, Public Health Service, Office of Population Affairs, Family Life Information Exchange, PO Box 30436, Bethesda, MD 20814.

**Provider Resources**

*The Intrauterine Device* (technical bulletin 164); *Oral Contraception* (technical bulletin 106); *Sterilization* (technical bulletin 113). American College of Obstetricians and Gynecologists, 409 12th St. SW, Washington, DC 20024; 1-800 762-2264.

*Family Planning at Your Fingertips: From the Pages of Contraceptive Technology*. EMIS Publishers, Dallas, TX; 1-800 225-0694.

**Selected References**

American Academy of Family Physicians, Commission on Public Health and Scientific Affairs. *Age Charts for Periodic Health Examination*. Kansas City, Mo: American Academy of Family Physicians, 1993.
American College of Obstetricians and Gynecologists, Committee on Professional Standards. *Standards for Obstetric and Gynecology Services*. 7th ed. Washington, DC: American College of Obstetricians and Gynecologists; 1989;chap 4.
American College of Obstetricians and Gynecologists *The Obstetrician-Gynecologist and Primary-Preventive Health Care*. Washington, DC: American College of Obstetricians and Gynecologists; 1993.
Baird D, Glasier AF. Hormonal contraception. *N Engl J Med*. 1993;328:1543-1549.
Canadian Task Force on the Periodic Health Examination. The periodic health examination: 2. 1987 update. *Can Med Assoc J*. 1988;138:618-626.
Hatcher RA, Stewart F, Trussell J, et al. *Contraceptive Technology 1990-1992*. New York, NY: Irvington Publishers; 1990.
Hatcher RA, Trussell J, Stewart F, et al. *Contraceptive Technology*. 16th Rev Ed. New York, NY: Irvington Publishers. In press.
Trussell J, Stewart F. The effectiveness of postcoital hormonal contraception. *Family Planning Perspectives*. 1992;24:262-264.
Trussell J, Stewart F, Guest F, Hatcher, RA. Emergency contraceptive pills: a simple proposal to reduce unintended pregnancies. *Family Planning Perspectives*. 1992;24:269-273.
US Preventive Services Task Force. Counseling to prevent unintended pregnancy. In: *Guide to Clinical Preventive Services*. Baltimore, Md: Williams & Wilkins; 1989:chap 54.

# Clinician's Handbook of Preventive Services

## Appendices/Index

# APPENDICES

# A. Major Authorities Cited

(In Alphabetical Order)

American Academy of Dermatology
930 N. Meacham Road
Schaumberg, Il 60618
Tel: (708) 330-0230
Fax: (708) 330-0050

American Academy of Family Physicians
8880 Ward Parkway
Kansas City, MO 64114-2797
Tel: 1-800 944-0000
Fax: (816) 822-0580

American Academy of Ophthalmology
P.O. Box 7424
San Francisco, CA 94120
Tel: (415) 561-8500
Fax: (415) 561-8533

American Academy of Otolaryngology-
Head and Neck Surgery
1 Prince Street
Alexandria, VA 22314
Tel: (703) 836-4444
Fax: (703) 683-5100

American Academy of Pediatric Dentistry
211 E. Chicago Avenue
Suite 700
Chicago, Il 60611
Tel: (312) 337-2169
Fax: (312) 337-6329

American Association of Pediatric
Ophthalmology and Strabismus
P.O. Box 193832
San Francisco, CA 94119
Tel: (415) 561-8505
Fax: (415) 561-8575

American Academy of Pediatrics
141 Northwest Point Boulevard
P.O. Box 927
Elk Grove, IL 60009-0927
Tel: 1-800 433-9016
Fax: (708) 228 5097

American Cancer Society
1559 Clifton Road NE.
Atlanta, GA 30329-4251
Tel: 1-800 ACS-2345

American College of Obstetricians and
Gynecologists
409 12th Street SW.
Washington, DC 20024
Tel: (202) 863-2502
Fax: (202) 488-3985

American College of Physicians
Independence Mall West
Sixth Street at Race
Philadelphia, PA 19104
Tel: (215) 351-2400
Fax: (215) 351-2829

American College of Sports Medicine
P.O. Box 1440
Indianapolis, IN 46202-1440
Tel: (317) 637-9200
Fax: (317) 634-7817

American Dental Association
211 E. Chicago Avenue
Chicago, IL 60611
Tel: 1-800 947-4746
Fax: (312) 440-3542

# Appendix A — Major Authorities Cited

American Diabetes Association
1660 Duke Street
Alexandria, VA 22314
Tel: (703) 549-1500
　　1-800 ADA-DISC

American Dietetic Association
216 W. Jackson Boulevard
Suite 800
Chicago, IL 60606-6995
Tel: (312) 899-0040
Fax: (312) 899-1979

American Gastroenterological Association
6900 Grove Road
Thoroughfare, NJ 08086
Tel: (609) 848-1000
Fax: (609) 848-5274

American Geriatrics Society
770 Lexington Avenue #300
New York, NY 10021
Tel: (212) 308-1414
Fax: (212) 832-8646

American Heart Association
7320 Greenville Avenue
Dallas, TX 75231
Tel: 1-800 242-1793
Fax: (214) 706-1341

American Medical Association
515 N. State Street
Chicago, IL 60610
Tel: (312) 464-4804
Fax: (312) 464-4184

American Nurses Association
600 Maryland Avenue SW. #100W
Washington, DC 20024-2571
Tel: (202) 554-4444
Fax: (202) 554-2262

American Optometric Association
243 N. Lindbergh Boulevard
St. Louis, MO 63141
Tel: (314) 991-4100
Fax: (314) 991-4101

American Society of Colon and Rectal Surgeons
800 E. Northwest Highway
Suite 1080
Palatine, IL 60067
Tel: (708) 290-9184

American Society of Dentistry for Children
211 E. Chicago Avenue
Suite 1430
Chicago, IL 60611
Tel: (312) 943-1244
Fax: (312) 943-5341

American Society for Gastrointestinal Endoscopy
13 Elm Street
Manchester, MA 01944
Tel: (508) 526-8330
Fax: (508) 526-4018

American Speech-Language-Hearing Association
10801 Rockville Pike
Rockville, MD 20852
Tel: 1-800 638-8255
　　(301) 897-5700
Fax: (301) 571-0457

American Thoracic Society
1740 Broadway
14th Floor
New York, NY 10019
Tel: (212) 315-8700
Fax: (212) 315-6498

# Appendix A — Major Authorities Cited

American Thyroid Association
Montefiore Medical Center
111 E. 210th Street
Bronx, NY 10467
Tel: (718) 882-6047
Fax: (718) 882-6085

American Urological Association
1120 N. Charles Street
Baltimore, MD 21201-5559
Tel: (410) 727-1100
Fax: (410) 625-2390

Canadian Task Force on Periodic Health Examination
Department of Pediatrics
Faculty of Medicine
Dalhousie University
Halifax, Nova Scotia B3H 1V7
Canada
Tel: (902) 428-8115
Fax: (902) 422-9229

Council for Education of the Deaf
Gallaudet University
800 Florida Avenue NE.
Washington, DC 20002
Tel: (202) 651-5020
Fax: (202) 651-5708

National Medical Association
1012 10th Street NW.
Washington, DC 20001
Tel: (202) 347-1895
Fax: (202) 842-3293

Skin Cancer Foundation
P.O. Box 561
New York, NY 10156
Tel: (212) 725-5176
Fax: (212) 725-5751

Society of General Internal Medicine
700 13th Street NW.
Suite 250
Washington, DC 20005
Tel: (202) 393-1662
Fax: (202) 783-1347

## U.S. Federal Agencies

Agency for Health Care Policy and Research
Publications Clearinghouse
P.O. Box 8547
Silver Spring, MD 20907
Tel: 1-800 358-9295

Advisory Committee on Immunization Practices
Centers for Disease Control and Prevention
Mailstop A-20
Atlanta, GA 30333
Tel: (404) 639-3851

Centers for Disease Control and Prevention
Division of Immunization
Mailstop E-52
Atlanta, GA 30333
Tel: (404) 639-8226
Fax: (404) 639-8626

Centers for Disease Control and Prevention
Division of Tuberculosis Elimination
Mailstop E-10
Atlanta, GA 30333
Tel: (404) 639-8125
Fax: (404) 639-8254

National Cancer Institute
Building 31, Room 10A24
Bethesda, MD 20892
Tel: 1-800 4-CANCER

National Eye Institute
Box 20/20
Bethesda, MD 20892
Tel: (301) 496-5248

# Appendix A — Major Authorities Cited

National Heart, Lung, and Blood Institute
P.O. Box 30105
Bethesda, MD 20824-0105
Tel: (301) 251-1222

National Institute of Dental Research
9000 Rockville Pike
Bethesda, MD 20892
Tel: (301) 496-4261
Fax: (301) 496-9988

National Institutes of Health Consensus
Development Conferences
NIH Consensus Program Clearing House
P.O. Box 2577
Kensington, MD 20891
Tel: 1-800 644-6627
Fax: (301) 816-2494

National Transportation Safety Board
490 L'Enfant Plaza East
Washington, DC 20594
Tel: (202) 382-0660

U.S. Preventive Services Task Force
c/o Office of Disease Prevention
    and Health Promotion
Switzer 2132
330 C Street SW.
Washington, DC 20201
Tel: (202) 205-8660
Fax: (202) 205-9478

# APPENDICES

# B. Summary Risk-Factor Tables

Throughout this book, risk factors for given disorders have been listed in the introductory sections of the respective chapters. For example, low socioeconomic level is listed separately as a risk factor in the anemia, cervical and oral cancer, and tuberculosis chapters. The tables that follow reverse this process: here, disorders are grouped by their risk factors. Thus, the diseases above are all listed under low socioeconomic status.

These tables are intended to help clinicians determine the specific preventive care needs of their patients. Risk factors or groups of risk factors may be examined to determine if any leading authority has found the risk factor to be an indication either for performing a specific preventive service, or for performing it more frequently. All risk factors that have been cited by at least one authority in the *Clinician's Handbook* have been compiled into seven tables by risk factor category:

Table B-1. Ethnic and Geographic Origin
Table B-2. Family History
Table B-3. Medical History
Table B-4. Occupational and Recreational History
Table B-5. Sexual History
Table B-6. Social or Living Situation
Table B-7. Substance Abuse History

It is hoped that these tables will stimulate clinicians to think both of individual patients and of patient populations in terms of their risk factors, and to associate these risk factors with disorders having preventive interventions that should be considered. Creation of these tables from the recommendations in the *Clinician's Handbook* has necessarily required simplification and consolidation of information. From an epidemiologic perspective, they are incomplete: Patients possessing a risk factor may be at increased risk for many disorders not listed in these tables and, conversely, not all risk factors for a disorder are listed. Risk factors and disorders related to types of preventive care not covered in the *Clinician's Handbook*, such as most types of tertiary prevention, have also not been included.

Each table gives the risk factor, the disorder for which a patient with the risk factor may be at risk, and the number of the relevant chapter in the *Clinician's Handbook*. Readers are urged to refer to the referenced chapter for details about specific preventive services for the listed disorder.

Appendix B — Summary Risk-Factor Tables

**Table B-1. Summary Risk Factors: Ethnic and Geographic Origin**

| Risk Factor | Disorder | Chapter No. Children/Adolescents | Chapter No. Adults/Older Adults |
|---|---|---|---|
| Asian, African, Mediterranean, Caribbean, Latin American descent | Hemoglobinopathy | 8 | 26 |
| Native American | Diabetes mellitus |  | 37 |
|  | Tuberculosis | 9 | 42 |
| Hispanic | Diabetes mellitus |  | 37 |
| African American | Diabetes mellitus |  | 37 |
|  | Glaucoma |  | 44 |
|  | Hypertension |  | 27 |
| Foreign-born individuals from countries with high tuberculosis prevalence (Africa, Asia, Latin America) | Tuberculosis | 9 | 42 |

# Appendix B  Summary Risk-Factor Tables

### Table B-2. Summary Risk Factors: Family History

| Risk Factor | Disorder | Chapter No. Children/Adolescents | Chapter No. Adults/Older Adults |
|---|---|---|---|
| Child ≥2 years with: parent with cholesterol level of ≥240 mg/dL; parent or grandparent who at age ≤55 years had myocardial infarction, angina pectoris, peripheral vascular disease, cerebrovascular disease, sudden cardiac death, or underwent coronary artery bypass surgery or angioplasty | Hypercholesterolemia | 4 | |
| Infant born of an iron-deficient mother | Anemia | 1 | |
| Child with sibling being followed or treated for lead poisoning (blood lead level ≥15 µg/dL) | Lead poisoning | 7 | |
| Child with family history of eye or vision problem | Vision loss | 11 | |
| Breast cancer in first-degree relative, especially if diagnosed before menopause | Breast cancer | | 29,35 |
| Colorectal cancer, endometrial cancer, adenomatous polyps, familial polyposis, cancer family syndrome | Colorectal cancer | | 29,33,40 |
| Prostate cancer | Prostate cancer | | 29,38 |
| Skin cancer | Skin cancer | | 29 |
| Depression | Depression | 5 | 32 |
| Hearing loss | Hearing loss | 6 | 34 |
| Diabetes mellitus, hypertension, hyperlipidemia | Diabetes mellitus | | 37 |
| Thyroid disease | Thyroid disease | | 41 |
| Multiple endocrine neoplasia type II | Thyroid cancer | | 29 |
| Hypertension | Hypertension | | 27 |

## Table B-3. Summary Risk Factors: Medical History

|  |  | Chapter No. ||
|---|---|---|---|
| Risk Factor | Disorder | Children/ Adolescents | Adults/ Older Adults |
| Infant with low birth weight, prematurity | Anemia<br>Hearing loss<br>Vision loss | 1<br>6<br>11 | |
| Newborn with severe depression at birth, craniofacial anomalies, congenital infections (toxoplasmosis, syphilis, rubella, cytomegalovirus, herpes, bacterial meningitis) hyperbilirubinemia, ototoxic medications | Hearing loss | 6 | |
| Infant with slow language development, bacterial meningitis, temporal bone fracture, measles, mumps, neurodegenerative disorders | Hearing loss | 6 | |
| Recurring ear infections or other ear problems | Hearing loss | 6 | 34 |
| Excessive menstrual flow | Anemia | 1 | 26 |
| Inflammatory bowel disease; colorectal adenomatous polyps; colorectal, breast, or ovarian cancer | Colorectal cancer | | 29,33,40 |
| Skin cancer or precursor lesions (e.g., dysplastic nevi and certain congenital nevi) | Skin cancer | 29 | 29 |
| Cryptorchidism, orchiopexy, infertile or atrophic testes, ambiguous genitalia, gonadal dysgenesis, Klinefelter's Syndrome | Testicular cancer | 29 | 29 |
| Vasectomy at least 20 years previously, vasectomy at 40 years of age or older | Prostate cancer | | 29,38 |
| Chronic illness, history of depression | Depression | 5 | 32 |
| Overweight, gestational diabetes, birth of infants weighing more than 9 pounds, circulatory dysfunction or frank vascular impairment | Diabetes mellitus | | 37 |
| Underweight | Tuberculosis | 9 | 42 |
| Prior STD episodes, attendance at STD or family planning clinics | Hepatitis B<br>HIV/STD | 14<br>22 | 47<br>39,58 |

# Appendix B — Summary Risk-Factor Tables

Table B-3. Summary Risk Factors: Medical History—Continued

| | | Chapter No. | |
|---|---|---|---|
| Risk Factor | Disorder | Children/ Adolescents | Adults/ Older Adults |
| Blood transfusion between 1978 and 1985 | HIV | 22,39 | 39,58 |
| Hemophiliacs and other recipients of certain blood products | HIV<br>Hepatitis B | 22<br>14 | 39,58<br>47 |
| Hemoglobinopathy | Influenza<br>Pneumococcus | 48<br>49 | 48<br>49 |
| Irradiation:<br>■ Upper body<br>■ For gynecologic cancer | Thyroid cancer<br>Colorectal cancer | | 29<br>29,40 |
| Gastrointestinal bypass or gastrectomy, chronic malabsorption syndromes, cancer of the upper gastrointestinal tract or oropharynx | Tuberculosis | 9 | 42 |
| Silicosis | Tuberculosis | 9 | 42 |
| Diabetes mellitus | Tuberculosis<br>Urinary tract infection<br>Influenza<br>Pneumococcal infection<br>Vision loss | 9<br>10<br>48<br>49<br>11 | 42<br>43<br>48<br>49<br>44 |
| Renal dysfunction or failure<br>■ Hemodialysis patients<br><br>■ All | Hepatitis B<br>Influenza<br>Pneumococcal infection<br>Tuberculosis | 14<br>48<br>49<br>9 | 47<br>48<br>49<br>42 |
| Chronic pulmonary or cardiovascular disorders | Influenza<br>Pneumococcal infection | 48<br>49 | 48<br>49 |
| At risk for coronary artery disease<br>■ Men over 40 years of age<br>■ Postmenopausal women | Coronary artery disease | | 45<br>46 |
| Certain types of structural heart disease and dental procedures | Endocarditis | 53 | 53 |
| Splenectomy, splenic dysfunction | Pneumococcal infection | 49 | 49 |

*(Continued)*

Table B-3. Summary Risk Factors: Medical History—Continued

| Risk Factor | Disorder | Children/ Adolescents | Adults/ Older Adults |
|---|---|---|---|
| Cirrhosis | Pneumococcal infection | 49 | 49 |
| | Influenza | 48 | 48 |
| Cerebrospinal fluid leaks | Pneumococcal infection | 49 | 49 |
| Lack of documented evidence of rubella immunity or prior immunization, especially women of childbearing age | Rubella | 15 | 50 |
| Lack of evidence of immunity to measles and born after 1956 | Measles | 15 | 15 |
| Immunosuppression (including HIV, organ transplantation, medication-induced) | Tuberculosis | 9 | 42 |
| | Influenza | 48 | 48 |
| | Pneumococcal infection | 49 | 49 |
| Autoimmune disease (women) | Thyroid dysfunction | | 41 |
| Postpartum state (women) | Thyroid dysfunction | | 41 |
| | Depression | 5 | 32 |

## Table B-4. Summary Risk Factors: Occupational and Recreational History

| Risk Factor | Disorder | Children/ Adolescents | Adults/ Older Adults |
|---|---|---|---|
| Increased occupational or recreational exposure to: | | | |
| ▪ Sunlight | Skin cancer | 29 | 29 |
| ▪ Noise | Hearing impairment | 6 | 34 |
| Exposure to polycyclic aromatic hydrocarbons | Skin cancer | | 29 |
| Prostitution, trading sex for money or drugs | HIV/STD | 22 | 39,58 |
| | Hepatitis B | 14 | 47 |
| Health care workers: | | | |
| ▪ Who have contact with blood or blood products; staff of institutions for the developmentally disabled | Hepatitis B | 14 | 47 |
| ▪ Who might transmit influenza to persons at increased risk of complications from influenza | Influenza | 48 | 48 |
| ▪ All | Tuberculosis | 9 | 42 |
| Staff of residential care facilities (e.g., hospitals, prisons) | Tuberculosis | 9 | 42 |
| Migrant laborers | Tuberculosis | 9 | 42 |

## Table B-5. Summary Risk Factors: Sexual History

|  |  | Chapter No. | |
| --- | --- | --- | --- |
| Risk Factor | Disorder | Children/ Adolescents | Adults/ Older Adults |
| Early age of sexual activity | Cervical cancer | 29,36 | 29,36 |
| Multiple sexual partners | Cervical cancer<br>HIV/STD<br>Hepatitis B | 29,36<br>22,39<br>14 | 29,36<br>39,58<br>47 |
| Homosexual or bisexual males | HIV/STD<br>Hepatitis B | 22,39<br>14 | 39,58<br>47 |
| Past or present sexual partners that have been HIV-infected | HIV | 22,39 | 39,58 |
| Sex partners of HBsAg-positive individuals | Hepatitis B | 14 | 47 |
| Heterosexuals who do not want to have children; adolescents | Unintended pregnancy | 24 | 60 |
| International travelers who have sexual contact (or blood contact) with residents in areas at high- or intermediate-risk for hepatitis B | Hepatitis B | 14 | 47 |
| History of sexual abuse | Depression | 5 | 32 |

Appendix B — Summary Risk-Factor Tables

### Table B-6. Summary Risk Factors: Social or Living Situation

| Risk Factor | Disorder | Chapter No. Children/Adolescents | Chapter No. Adults/Older Adults |
|---|---|---|---|
| Low socioeconomic level | Anemia | 1 | 26 |
|  | Cervical cancer | 29,36 | 29,36 |
|  | Oral cancer | 18 | 29,53 |
|  | Tuberculosis | 9 | 42 |
| Lack of social support, stressful life events, recent loss | Depression | 5 | 32 |
| Homeless | Tuberculosis | 9 | 42 |
| Child with residence in or regular visits to a house built before 1960 with recent, ongoing, or planned renovation or remodeling, or peeling or chipping paint | Lead poisoning | 7 |  |
| Residence in areas or populations with: |  |  |  |
| ■ High prevalence of HIV/STDs | HIV/STD | 22,39 | 39,58 |
| ■ Increased risk of pneumococcal disease or its complications (e.g., certain Native American populations) | Pneumococcal infection | 49 | 49 |
| ■ Prevalence of tuberculosis >10% (injection drug users, homeless, migrant labors, first-generation immigrants from Asia, Africa, Latin America) | Tuberculosis | 9 | 42 |
| ■ Inadequately fluoridated water supply (child—<0.3 ppm if <2 years old, <0.7 ppm if ≥2 years old) | Dental caries | 18 |  |
| ■ Nearby smelter, battery recycling plant or other industry likely to release lead | Lead poisoning | 7 |  |
| Residence in institutions for: |  |  |  |
| ■ Long-term care of chronic medical conditions | Influenza | 48 | 48 |
| ■ Care of the developmentally disabled | Hepatitis B | 14 | 47 |
| ■ Long-term correctional incarceration | Hepatitis B | 14 | 47 |
| ■ Elderly persons | Influenza |  | 48 |
|  | Cognitive/functional impairment |  | 31 |
| ■ Long-term care (all) | Tuberculosis | 9 | 42 |
| Firearm in home | Injuries and violence | 21,25 | 54 |

*(Continued)*

Table B-6. Summary Risk Factors: Social or Living Situation—Continued

| Risk Factor | Disorder | Children/ Adolescents | Adults/ Older Adults |
|---|---|---|---|
| Household: | | | |
| ■ Member or playmate being followed or treated for lead poisoning (blood lead level ≥15 µg/dL); adult member with hobby or job working with lead | Lead poisoning | 7 | |
| ■ Contact of HBsAg-positive person | Hepatitis B | 14 | 47 |
| ■ Member who might transmit influenza to individuals at increased risk of complications from influenza | Influenza | 48 | 48 |
| ■ Child with Hib contact | *Haemophilus influenzae* | 13 | |
| ■ Tuberculosis contact | Tuberculosis | 9 | 42 |
| Adolescents living in areas with high rates of injection drug use, teenage pregnancy, or sexually transmitted diseases | Hepatitis B | 14 | |
| International travelers who spend more than 6 months in areas with high rates of hepatitis B infection and who will have close contact with the local population; short-term travelers who have contact with blood or sexual contact with residents in high- or intermediate-risk areas | Hepatitis B | 14 | 47 |

# Appendix B — Summary Risk-Factor Tables

Table B-7. Summary Risk Factors: Substance Abuse History

| Risk Factor | Disorder | Children/ Adolescents | Adults/ Older Adults |
|---|---|---|---|
| Alcohol abuse | Depression | 5 | 32 |
|  | Injuries | 17,21 | 52,54 |
|  | Oral cancer | 17,29 | 29,52 |
|  | Tuberculosis | 9,17 | 42,52 |
|  | Pneumococcal infection | 17,49 | 49,52 |
| Illicit drug use | Depression | 5 | 32 |
|  | HIV | 17,22,39 | 39,52,58 |
|  | Tuberculosis | 9,17 | 42,52 |
|  | Hepatitis B | 14,17 | 47,52 |
| Tobacco use | Cervical cancer | 29,36 | 29,36 |
|  | Oral cancer | 18,23,29 | 29,53,59 |

# APPENDICES

# C. Varicella Immunization

Varicella disease—chickenpox—is a highly contagious childhood disease caused by varicella zoster virus (VZV). Although chickenpox is usually a mild disease that resolves without sequelae, in recent years an average of 92 deaths per year have been attributed to complications of the disease. A vaccine to prevent chickenpox is expected to be licensed in 1994 for use in the United States. One dose has been proven 97 percent effective in children 12 months through 12 years of age. The Advisory Committee on Immunization Practices (ACIP) and other major authorities are likely to recommend its use for all susceptible children 12 months through 12 years of age and for some high-risk older persons. Preliminary information on the vaccine and its use follows.

**Basics of VZV Immunization**

1. *Vaccine Types.* The single vaccine that will be available in the United States (Varivax®—Merck, Sharp and Dohme) is a live, cell-free preparation. (A multiple antigen measles-mumps-rubella-varicella vaccine is currently being tested.)

2. *Indications.* It is anticipated that VZV vaccine will be recommended to prevent varicella disease in healthy children aged 12 months through 12 years of age. It need not be given to children with a history of chickenpox, as they may be assumed to be immune. Children with an uncertain history of chickenpox should be considered susceptible.

   It is expected that VZV vaccine will also be recommended for susceptible persons 13 years of age and older who have close contact with those at high risk for serious complications from VZV disease (e.g., health care workers and those in contact with immunocompromised individuals).

3. *Schedule.* It is anticipated that ACIP will recommend that all children be routinely vaccinated between 12 and 18 months of age, preferably at the same time as the measles-mumps-rubella immunization. Limited data are available on the simultaneous administration of VZV vaccine with vaccines other than MMR.

   Children 18 months through 12 years of age who do not have a history of chickenpox should be immunized at any time during childhood. This "catch-up" immunization should occur before age 13, as adolescents and adults are at risk for more severe disease from varicella, and two doses of the VZV vaccine are needed after this age.

3. *Dosage and Administration.* The recommended dosage of VZV vaccine in children aged 12 months through 12 years is 0.5 mL in a single vaccination. In persons 13 years of age or older, two injections of 0.5 mL are given four to eight weeks apart. The injection

should be given subcutaneously into the thigh in infants and in the deltoid area in older children, using a ⅝- to ¾-inch 23-25 gauge needle.

4. *Precautions.* VZV vaccine is contraindicated in persons with a history of an anaphylactic reaction to neomycin. It does not contain preservatives or egg protein, substances that have caused hypersensitivity reactions to other vaccines. In general, VZV vaccine should not be given to persons with blood dyscrasias, leukemia, lymphomas, primary or acquired immunodeficiency (including AIDS), those on immunosuppressive therapy, or women who are pregnant or intend to become pregnant within three months.

   Persons with severe illness should not be vaccinated until they recover, but the vaccine may be given to children with mild illnesses with or without low-grade fever.

   Children receiving the vaccine should avoid use of salicylates for six weeks following vaccination, due to the theoretical risk of developing Reye's syndrome.

5. *Adverse Reactions.* The vaccine is well tolerated. Pain and redness at the injection site is reported by up to 20 percent of vaccinees. A mild rash, either local or generalized, has also been reported. Inadvertent administration of vaccine to individuals immune to varicella has not resulted in an increase in any adverse reactions.

7. *Vaccine Storage and Handling.* The lyophilized vaccine must be stored frozen at an average temperature of -15°C (8°F) or colder. The diluent is stored separately at room temperature or in the refrigerator. The vaccine should be used within 30 minutes of reconstitution with the supplied diluent. If not, it should be discarded. Handle all vaccine preparations according to manufacturers' instructions.

**Reference**

Advisory Committee on Immunization Practices. Varicella prevention. *MMWR*. In press.

# APPENDICES

## D. Copyright Considerations

The *Clinician's Handbook of Preventive Services* contains information that is subject to copyright; that information has been included in this publication subject to the specific terms of permission received from the copyright holders, who reserve all other rights. All such information is clearly marked in the text of the *Handbook*. It is a violation of copyright law to reproduce any copyrighted information from this publication without first obtaining separate permission from the copyright holder or holders, except as detailed herein.

That portion of the content of the *Handbook* produced by the Federal Government is in the public domain, although it is subject to certain legal restrictions: any portion reproduced must be clearly identified as Federal information produced by the U.S. Department of Health and Human Services, Public Health Service; and the following disclaimer must appear on any information product that is linked in a substantive way with the Put Prevention Into Practice campaign or the *Handbook*—"Neither the Public Health Service nor the U.S. Department of Health and Human Services endorses any particular organization or its activities, products, or services." If supplemental information, such as a preface or appendix, is incorporated in a reprint, all supplemental pages must be clearly labeled as such.

The *Handbook* has been published by the U.S. Department of Health and Human Services (DHHS) through the U.S. Government Printing Office (GPO) and is available to the public through the GPO Sales Program, which markets Federal publications on a revolving-fund basis, and Federal Depository Libraries, which provide access to collections of Federal documents.

DHHS received permission to reproduce the copyrighted information in this publication subject to the following conditions:

1. Permission was granted for publication of a single edition of the *Handbook* for distribution by DHHS and GPO.
2. This edition of the *Handbook* may be reprinted only in its entirety.
3. DHHS's formal partners among voluntary and professional organizations in the Put Prevention Into Practice campaign may reprint this edition of the *Handbook*—again, only in its entirety—to promote its use in medical and educational settings, including sale to their individual members at a price not exceeding the price set by GPO for sale to the general public.

Any organization or individual intending to make commercial use of any of the copyrighted information in the *Handbook* must obtain separate permission from all copyright holders. ("Commercial use" is defined as incorporation of any portion of the *Handbook* that is subject to copyright in another publication or sale of reprints of the *Handbook* at a price higher than that set by GPO for sale to the general public.)

# Clinician's Handbook of Preventive Services

## Index

Achondroplasia, 10
Acquired immunodeficiency disease, 214
    mortality, 323
Activities of daily living, 171, 174-175
Adolescents. *see* Children and adolescents
Adult immunization
    diphtheria, 271-273
    hepatitis B, 251
    influenza, 257-260
    patient resources, 273-274
    pneumococcus, 263-265
    principles of, xxvii-xxviii, xxxi
    rubella, 267-269
    tetanus, 271-273
Adult screening
    alcohol/substance abuse, 275, 276-279
    anemia, 131, 132
    blood pressure, 135-139
    body measurement, 141-146
    breast cancer, 147-150, 191-193
    chlamydia, 211-213
    cholesterol levels, 163-169
    cognitive/functional impairment, 171-175
    depression, 177-179
    fecal occult blood, 183-185
    gonorrhea, 211-213
    hearing loss, 187-190
    hemoglobinopathies, 131, 132-133
    HIV infection, 214-216, 324
    oral examination, 150-151
    Papanicolaou smear for cervical cancer, 195-199
    pelvic examination, 152-153
    plasma glucose screening for diabetes, 201-202
    preventive care timeline, xix, xvii
    principles of, xxv-xxvi
    prostate cancer, 153-155, 205-207
    rubella immunity, 267
    sigmoidoscopy, 219-222
    skin examination, 155-156
    surveillance in estrogen supplementation, 248-249
    syphilis, 209-211
    testis examination, 156-158
    thyroid cancer, 158-160
    thyroid dysfunction, 223-225
    tuberculosis, 227-229
    urinalysis, 233-235
    vision impairment, 237-239
Advisory Committee on Immunization Practices, A-3
Agency for Health Care Policy and Research, A-3
Alcohol abuse in adults
    assessment, 275, 276-279
    counseling, 275-276, 279-281
    outcomes, 275
    patient resources, 281
Alcohol abuse in children/adolescents
    assessment, 85, 86-87
    counseling, 85-86, 87, 105
    family resources, 88
    incidence, 85
Alzheimer's disease, 171
Amblyopia, 49
American Academy of Dermatology, A-1
American Academy of Family Physicians, A-1
American Academy of Ophthalmology, A-1
American Academy of Otolaryngology-Head and Neck Surgery, A-1
American Academy of Pediatrics, A-1
American Academy of Pediatric Dentistry, A-1
American Association of Pediatric Ophthalmology and Strabismus, A-1
American Cancer Society, A-1

# Index

American College of Obstetricians and Gynecologists, A-1
American College of Sports Medicine, A-1
American Dental Association, A-1
American Diabetes Association, A-2
American Dietetic Association, A-2
American Gastroenterological Association, A-2
American Geriatrics Society, A-2
American Heart Association, A-2
American Medical Association, A-2
American Nurses Association, A-2
American Optometric Association, A-2
American Society for Gastrointestinal Endoscopy, A-2
American Society of Colon and Rectal Surgeons, A-2
American Society of Dentistry for Children, A-2
American Speech-Language-Hearing Association, A-2
American Thoracic Society, A-2
American Thyroid Association, A-3
American Urological Association, A-3
Anemia in adults
 causes, 131
 prevalence, 131
 risk factors, B-4, B-9
 screening for, 131, 132
Anemia in children
 causes, 1
 cut points, 2, 3
 risk factors, B-3, B-4, B-9, 1
 screening, 1-3
 symptoms, 1
Aspirin
 precautions, 242
 prophylactic use, 241-242
Athletics. *See* Physical activity
Audiometric testing, 21-2, 23
Automobile safety, 104, 105, 237, 291, 292-293

*Bacille Calmett-Guérin* vaccination, 39, 40, 42, 43, 228, 229, 231
 efficacy, 227
Bacteriuria, 45, 46, 233

BCG. *See Bacille Calmett-Guérin* vaccination
Bicycle safety, 105, 293
Blood pressure
 adult, 135-139
 child/adolescent, 5-8
Body mass index
 adult, 143
 child/adolescent, 11
Body measurement
 adult, 141-145
 child/adolescent, 9-11, 94-95
 family resources, 11
 patient resources, 145-146
 provider resources, 11
Breast cancer, B-3
 estrogen/progestin supplementation and, 245, 246, 249
 examination, 147-150
 high-risk women, 192
 incidence and mortality, 191
 mammography, 191-193
 patient resources, 193
 provider resources, 193
Breast feeding, 90, 93, 94

CAGE questionnaire, 276-277
Calcium, 301
Canadian Task Force on Periodic Health Examination, A-3
Cancer
 breast, B-3, 147-150, 191-193, 245
 cervical, B-8, B-9, B-11, 195-199
 colorectal, B-4, 153-155, 183-185, 219-222, 241
 endometrial, 245
 incidence, 147, 150, 152, 153, 155, 156, 158, 191, 195
 liver, 251
 mortality, 147, 150, 152, 153, 155, 156, 158, 191, 195
 obesity and, 141
 oral, B-9, B-11, 150-151
 pelvic, 152-153
 prostate, B-3, B-4, 153-155, 205-207

# Index

skin, B-3, B-4, B-7, 155-156
testicular, B-4, 156-158
thyroid, B-3, B-5, 158-160
Cataracts, 237
    in children, 49
Centers for Disease Control and Prevention, A-3
Cervical cancer, B-8, B-9, B-11
    Papanicolaou smear for, 195-199
Chickenpox, C-1, C-2
Children and adolescents
    AIDS/HIV in, 109
    anemia screening, 1-3
    blood pressure screening, 5-8
    body measurement, 9-11
    cholesterol screening, 13-15
    dental/oral health, 89-92
    depression in, 17-18
    DTP immunization for, 55-58
    *Haemophilus influenzae* immunization, 61, 62-63
    *Haemophilus influenzae* prophylaxis, 61-62, 64-65
    hearing assessment, 21-23
    hepatitis B infection/immunization, 65-70
    influenza immunization, 257-260
    lead poisoning screening, 25-27, 28, 29
    measles-mumps-rubella immunization, 73-77
    newborn screening, 31-35, 37-38
    nutrition counseling, 93-96
    physical activity, 97-102
    pneumococcus in, 263-265
    poliomyelitis immunization, 79-82
    pregnancy counseling, 119-122
    preventive care timeline, xvii, xviii
    principles of counseling, xxxii
    principles of immunization, xxvii-xxx
    principles of screening, xxv-xxvi
    sexually transmitted diseases in, counseling for, 109-112
    sexually transmitted diseases in, screening for, 45, 46
    substance abuse, 85-88
    suicide, 17
    tetanus prophylaxis, 58-59
    tobacco use, 91, 115-117
    tuberculosis prophylaxis, 39, 40, 42-43
    tuberculosis screening, 39-42
    urinalysis, 45-46
    varicella immunization, C-1-C-2
    violent behavior and firearms, risks of, 125-128
    vision screening, 49-53
Chlamydia, 45, 46, 109, 323
    adult screening, 211-213
    incidence, 211, 323
Cholesterol levels
    adult diet and, 303
    adult screening, 163-169
    childhood screening, 13-16
    coronary heart disease and, 163
    hypercholesterolemia risk factors, B-3
    patient resources, 166
    provider resources, 166
Cocaine, 275
Colon cancer, 241
Colorectal cancer, 153-155
    fecal occult blood screening for, 183-185
    patient resources, 185
    risk factors, B-4, B-5
    sigmoidoscopy for, 219-222
Condoms, 111, 324, 325, 326, 339
Confidentiality
    in adolescent pregnancy counseling, 120
    in adolescent substance abuse counseling, 86
    adolescents in violent situations and, 127
Contraception, 119, 120-121, 337-342
    patient resources, 342
    postcoital, 341-342
Coronary heart disease
    adolescent health and, 97
    adult prophylaxis, 241-242
    age as risk factor, B-5
    cholesterol and, 163
    estrogen/progestin prophylaxis for, 245
    hyperlipidemia in children and, 13
    mortality, 241, 245

physical activity and, 311, 312
smoking and, 329
Corticosteroids, contraindication to polio vaccine, 80
Council for Education of the Deaf, A-3
Counseling for adults
    alcohol/substance abuse, 275-281
    contraception, 337-342
    in hemoglobinopathy screening, 133
    nutrition, 299-305
    parents of newborns with abnormal test results, 35
    physical activity, 311-316
    polypharmacy, 319-321
    principles of, xxxii
    safety, 291-296
    sexually transmitted diseases, 323-327
    tobacco use, 329-334
Counseling for children/adolescents
    contraception, 120-121
    dental/oral health, 89-92
    eye safety, 53
    nutrition, 93-96
    physical activity, 97-99
    safety, 103-106
    sexually transmitted diseases, 109-112
    substance abuse, 85-88
    suicide intervention, 18
    tobacco use, 91, 115-117
    unintended pregnancy, 119-122
    violent behavior and firearms, 125-128
Cytomegalovirus, 323

Delivery of preventive services
    feasibility evaluation, xxi
    obstacles to, xvii
Dental/oral health
    adult patient resources, 288
    antibacterial prophylaxis, precautions in, 287-288
    counseling for adults, 285-287
    counseling for children/adolescents, 89-91
    family resources, 92
    oral cancer, B-9, B-11, 150-151

provider resources, 288
Depression in adults
    assessment, 177-179
    patient resources, 179
    provider resources, 181
    risk factors, B-3, B-4, B-6, B-8, B-9, B-11, 177
Depression in children/adolescents
    complications of, 17
    family resources, 18
    prevalence, 17
    risk factors, B-3, B-4, B-6, B-8, B-9, B-11, 17
    screening, 17-18
Diabetes mellitus, 93, 227
    mortality, 201
    patient resources, 202
    plasma glucose screening for, 201-202
    prevalence, 201
    risk factors, B-2, B-4, 201
Diabetic retinopathy, 237
Diet. *See* Nutrition
Diphtheria. *See also* DTP immunization
    adult immunization, 271-273
    incidence, 271
Down syndrome, 10
Drowning, accidental, 104
DTP immunization
    adverse reactions, 56-57
    contraindications, 56, 58
    family resources, 59
    informed consent, 57
    procedure, 55-58
    role of, 55
    vaccine storage and handling, 57

Eating disorders, 9
Encephalitis
    as complication of rubella, 73
    as mumps complication, 73
Endocarditis, B-5, 211

# Index

Estrogen supplementation
    adverse effects, 245, 248
    contraindications, 247-248
    dosage/administration, 247
    indications for, 246-247
    patient resources, 249
    progestin and, 245, 248-249
    role of, 245
    surveillance, 248-249
Ethnicity as risk factor, B-2
    for diabetes, 201
    in hemoglobinopathies, 131
    in tuberculosis, 227
    in unintended pregnancy, 337
Exercise. *See* Physical activity
Eye disease in children
    family resources, 53
    high-risk groups, 50
    incidence, 49
    provider resources, 53
    recommendations for screening, 49
    screening procedure, 50-53
Eye disease/vision impairment in adults
    assessment questionnaire, 238
    patient resources, 238
    prevalence, 237
    provider resources, 239
    treatment, 237

Families
    parents' role in adolescent sex counseling, 110
    parents' role in child safety, 103-105
    risk factors for child/adolescent depression in, 17
    risk factors for child/adolescent suicide in, 17
    in vision assessment for children, 50
Fecal occult blood screening, 183-185
Firearms, 125, 126-127, 293
Fluoride supplementation, 89-90, 94
Folic acid, 95, 301
Food Guide Pyramid, 301

Galactosemia, newborn screening for, 31
Glaucoma, B-2, 237
    in children, 49
Glucosuria, 45
Gonorrhea, 46, 109, 323
    adult screening, 211-213
    incidence, 211
Growth assessment, 9-11
Guillain-Barré syndrome, 68

*Haemophilus influenzae* type B immunization
    adverse reactions, 63
    disease risk factors, 61
    with DTP immunization, 56, 63
    family resources, 64
    procedure, 62-64
    prophylaxis, 61-62, 64-65
    role of, 61
    vaccine storage and handling, 63
Head circumference measurement, 9, 10, 11
Hearing impairment in children
    family resources, 23
    incidence, 21
    risk factors, B-4, B-7, 21-22
    screening, 21-23
Hearing loss in adults
    outcomes, 187
    patient resources, 190
    screening, 187-189
Height measurement
    adults, 141
    children, 9-10
Hematuria, 233
Hemoglobinopathies
    adult screening, 131, 132-133
    in anemia, 1
    newborn screening, 31, 32
    risk factors, B-2, 131
Hepatitis B in adults
    immunization, 251-253
    incidence, 251
    outcomes, 251
    patient resources, 255

precautions in immunization/prophylaxis, 253, 255
prophylaxis, 252, 254-255
risk factors, B-4, B-5, B-7, B-8, B-9, B-10
vaccine efficacy, 251
vaccine storage and handling, 253
Hepatitis B in children/adolescents
   adverse reactions in immunization/prophylaxis, 67-68, 69
   family resources, 69
   immunization, 66-69
   incidence, 65
   informed consent for immunization, 68
   prophylaxis, 66, 69
   provider resources, 69
   risk factors, B-3, B-5, B-7, B-8, B-9, B-10, 65
   vaccine storage and handling, 69
Herpes simplex virus, 109, 323
Honey, 94
Household safety
   children and, 103-105
   firearms and, 125, 126-127
   older adults and, 293-294
Human immunodeficiency virus. *See also* Sexually transmitted diseases
   adult screening, 214-216
   counseling for adolescents, 109, 110, 111-112
   counseling for adults, 323-327
   hepatitis B and, 251
   Hib immunization and, 61
   prevalence, 214
   preventive efforts, 209
   risk factors, B-4, B-5, B-7, B-8, B-9, B-11, 209, 323
   substance abuse and, 275
   tuberculosis and, 227, 230, 231
Human papilloma virus, 109, 323
Hydrocephalus, 9
Hypercholesterolemia risk factors, B-3
Hyperlipidemia
   in children, 13
   estrogen/progestin supplementation and, 247

Hypertension in adults
   estrogen/progestin supplementation and, 247
   lifestyle modifications for control of, 137
   outcomes, 135
   patient resources, 138
   provider resources, 139
   risk factors, B-2, B-3
   screening, 135-137
Hypertension in children
   algorithm, 8
   screening, 5-8
Hyperthyroidism, 223-225
Hypothyroidism, 223-225
   in newborn, 31, 32

Immunization/vaccination
   for adults. *See* Adult immunization
   DTP, 55-58
   family resources, 77-78
   hepatitis B, 65-70
   influenza, 257-260
   measles-mumps-rubella, 73-77
   pneumococcus, 263-265
   poliomyelitis, 79-82
   principles, xxvii-xxxi
   tetanus prophylaxis, 58-59
   varicella, C-1, C-2
Infant formulas, 1
Influenza
   adverse reactions to vaccine, 259
   immunization, 258-260
   mortality, 257
   patient resources, 260
   prophylaxis, 257, 260
   risk for complications in, B-5, B-6, B-7, B-10, 257
   vaccine efficacy, 257
   vaccine storage and handling, 260
Informed consent
   in adolescent pregnancy counseling, 120
   in DTP immunization, 57
   in hepatitis B immunization, 68

# Index

in measles-mumps-rubella immunization, 76-77
in poliomyelitis immunization, 82
Instrumental activities of daily living, 171, 174
Iron deficiency, 1, 93
  lead absorption and, 26
Isoniazid
  adverse reactions, 231
  efficacy, 227
  precautions, 230
  for tuberculosis prophylaxis, 39, 40, 42-43, 227, 228, 229-231

Lead poisoning in children
  family resources, 26-27
  iron deficiency and, 26
  outcomes, 25
  prevalence, 25
  provider resources, 27
  risk factors, B-3, B-9, B-10
  screening, 25-27, 28, 29
Leukemia, Hib immunization and, 61
Lipoprotein levels in children, 13, 15

Mammography, 191-193
Mantoux test, 40, 41-42, 228, 229
Marfan's syndrome, 10
Marijuana, 275
Measles
  adverse reactions in immunization/prophylaxis, 75, 76, 77
  family resources, 77-78
  high-risk groups, 74
  immunization, 73-77
  incidence, 73
  informed consent in immunization, 76-77
Medication(s)
  adult patient resources, 321
  aspirin prophylaxis, 241-242
  cholesterol screening and, 14
  household safety, 104
  polypharmacy counseling for adults, 319-321
  provider resources, 321

safety counseling for adults, 294
thyroid function screening and, 224-225
tuberculosis prophylaxis, 39, 40, 42-43
Meningitis, 61, 211
Mental health
  adult cognitive/functional impairment, 171-175
  adult depression, 177-179
  depression in children/adolescents, 17-18
  hearing loss and, 187
  unintended pregnancy and, 337
Microhematocrit analysis, for childhood anemia, 1-2
Mumps
  adverse reactions in immunization/prophylaxis, 75, 76, 77
  family resources, 77-78
  high-risk groups, 74
  immunization, 73-77
  incidence, 73
  informed consent in immunization, 76-77
Myocardial infarction. *See* Coronary heart disease

National Cancer Institute, A-3
National Eye Institute, A-3
National Heart, Lung, and Blood Institute, A-4
National Institute of Dental Research, A-4
National Institutes of Health Consensus Development Conferences, A-4
National Medical Association, A-3
National Transportation Safety Board, A-4
Neurofibromatosis, 10
Newborn screening, 31-35
  documentation, 33, 34
  family resources/counseling, 35
  follow-up, 34-35
  provider resources, 35
  state mandates, 31, 33, 37-38
Nutrition
  adult counseling, 299-305
  adult patient resources, 305
  anemia and, 1
  child/adolescent counseling, 93-96

## Index

concerns of women, 301
dental health and, 91
family resources, 95-96
provider resources, 305

Obesity
in adults, 141, 299, 301
in children, 9, 93
as diabetes risk factor, 201, 202
physical activity and, 97
as risk factor, 141
Occupational safety, 293
Orchitis, 73
Osteoporosis, estrogen prophylaxis for, 245, 294
Otitis media, 21

Pelvic cancer, 152-153
Pelvic inflammatory disease, 211, 323
Pertussis. *See* DTP immunization
Pharyngitis, 211
Phenylketonuria (PKU) screening, 31, 32
Physical activity
counseling for adults, 311-316
counseling for children/adolescents, 97-99
family resources, 102
health and, 97, 311
medical conditions of children and, 98, 100-101
for overweight children, 95
PKU. *See* Phenylketonuria
Plasma glucose screening, 201-202
Pneumococcus
adverse reactions in immunization, 265
immunization, 263-265
outcomes, 263
patient resources, 265
risk factors, B-5, B-6, B-9, B-11
vaccine efficacy, 263
vaccine storage and handling, 265
Poliomyelitis
adverse reactions in immunization, 80-82
contraindications, 80, 81
family resources, 82

immunization, 79-82
incidence, 79
informed consent in immunization, 82
vaccine storage and handling, 82
Pregnancy
alcohol consumption in, 301
anemia screening in, 132
family resources, 121
folic acid intake in, 95
lead poisoning risk assessment in, 26
provider resources for counseling, 122, 342
rubella and, 267, 268
teenage incidence, 119
tuberculosis in, 230
unintended, counseling for adults, 337-342
unintended, counseling for children/adolescents, 119-121
urinalysis, 233
Preventive services protocol, xx-xxii
implementation, xxii-xxiv
Proctitis, 211
Progestin prophylaxis, 245-249
Prostate cancer, B-3, B-4, 153-155
clinical course, 205
incidence, 205
mortality, 205
risk factors, 205
Proteinuria, 233

Record keeping, xxiii-xxiv, 33, 34
Reimbursement issues, xxii
Retinoblastoma, in children, 49
Rifampin
adverse reactions, 64
contraindications, 64
in Hib prophylaxis in children, 61-62, 63-64
Rubella in adults
adverse reactions in immunization, 268-269
immunization, 267-269
outcomes, 267
postpartum vaccination, 268
risk factors, B-6

# Index

Rubella in children
    adverse reactions in immunization/prophylaxis, 75, 76, 77
    congenital syndrome, 73, 267
    family resources, 77-78
    high-risk groups, 74
    immunization, 73-77
    incidence, 73, 267
    informed consent in immunization, 76-77

Safety
    adult patient resources, 297
    concerns of women, 291, 294-296
    counseling for adults, 291-296
    counseling for children/adolescents, 103-105
    counselor resources, 297-298
    family resources, 105-106
    firearm, 125, 126-127
    in pharmacotherapy, 319-321
    provider resources, 106
    sources of child injuries, 103

Schiotz test, 237

Sexually transmitted diseases. *See also* Human immunodeficiency virus
    adult counseling, 323-327
    adult patient resources, 216-217, 327
    adult screening, 209
    child/adolescent counseling, 109-112
    child/adolescent screening, 45, 46
    chlamydia in adults, 211-214
    concerns of women, 323
    family resources, 112
    gonorrhea in adults, 211-213
    high risk groups, 109, 323
    incidence, 323
    provider resources, 112-113, 217, 327
    syphilis in adults, 209-210
    types of, 323

Sickle cell disease, 1, 10. *See also* Hemoglobinopathies
    Hib immunization and, 61
    in newborns, 31, 35

Skin cancer, B-3, B-4, B-7, 155-156, 286

Skin Cancer Foundation, A-3

Smoke detectors, 293

Society of General Internal Medicine, A-3

Splenectomy, Hib immunization and, 61

Sports. *See* Physical activity

Strabismus, 49

Substance abuse in adults
    assessment, 275, 276-279
    counseling, 275-276, 279-281, 326
    outcomes, 275
    patient resources, 281

Substance abuse in children
    assessment, 85, 86-87
    counseling, 85-86, 87, 105
    family resources, 88
    incidence, 85
    sexually transmitted diseases and, 109-110

Sudden infant death syndrome, 105

Suicide
    assessment/intervention with children/adolescents, 18
    child/adolescent risk factors, 17
    family resources, 18
    prevalence in children/adolescents, 17

Syphilis, 109
    adult screening, 210, 214
    clinical course, 209-210
    incidence, 209

Tenosynovitis, 211

Testicular cancer, B-4, 156-158

Tetanus. *See also* DTP immunization
    adult immunization, 271-273
    incidence, 55, 271
    prophylaxis, 58-59, 271, 273

Thalassemia, 1, 31. *See also* Hemoglobinopathies

Thrombocytopenia, 73

Thumb-sucking, 91

Thyroid cancer, 158-160

Thyroid dysfunction
    adult screening, 223-225
    incidence, 223
    risk factors, B-3, B-5, B-6, 223

# Index

Tobacco use
- in children/adolescents, 115-117
- counseling for adults, 329-334
- dental health and, 91
- family resources, 117
- nicotine patches for, 117
- outcomes, 329
- passive exposure, 115
- patient resources, 333-334
- provider resources, 117, 334-336
- smokeless tobacco, 115

Tuberculosis in adults
- antibiotic resistance, 227
- BCG vaccination, 227, 228, 229, 231
- incidence, 227
- preventive services, 231
- prophylaxis, 227, 228, 229-231
- provider resources, 231
- risk factors, B-2, B-4, B-5, B-6, B-7, B-9, B-11, 227
- screening, xx, 227-229

Tuberculosis in children
- adverse testing effects, 42
- family resources, 43
- high-risk populations, 39
- prevalence, 39
- prophylaxis, 39, 40, 42-43
- provider resources, 44
- risk factors, B-2, B-4, B-5, B-6, B-7, B-9, B-11, 39, 40
- screening, xx, 39-42

Turner's syndrome, 10

Urinalysis for adults
- procedure, 234-235
- role of, 233

Urinalysis for children
- procedure, 46
- role of of, 45-46

U.S. Preventive Services Task Force, A-4

Vaccine Adverse Event Reporting System, 57, 63, 68, 76, 81, 268-269, 273
Varicella, C-1-C-2

Violence, child/adolescent exposure to
- counseling interventions, 125-128
- provider resources for counseling, 128
- statistics, 125

Violence toward women, 291, 294-296

Vision screening
- for adults, 237-239
- for children, 49-53

Vitamins
- deficiency risk factors, B-6
- needs of women, 301301
- supplements, 94, 95

Weight measurement
- adults, 142-145
- children/adolescents, 9, 10, 94-95

☆ U.S. G.P.O.: 1994-365-753 (ITEM #4)

# Superintendent of Documents Order Form

Order Processing Code:
**\* 7378**

*Charge your order. It's easy!* MasterCard  VISA

**Fax orders to (202) 512-2250**

☐ **YES,** send me the following publications from the U.S. Public Health Service, so I can continue to *Put Prevention Into Practice!*

| Qty. | Stock Number | Title | Price Each | Total Price |
|---|---|---|---|---|
|  | 017-001-00492-8 | Put Prevention Into Practice Education and Action Kit* | $ 57.00 |  |
|  | 017-001-00493-6 | Personal Health Guide – doctor version (Adult), package of 25 | $ 20.00 |  |
|  | 017-001-00494-4 | Personal Health Guide – clinician version (Adult), package of 25 | $ 19.00 |  |
|  | 017-001-00495-2 | Child Health Guide, package of 25 | $ 23.00 |  |
|  | 017-001-00496-1 | Clinician's Handbook, package of 1 | $ 20.00 |  |
|  | 017-001-00497-9 | Flow Sheets (10 each of 3), package of 30 | $ 4.00 |  |
|  | 017-001-00501-1 | Reminder Post Cards (Adult), package of 50 | $ 8.00 |  |
|  | 017-001-00521-5 | Reminder Post Cards (Child), package of 50 | $ 8.00 |  |
|  | 017-001-00505-3 | Chart Stickers (Blank), package of 25 (500 stickers) | $ 6.50 |  |
|  | 017-001-00506-1 | Chart Stickers (Blood Pressure), package of 25 (500 stickers) | $ 6.50 |  |
|  | 017-001-00507-0 | Chart Stickers (Cholesterol), package of 25 (500 stickers) | $ 6.50 |  |
|  | 017-001-00508-8 | Chart Stickers (Diet), package of 25 (500 stickers) | $ 6.50 |  |
|  | 017-001-00509-6 | Chart Stickers (Exercise), package of 25 (500 stickers) | $ 6.50 |  |
|  | 017-001-00510-0 | Chart Stickers (EtOH), package of 25 (500 stickers) | $ 6.50 |  |
|  | 017-001-00511-8 | Chart Stickers (Firearms), package of 25 (500 stickers) | $ 6.50 |  |
|  | 017-001-00512-6 | Chart Stickers (Flu Shot), package of 25 (500 stickers) | $ 6.50 |  |
|  | 017-001-00513-4 | Chart Stickers (Lead), package of 25 (500 stickers) | $ 6.50 |  |
|  | 017-001-00514-2 | Chart Stickers (Mammogram), package of 25 (500 stickers) | $ 6.50 |  |
|  | 017-001-00515-1 | Chart Stickers (Obesity), package of 25 (500 stickers) | $ 6.50 |  |
|  | 017-001-00516-9 | Chart Stickers (Pap Smear), package of 25 (500 stickers) | $ 6.50 |  |
|  | 017-001-00517-7 | Chart Stickers (Safety), package of 25 (500 stickers) | $ 6.50 |  |
|  | 017-001-00518-5 | Chart Stickers (Smoking), package of 25 (500 stickers) | $ 6.50 |  |
|  | 017-001-00519-3 | Chart Stickers (Sun Exposure), package of 25 (500 stickers) | $ 6.50 |  |
|  | 017-001-00520-7 | Chart Stickers (STD/HIV Risk), package of 25 (500 stickers) | $ 6.50 |  |
|  | 017-001-00499-5 | Prevention Prescription Pads, package of 10 | $ 24.00 |  |
|  | 017-001-00500-2 | Post-it ™ Note Pads, package of 10 | $ 20.00 |  |
|  | 017-001-00502-9 | Waiting Room Poster (1) Examination Room Charts (2: Adult/Child)† | $ 5.50 |  |

\* Kit contains 5 of each Health Guide, 1 Clinician's Handbook, and samples of all other materials.
† Posters come in sets of 3.

**Total**

*Thank you for your order!*

Price includes regular shipping and handling and is subject to change. International customers please add 25%.

**Check method of payment:**
☐ Check payable to Superintendent of Documents
☐ GPO Deposit Account ☐☐☐☐☐☐☐-☐
☐ VISA ☐ MasterCard

☐☐☐☐ ☐☐☐☐ ☐☐☐☐ ☐☐☐☐
☐☐☐☐ (expiration date)

Company or personal name (Please type or print)

Additional address/attention line

Street address

City, State, Zip code

Daytime phone including area code

Purchase order number (optional)

Authorizing signature                    5/94

**Mail To:**
Superintendent of Documents
P.O. Box 371954, Pittsburgh, PA 15250-7954

*Also meeting your information needs at convenient locations nationwide are these 24 U.S. Government Bookstores*

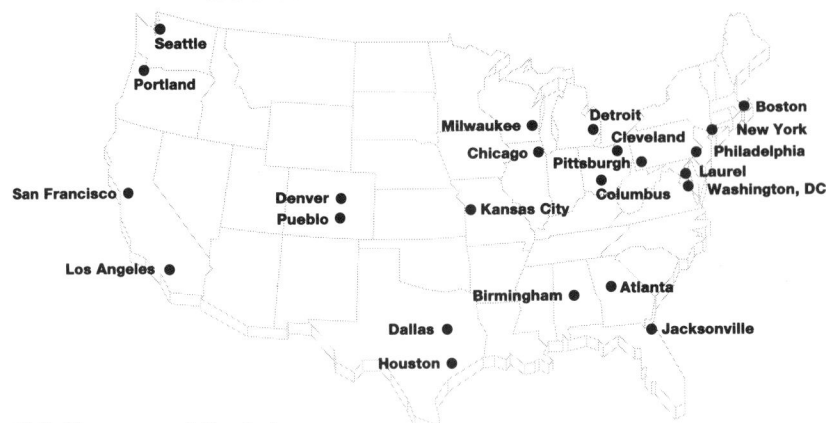

## Your U.S. Government Bookstores

GPO operates U.S. Government bookstores all around the country where you can browse through the shelves and take your books home with you. Naturally, these stores can't stock all of the more than 12,000 titles in our inventory, but they do carry the ones you're most likely be looking for. And they'll be happy to order any government book currently offered for sale and have it sent directly to you. All of our bookstores accept VISA, MasterCard, and Superintendent of Documents deposit account orders. For more information, please contact your nearest U.S. Government Bookstore.

U.S. Government Bookstore
First Union Plaza
999 Peachtree Street, NE
Suite 120
**Atlanta, GA** 30309-3964
(404) 347-1900
FAX: (404) 347-1897

U.S. Government Bookstore
O'Neill Building
2021 Third Ave., North
**Birmingham, AL** 35203
(205) 731-1056
FAX: (205) 731-3444

U.S. Government Bookstore
Thomas P. O'Neill Building
Room 169
10 Causeway Street
**Boston, MA** 02222
(617) 720-4180
FAX: (617) 720-5753

U.S. Government Bookstore
One Congress Center
401 South State St., Suite 124
**Chicago, IL** 60605
(312) 353-5133
FAX: (312) 353-1590

U.S. Government Bookstore
Room 1653, Federal Building
1240 E. 9th Street
**Cleveland, OH** 44199
(216) 522-4922
FAX: (216) 522-4714

U.S. Government Bookstore
Room 207, Federal Building
200 N. High Street
**Columbus, OH** 43215
(614) 469-6956
FAX: (614) 469-5374

U.S. Government Bookstore
Room IC50, Federal Building
1100 Commerce Street
**Dallas, TX** 75242
(214) 767-0076
FAX: (214) 767-3239

U.S. Government Bookstore
Room 117, Federal Building
1961 Stout Street
**Denver, CO** 80294
(303) 844-3964
FAX: (303) 844-4000

U.S. Government Bookstore
Suite 160, Federal Building
477 Michigan Avenue
**Detroit, MI** 48226
(313) 226-7816
FAX: (313) 226-4698

U.S. Government Bookstore
Texas Crude Building,
801 Travis Street, Suite 120
**Houston, TX** 77002
(713) 228-1187
FAX: (713) 228-1186

U.S. Government Bookstore
100 West Bay Street
Suite 100
**Jacksonville, FL** 32202
(904) 353-0569
FAX: (904) 353-1280

U.S. Government Bookstore
120 Bannister Mall
5600 E. Bannister Road
**Kansas City, MO** 64137
(816) 765-2256
FAX: (816) 767-8233

U.S. Government Bookstore
U.S. Government Printing Office
Warehouse Sales Outlet
8660 Cherry Lane
**Laurel, MD** 20707
(301) 953-7974
(301) 792-0262
FAX: (301) 498-8995

U.S. Government Bookstore
ARCO Plaza, C-Level
505 South Flower Street
**Los Angeles, CA** 90071
(213) 239-9844
FAX: (213) 239-9848

U.S. Government Bookstore
Suite 150, Reuss Federal Plaza.
310 W. Wisconsin Avenue
**Milwaukee, WI** 53203
(414) 297-1304
FAX: (414) 297-1300

U.S. Government Bookstore
Room 110, Federal Building
26 Federal Plaza
**New York, NY** 10278
(212) 264-3825
FAX: (212) 264-9318

U.S. Government Bookstore
Robert Morris Building
100 North 17th Street
**Philadelphia, PA** 19103
(215) 636-1900
FAX: (215) 636-1903

U.S. Government Bookstore
Room 118, Federal Building
1000 Liberty Avenue
**Pittsburgh, PA** 15222
(412) 644-2721
FAX: (412) 644-4547

U.S. Government Bookstore
1305 SW First Avenue
**Portland, OR** 97201-5801
(503) 221-6217
FAX: (503) 225-0563

U.S. Government Bookstore
Norwest Banks Building
201 West 8th Street
**Pueblo, CO** 81003
(719) 544-3142
FAX: (719) 544-6719

U.S. Government Bookstore
Room 1023, Federal Building
450 Golden Gate Avenue
**San Francisco, CA** 94102
(415) 252-5334
FAX: (415) 252-5339

U.S. Government Bookstore
Room 194, Federal Building
915 Second Avenue
**Seattle, WA** 98174
(206) 553-4270
FAX: (206) 553-6717

U.S. Government Bookstore
U.S. Government Printing Office
710 N. Capitol Street, NW
**Washington, DC** 20401
(202) 512-0132
FAX: (202) 512-1355

U.S. Government Bookstore
1510 H Street, NW
**Washington, DC** 20005
(202) 653-5075
FAX: (202) 376-5055

ISBN 0-16-043115-8

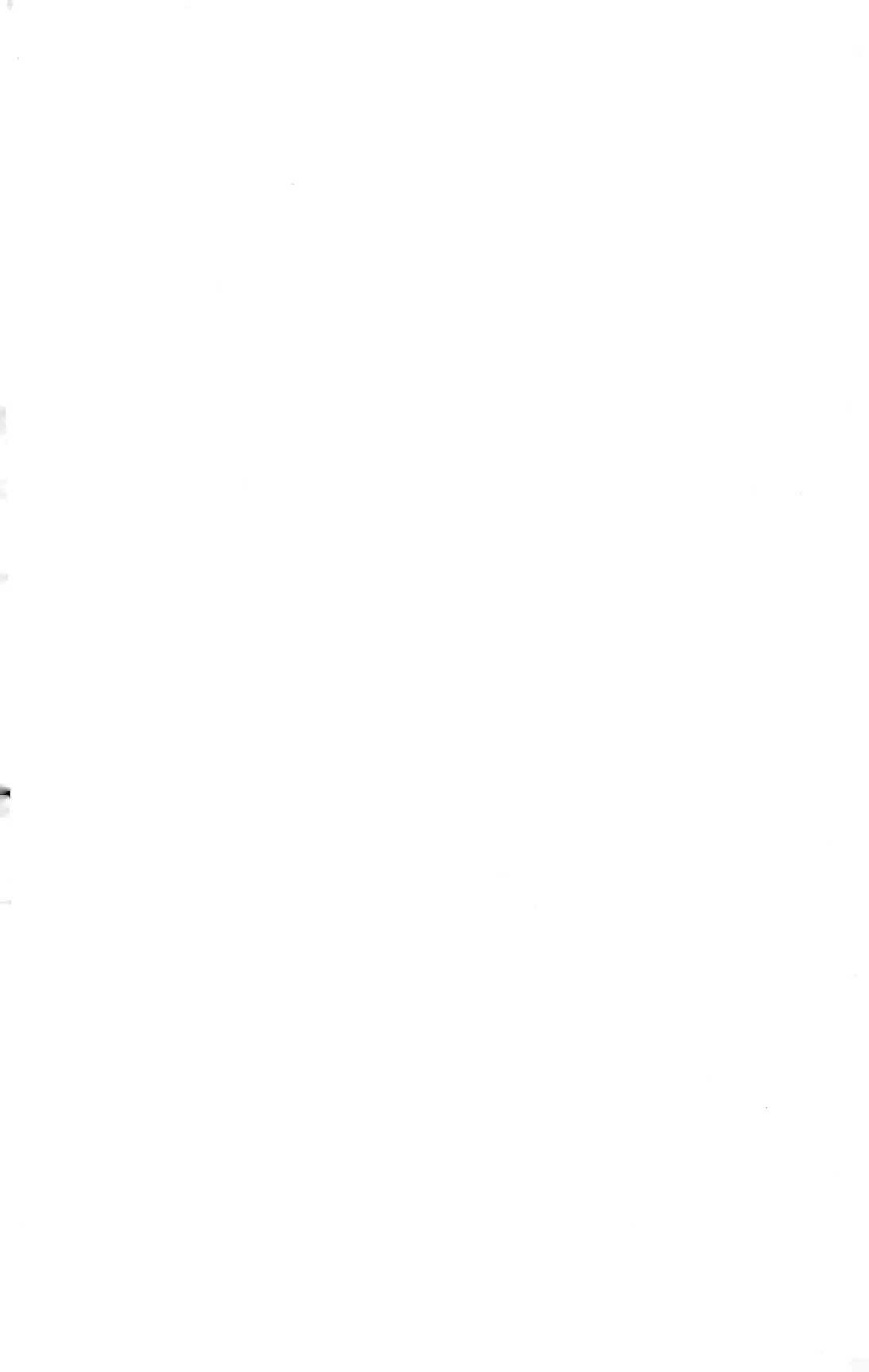

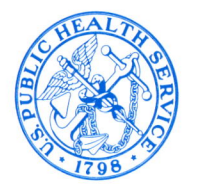